Updates in Thyroidology

Editors

MEGAN R HAYMART
MARIA PAPALEONTIOU

ENDOCRINOLOGY AND METABOLISM CLINICS OF NORTH AMERICA

www.endo.theclinics.com

Consulting Editor
ADRIANA G. IOACHIMESCU

June 2022 • Volume 51 • Number 2

ELSEVIER

1600 John F. Kennedy Boulevard • Suite 1800 • Philadelphia, Pennsylvania, 19103-2899

http://www.theclinics.com

ENDOCRINOLOGY AND METABOLISM CLINICS OF NORTH AMERICA Volume 51, Number 2
June 2022 ISSN 0889-8529, ISBN 13: 978-0-323-84983-8

Editor: Katerina Heidhausen
Developmental Editor: Jessica Cañaberal

Endocrinology and Metabolism Clinics of North America (ISSN 0889-8529) is published quarterly by Elsevier Inc., 360 Park Avenue South, New York, NY 10010-1710. Months of issue are March, June, September, and December. Periodicals postage paid at New York, NY and additional mailing offices. Subscription prices are USD 394.00 per year for US individuals, USD 1058.00 per year for US institutions, USD 100.00 per year for US students and residents, USD 467.00 per year for Canadian individuals, USD 1079.00 per year for Canadian institutions, USD 512.00 per year for international individuals, USD 1079.00 per year for international institutions, USD 100.00 per year for Canadian students/residents, and USD 245.00 per year for international students/residents. To receive student/resident rate, orders must be accompanied by name of affiliated institution, date of term, and the signature of program/residency coordinator on institution letterhead. Orders will be billed at individual rate until proof of status is received. Foreign air speed delivery is included in all *Clinics* subscription prices. All prices are subject to change without notice. **POSTMASTER:** Send address changes to *Endocrinology and Metabolism Clinics of North America*, Elsevier Health Sciences Division, Subscription Customer Service, 3251 Riverport Lane, Maryland Heights, MO 63043. **Customer Service: Telephone: 1-800-654-2452** (U.S. and Canada); **1-314-447-8871** (outside U.S. and Canada). **Fax: 1-314-447-8029. E-mail: journalscustomerservice-usa@elsevier.com (for print support); journalsonlinesupport-usa@elsevier.com (for online support)**.

Reprints. For copies of 100 or more, of articles in this publication, please contact the Commercial Rights Department, Elsevier Inc., 360 Park Avenue South, New York, NY 10010-1710; phone: +1-212-633-3874; fax: +1-212-633-3820; E-mail: reprints@elsevier.com.

Endocrinology and Metabolism Clinics of North America is covered in *MEDLINE/PubMed (Index Medicus)*, *EMBASE/Excerpta Medica, Current Contents/Clinical Medicine, Current Contents/Life Sciences, Science Citation Index, ISI/BIOMED, BIOSIS,* and *Chemical Abstracts*.

Contributors

CONSULTING EDITOR

ADRIANA G. IOACHIMESCU, MD, PhD
Professor, Departments of Medicine: Endocrinology and Metabolism, and Neurosurgery, Emory University, Emory University School of Medicine, Atlanta, Georgia, USA

EDITORS

MEGAN R. HAYMART, MD
Nancy Wigginton Endocrinology Research Professor of Thyroid Cancer and Professor of Medicine, Division of Metabolism, Endocrinology and Diabetes, Division of Hematology/Oncology, Department of Internal Medicine, University of Michigan, Ann Arbor, Michigan, USA

MARIA PAPALEONTIOU, MD
Assistant Professor, Division of Metabolism, Endocrinology and Diabetes, Department of Internal Medicine, Research Assistant Professor, Institute of Gerontology, University of Michigan, Ann Arbor, Michigan, USA

AUTHORS

CHELSEY K. BALDWIN, MD, ECNU
Assistant Professor, Department of Medicine, Diabetes and Endocrinology Section, NYU Grossman School of Medicine, New York, New York, USA

KRISTIEN BOELAERT, MD, PhD, FRCP
Institute of Applied Health Research, University of Birmingham, Birmingham, United Kingdom

HENRY B. BURCH, MD
Division of Diabetes, Endocrinology and Metabolic Diseases, National Institute of Diabetes and Digestive and Kidney Diseases, National Institutes of Health, Professor of Medicine, Uniformed Services University of the Health Sciences, Bethesda, Maryland, USA

NYDIA BURGOS, MD
Division of Endocrinology, Diabetes and Metabolism, Department of Medicine, University of Puerto Rico, Medical Sciences Campus, San Juan, Puerto Rico

NAIFA BUSAIDY, MD
Department of Endocrine Neoplasia, The University of Texas MD Anderson Cancer Center, Houston, Texas, USA

MARIA E. CABANILLAS, MD
Department of Endocrine Neoplasia and Hormonal Disorders, Division of Internal Medicine, Professor, The University of Texas MD Anderson Cancer Center, Houston, Texas, USA

DEBBIE W. CHEN, MD
Clinical Instructor, Department of Internal Medicine, Division of Metabolism, Endocrinology, and Diabetes, University of Michigan, Ann Arbor, Michigan, USA

EVA L. CHOU, MD
Department of Ophthalmology, Oculoplastic Service, Walter Reed National Military Medical Center, Assistant Professor of Surgery, Uniformed Services University of the Health Sciences, Bethesda, Maryland, USA

RIMA K. DHILLON-SMITH, MBChB, PhD, MRCOG
Institute of Metabolism and Systems Research, Tommy's National Centre for Miscarriage Research, University of Birmingham, Birmingham, United Kingdom

THANH D. HOANG, DO
Division of Diabetes, Endocrinology and Metabolism, Walter Reed National Military Medical Center, Professor of Medicine, Uniformed Services University of the Health Sciences, Bethesda, Maryland, USA

STEVEN P. HODAK, MD, ECNU
Professor, Department of Medicine, Diabetes and Endocrinology Section, NYU Grossman School of Medicine, New York, New York, USA

JACQUELINE JONKLAAS, MD, PhD
Professor of Medicine, Division of Endocrinology, Georgetown University, Washington, DC, USA

TIM I.M. KOREVAAR, MD, PhD
Department of Internal Medicine, Erasmus Medical Center, Academic Center for Thyroid Diseases, Rotterdam, the Netherlands

ANUPAM KOTWAL, MD
Assistant Professor, Division of Diabetes, Endocrinology and Metabolism, Department of Internal Medicine, University of Nebraska Medical Center, Omaha, Nebraska, USA

ANGELA M. LEUNG, MD, MSc
Division of Endocrinology, Diabetes, and Metabolism, Department of Medicine, UCLA David Geffen School of Medicine, Division of Endocrinology, Diabetes, and Metabolism, Department of Medicine, VA Greater Los Angeles Healthcare System, Los Angeles, California, USA

LEEDOR LIEBERMAN, MD
Department of Metabolism, Endocrinology and Diabetes, University of Michigan, Ann Arbor, Michigan, USA

ANASTASIOS MANIAKAS, MD, MSc
Division of Otolaryngology–Head and Neck Surgery, Hôpital Maisonneuve-Rosemont, Université de Montréal, Montreal, Québec, Canada; Department of Head and Neck Surgery, The University of Texas MD Anderson Cancer Center, Houston, Texas, USA

DONALD S. A. MCLEOD, MBBS (Hon I), FRACP, MPH, PhD
Senior Staff Specialist, Department of Endocrinology and Diabetes, Royal Brisbane and Women's Hospital, Senior Honorary Research Officer, Population Health Department, QIMR Berghofer Medical Research Institute, Brisbane, Queensland, Australia

MICHAEL B. NATTER, MD
Endocrinology Fellow, Department of Medicine, Diabetes and Endocrinology Section, NYU Grossman School of Medicine, New York, New York, USA

JOANA OCHOA, MD
Department of Surgery, University of Florida College of Medicine–Jacksonville, Jacksonville, Florida, USA

NAYKKY SINGH OSPINA, MD, MS
Associate Professor, Division of Endocrinology, Diabetes and Metabolism, Department of Medicine, University of Florida, Gainesville, Florida, USA

KEPAL N. PATEL, MD, FACS
Associate Professor of Surgery, Otolaryngology and Biochemistry, Chief, Division of Endocrine Surgery, Department of Surgery, NYU Grossman School of Medicine, New York, New York, USA

SUSAN C. PITT, MD, MPHS
Division of Endocrine Surgery, Department of Surgery, University of Michigan, Ann Arbor, Michigan, USA

JENNIFER A. SIPOS, MD
Professor of Medicine, Division of Endocrinology, Diabetes and Metabolism, Department of Medicine, The Ohio State University Wexner Medical Center, Columbus, Ohio, USA

DEREK J. STOCKER, MD
Department of Radiology, Nuclear Medicine Service, Walter Reed National Military Medical Center, Associate Professor, Departments of Internal Medicine, Pathology, and Radiologic Sciences, Uniformed Services University of the Health Sciences, Bethesda, Maryland, USA

EVERT F.S. VAN VELSEN, MD, MSc
Department of Internal Medicine, Erasmus Medical Center, Academic Center for Thyroid Diseases, Rotterdam, the Netherlands

EVAN WALGAMA, MD
Saint John's Cancer Institute and Pacific Neuroscience Institute, Providence Health System, Santa Monica, California, USA

FRANCIS WORDEN, MD
Department of Hematology and Oncology, University of Michigan, Ann Arbor, Michigan, USA

MICHAEL W. YEH, MD, FACS
Professor of Surgery and Medicine, Section of Endocrine Surgery, UCLA David Geffen School of Medicine, Los Angeles, California, USA

MARK ZAFEREO, MD
Department of Head and Neck Surgery, The University of Texas MD Anderson Cancer Center, Houston, Texas, USA

Contents

Thyroid disease affects an estimated 20 million Americans, with 1 in 8 women developing a thyroid disorder during her lifetime. Although most patients with thyroid cancer have a good prognosis and effective treatments for benign thyroid disease are available, disparities exist in thyroid care and result in worse outcomes for racial and ethnic minorities. Inequities in the diagnosis and treatment of thyroid disease are due to the complex interplay of systems-, physician-, and patient-level factors. Thus, innovative strategies that take an ecological approach to addressing racial disparities are needed to achieve equitable care for all patients with thyroid disease.

Diverse causes potentially underlie decreased quality of life in biochemically euthyroid patients treated for hypothyroidism with levothyroxine. Once these contributing factors are addressed, if symptoms persist, there may be benefit to personalized use of combination therapy adding liothyronine. This approach should be carefully monitored: avoiding overtreatment and ensuring that therapy is only continued if it improves patient-reported quality of life. Most randomized clinical trials have not shown benefits, perhaps because of not targeting the most symptomatic patients. Sustained-release liothyronine preparations may soon be available for optimally designed studies assessing whether combination therapy provides superior therapy for hypothyroidism in select patients.

In recent years, cancer care has been transformed by immune-based and targeted treatments. Although these treatments are effective against various solid organ malignancies, multiple adverse effects can occur, including thyroid dysfunction. In this review, the authors consider treatments for solid organ cancers that affect the thyroid, focusing on immune checkpoint inhibitors, kinase inhibitors, and radioactive iodine-conjugated treatments (I-131-metaiodobenzylguanidine). They discuss the mechanisms causing thyroid dysfunction, provide a framework for their diagnosis and management, and explore the association of thyroid dysfunction from these agents with patient survival.

The management of hyperthyroidism and extrathyroidal manifestations of Graves disease remains complex. Considerations that include patient preference, age, comorbidity, pregnancy, tobacco smoking, and social determinants of health must all be weaved into a cohesive management plan. A multidisciplinary team is required to manage all aspects of Graves disease, particularly thyroid eye disease, for which new therapeutic options are now available.

Clinical evidence supports the association of ultrasound features with benign or malignant thyroid nodules and serves as the basis for sonographic stratification of thyroid nodules, according to an estimated thyroid cancer risk. Contemporary guidelines recommend management strategies according to thyroid cancer risk, thyroid nodule size, and the clinical scenario. Yet, reproducible and accurate thyroid nodule risk stratification requires expertise, time, and understanding of the weight different ultrasound features have on thyroid cancer risk. The application of artificial intelligence to overcome these limitations is promising and has the potential to improve the care of patients with thyroid nodules.

Image-guided interventional techniques have emerged as promising treatments for thyroid disease. Percutaneous ethanol ablation, radiofrequency ablation, laser ablation, high intensity focused ultrasound, and microwave ablation have shown efficacy in treating benign thyroid disease. There is increasing evidence that these techniques may effectively treat papillary thyroid microcarcinomas, recurrent and metastatic disease, follicular neoplasms, and parathyroid lesions. They are performed in an outpatient setting, well-tolerated, with negligible risk for thyroid hormone supplementation, making them a popular alternative to surgical resection. In this comprehensive review, we discuss the devices, techniques, advantages, and disadvantages of each intervention, and summarize the published outcomes.

The incidence of thyroid cancer is increasing, whereas mortality remains relatively stable. An increasing body of research supports the use of less-intensive treatment for low-risk thyroid cancer, as the overall prognosis is excellent. Although total thyroidectomy was the gold standard for many years, the options of lobectomy alone, active surveillance, and other ablative modalities are increasingly being used. The clinicohistologic features of any thyroid cancer are important to help determine the optimal management for a given tumor. However, the patient's own desires and goals in their cancer treatment must be evaluated.

questions about thyroid cancer prognosis and treatment, but also fertility and risk for adverse obstetric and/or fetal and neonatal outcomes. The benefits of thyroid cancer treatment should be weighed against its harms, as various options may adversely impact maternal and fetal health. In the current review, the authors focus on perinatal-specific clinical considerations related to the care of patients with thyroid cancer.

Thyroid disease is associated with adverse maternal and fetal outcomes. Appropriate reference ranges should be used for the interpretation of test results, although universal screening for thyroid dysfunction is not warranted. Overt thyroid dysfunction requires careful consideration of medication adjustments and close monitoring. Mild thyroid hypofunction has been linked to adverse pregnancy outcomes including preterm delivery, and poor neurocognition in the offspring. This review summarizes the most recent evidence on the counseling and management of women with thyroid disease before and during pregnancy and highlights the areas of controversy in need of further research.

ENDOCRINOLOGY AND METABOLISM CLINICS OF NORTH AMERICA

SERIES OF RELATED INTEREST

Medical Clinics
https://www.medical.theclinics.com
Primary Care: Clinics in Office Practice
https://www.primarycare.theclinics.com/

VISIT THE CLINICS ONLINE!
Access your subscription at:
www.theclinics.com

Foreword

Thyroid Disorders: An Update

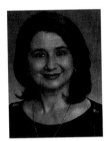

Adriana G. Ioachimescu, MD, PhD, FACE
Consulting Editor

The "Updates in Thyroidology" issue of the *Endocrinology and Metabolism Clinics of North America* reflects the progress in clinical management of patients with thyroid disorders in the past decade. The guest editors are Dr Megan Haymart and Dr Maria Papaleontiou from University of Michigan in Ann Arbor, Michigan, both endocrinologists with extensive clinical and research experience in this field.

Thyroid disorders are prevalent in the general population and can be diagnosed by primary care physicians, endocrinologists, obstetricians, or other health care professionals. Management of some thyroid conditions, such as Graves disease and thyroid nodules, entails multidisciplinary care by endocrinologists, thyroid surgeons, radiologists, ophthalmologists, and medical oncologists. Our collection of articles provides evidence-based information to guide the management of patients with thyroid disorders.

It is important to understand the racial and ethnic disparities in diagnosis, management, and prognosis of thyroid conditions. Proposed strategies to improve the prognosis of black and Hispanic patients include physician education, use of medical interpreters and multilingual and culturally sensitive written patient educational information, community engagement, and public policy changes to expand the medical insurance coverage.

A hot topic in hypothyroidism is combination therapy with levothyroxine and liothyronine for some patients with persistently low quality of life despite biochemical control on levothyroxine alone. If combination therapy is started, patients should be monitored closely to avoid iatrogenic hyperthyroidism and to ensure they experience health benefits. Other factors that may affect the quality of life should be evaluated, including other medical conditions, stress, and lifestyle.

Pregnancy is an important topic to discuss with female patients of reproductive age, including tailored preconception counseling for overt or subclinical thyroid dysfunction and expected changes in management during the perinatal period.

Endocrinol Metab Clin N Am 51 (2022) xiii–xiv
https://doi.org/10.1016/j.ecl.2022.02.007
0889-8529/22/© 2022 Published by Elsevier Inc.

endo.theclinics.com

Regarding thyroid nodules, the authors discuss the sonographic risk stratification systems and the potential role of artificial intelligence for early detection of thyroid cancer and avoidance of unnecessary biopsies.

Immune checkpoint inhibitors and kinase inhibitors have been increasingly used for solid organ malignancies, and these drugs can cause thyroiditis, hypothyroidism, or hyperthyroidism. A careful multidisciplinary approach is recommended, monitoring of thyroid function tests, and individualized management depending on clinical and biochemical parameters.

For patients with Graves disease who experience ophthalmopathy, new therapeutics with insulin-like growth factor 1 receptor inhibitors have recently become available. The authors present a comprehensive update in management of Graves thyroid and eye disease and their interplay.

Another area of recent development consists of minimally invasive techniques, such as radiofrequency or laser or percutaneous ethanol ablation, as nonsurgical options for patients with benign and malignant thyroid nodules. The authors present useful criteria to identify patients who might benefit from these procedures.

For patients with thyroid cancer, personalized treatment is emphasized, especially with the increased incidental detection in the past three decades. Less-intensive treatment options for low-risk thyroid cancer are discussed along with their influence on patients' quality of life. Preconception counseling is important for young women with thyroid cancer, and careful monitoring during pregnancy is recommended. For advanced differentiated cancer, the authors discuss novel targeted therapies (multi-targeted tyrosine kinase inhibitors and other agents currently under study) and radioactive iodine therapy. Medullary and anaplastic thyroid cancers are rare but have a significantly worse prognosis. These patients require careful evaluation (which includes genetic studies) and management at specialized tertiary referral centers.

I hope you will find this issue of the *Endocrinology and Metabolism Clinics of North America* an exciting reading and a helpful resource in your practice. I would like to thank our guest editors for orchestrating this important project, the authors for their excellent contributions, and the Elsevier editorial staff for their continuous support.

Adriana G. Ioachimescu, MD, PhD, FACE
Emory University School of Medicine
1365 B Clifton Road, Northeast, B6209
Atlanta, GA 30322, USA

E-mail address:
aioachi@emory.edu

Preface

Hot Topics and Advances in Thyroidology: Looking into the Future

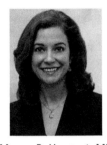
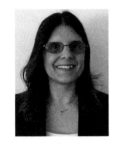

Megan R. Haymart, MD   Maria Papaleontiou, MD
Editors

Over the past decade, we have witnessed tremendous and exciting scientific advances in the field of thyroidology. These advances have been driven by scholarly inquisition, recognition of unmet patient needs, and researchers' drive to optimize patient care. In this special issue of *Endocrinology and Metabolism Clinics of North America*, our objective was to provide a contemporary view of the recent advances in the diagnosis and management of thyroid conditions, addressing topics that directly impact patient care. We have assembled a collection of 12 superb articles skillfully written by a distinguished panel of internationally renowned experts in the field and spanning a diverse array of topics focusing on both benign thyroid disease and thyroid cancer.

Commencing this issue, Drs Chen and Yeh discuss the important topic of disparities in thyroid care, including diagnosis and management, and underscore the need for innovative interventions to address these inequities. Dr Jonklaas addresses the role of LT4/LT3 combination therapy in the management of patients treated for hypothyroidism, provides insights on its personalized use, and delivers a glimpse into clinical trials underway. Drs Kotwal and McLeod expand on the hot topic of immune checkpoint inhibitors and kinase inhibitors used in the treatment of solid organ cancers and their association with thyroid dysfunction. Drs Hoang, Stocker, Chou, and Burch provide an exciting update on recent progress in the clinical management of Graves disease, with a particular focus on the rollout of promising new therapeutics for thyroid eye disease. Subsequently, in an era where artificial intelligence technologies are rapidly evolving into applicable solutions in clinical practice, Drs Burgos, Singh Ospina, and Sipos delve into the potential of such technologies to improve thyroid nodule risk stratification. Drs Baldwin, Natter, Patel, and Hodak skillfully discuss the

Endocrinol Metab Clin N Am 51 (2022) xv–xvi
https://doi.org/10.1016/j.ecl.2022.01.002
0889-8529/22/© 2022 Published by Elsevier Inc.

advent of innovative, emerging, minimally invasive techniques, such as radiofrequency ablation, as exciting nonsurgical options and patient-tailored approaches for the treatment of structural thyroid disease. In line with the shifting paradigm of thyroid cancer management to "less is more," Drs Ochoa and Pitt outline less-intensive treatment options for low-risk thyroid cancer while exploring the benefits and limitations of each treatment. On the other side of the thyroid cancer spectrum, Drs Lieberman and Worden discuss novel targeted therapies for advanced differentiated thyroid cancer, which have evolved based on our improved understanding of cancer genomics. Advances in medullary thyroid cancer and in anaplastic thyroid cancer are closely examined by Drs Walgama, Busaidy, and Zafereo, and Drs Maniakas, Zafereo, and Cabanillas, respectively. Finally, shifting the focus to thyroid and pregnancy, Drs van Velsen, Leung, and Korevaar address diagnostic and treatment considerations for thyroid cancer in women of reproductive age and the perinatal period, while Drs Dhillon-Smith and Boelaert review preconception counseling and care for pregnant women with benign thyroid disease.

We are honored to be invited by Elsevier to assemble and edit this timely series dedicated to thyroidology and are extremely grateful to all the authors and esteemed colleagues for their valuable, generous, and clinically relevant contributions. We are also thankful to the editorial staff for their continuous support during the preparation of this issue. We are delighted to present this issue on "Updates in Thyroidology," which we are certain will enhance the readers' care for their thyroid patients.

Megan R. Haymart, MD
Division of Metabolism
Endocrinology and Diabetes
Department of Internal Medicine
University of Michigan
North Campus Research Complex
2800 Plymouth Road
Building 16, Room 408E
Ann Arbor, MI 48109, USA

Maria Papaleontiou, MD
Division of Metabolism
Endocrinology and Diabetes
Department of Internal Medicine
University of Michigan
North Campus Research Complex
2800 Plymouth Road
Building 16, Room 453S
Ann Arbor, MI 48109, USA

E-mail addresses:
meganhay@med.umich.edu (M.R. Haymart)
mpapaleo@med.umich.edu (M. Papaleontiou)

Disparities in Thyroid Care

Debbie W. Chen, MD[a,*], Michael W. Yeh, MD[b]

KEYWORDS

- Health care disparity • Minority groups • Thyroid disease • Thyroid cancer
- Graves disease • Hypothyroidism

KEY POINTS

- Disparities exist in the diagnosis and treatment of malignant and benign thyroid disease, with racial and ethnic minorities experiencing worse clinical outcomes.
- Racial and ethnic minorities with thyroid cancer present with more advanced disease and experience more surgical complications, likely a result of care delivered by lower-volume surgeons.
- Black patients with Graves disease are more likely to receive surgical treatment, and have worse surgical outcomes compared with their White counterparts.
- Ethnic differences exist in the treatment of hypothyroidism, with Hispanic ethnicity associated with undertreatment compared with non-Hispanic Whites.
- Inequities in thyroid care are due to the complex interplay of systems-, physician-, and patient-level factors. Thus, innovative multilevel interventions are necessary to address racial disparities and ultimately to achieve more equitable care for all patients with thyroid disease.

INTRODUCTION

The 1985 landmark Report of the Secretary's Task Force on Black and Minority Health, commonly referred to as the Heckler Report, elevated minority health into the national consciousness. The first comprehensive study of racial and ethnic minority health conducted by the US government, the Heckler Report detailed persistent health disparities that accounted for 60,000 excess deaths each year.[1] It served as a driving force for change in research, policy, and initiatives aimed at advancing health equity at the local, state, and national levels. Almost 2 decades later in 2003, the Institute of Medicine (IOM) published its groundbreaking report, *Unequal Treatment: Confronting Racial and Ethnic Disparities in Healthcare*, which found that racial and ethnic

Disclosure: Dr D.W. Chen receives support from grant T32DK07245 from the National Institutes of Diabetes and Digestive and Kidney Diseases.
[a] Department of Internal Medicine, Division of Metabolism, Endocrinology, and Diabetes, University of Michigan, 24 Frank Lloyd Wright Drive, PO Box 451, Ann Arbor, MI 48106, USA;
[b] Section of Endocrine Surgery, UCLA David Geffen School of Medicine, 10833 Le Conte Avenue, Los Angeles, CA 90095, USA
* Corresponding author.
E-mail address: chendeb@med.umich.edu

minorities tended to receive lower-quality health care than nonminorities with resultant worse outcomes.[2] The IOM report also offered recommendations regarding interventions to eliminate health care disparities that were targeted to a broad audience. Although significant progress has been made in reducing health care disparities, defined by the IOM study committee as racial or ethnic differences in the quality of health care that are not due to access-related factors or clinical needs, preferences, and appropriateness of intervention, the elimination of disparities has yet to be achieved.[2]

Disparities continue to exist in the diagnosis and treatment of thyroid disease, which affects an estimated 20 million Americans, with patients of racial and ethnic minorities experiencing worse outcomes for both malignant and benign thyroid disease.[3] The interaction between race, culture, and health care is complex, with disparities in thyroid care arising from the complex interplay of systems-, physician-, and patient-level factors. Research has suggested that in addition to socioeconomic factors and insurance status, poor access to adequate medical and surgical care for thyroid disease in minority populations plays a contributing role.[4–8] This review will provide a comprehensive summary of the evidence describing health care disparities in thyroid disease, examine contributing factors, and provide recommendations for multilevel strategies to reduce disparities in thyroid care.

DISPARITIES IN THYROID CANCER CARE
Evidence of Inequitable Care Across the Thyroid Cancer Continuum

Racial and ethnic minorities with thyroid cancer experience a substantial burden of disease. Thyroid cancer is the second most common cancer among Hispanic and Asian/Pacific Islander women in the United States, and both patient populations have the highest thyroid cancer mortality rates.[9–11] From the time of thyroid cancer diagnosis and into the survivorship period, racial and ethnic minorities experience disparities in care with resultant worse patient outcomes.[12]

Studies have consistently demonstrated that racial and ethnic minorities with thyroid cancer are more likely to present with larger tumors and more advanced diseases compared with their White counterparts.[4,13–16] With regards to thyroid surgery, higher surgeon volume predicts lower complication rates and shorter length of stay.[8,17–19] In a nationwide sample of 16,878 patients who underwent thyroid surgery between 1999 and 2004, Sosa and colleagues[7] revealed that most Hispanic and Black patients had surgery by the lowest-volume surgeons and that in-hospital mortality was higher for Black patients. Al-Qurayshi et al reported similar findings using data from 2010 to 2011, with Hispanic and Black patients with thyroid cancer more likely to receive treatment by low-volume surgeons compared with their White counterparts.[17] Non-White patients with thyroid cancer are more likely to experience surgical complications, possibly secondary to care by lower-volume surgeons, and more likely to not receive radioactive iodine (RAI) treatment when it was clinically indicated based on the 2015 American Thyroid Association (ATA) management guidelines for thyroid cancer.[20,21]

Even in the management of anaplastic thyroid cancer, an aggressive cancer that is associated with a poor prognosis and high mortality rate, disparities exist.[22] In a study of 719 patients with anaplastic thyroid cancer between 1998 and 2011, Roche and colleagues[23] revealed that non-White patients were more likely to receive no treatment and have a poorer overall survival.

Beyond the initial treatment of thyroid cancer, racial and ethnic minorities continue to have different experiences from that of their White counterparts. In a survey of 2215 disease-free thyroid cancer survivors 2 to 4 years after their diagnosis, Papaleontiou and colleagues[24] found that thyroid cancer-related worry was associated with being Hispanic or Asian. Hispanic ethnicity was also found to be associated with overestimating thyroid cancer recurrence risk in a population-based study of 1597 patients with low-risk differentiated thyroid cancer.[25] Furthermore, survey-based studies have found that among Hispanic patients with thyroid cancer, differences exist based on the level of acculturation. Chen and colleagues[26] demonstrated that although financial hardship decreased with older age for high-acculturated Hispanic women with thyroid cancer, financial hardship remained elevated across all age groups for low-acculturated Hispanic women.

Factors that Contribute to Inequitable Care for Racial/Ethnic Minorities with Thyroid Cancer

Thyroid cancer patient outcomes are influenced by multilevel factors that can be visualized as a hierarchy of needs, with the most critical need, access to high-volume physicians, at the bottom to the hierarchy (**Fig. 1**). Disparities exist in thyroid cancer care when these needs are unmet because of the interplay of multiple systems-, physician-, and patient-level factors. Systems-level factors include health insurance and socioeconomic status, and differences in where patients seek medical care. In a retrospective study of 190,298 patients with papillary thyroid cancer diagnosed between 2004 and 2015, Ullmann and colleagues[27] revealed that a significant inverse correlation exists between the percentage of uninsured 18- to 64-year-old adults in each state and the state-by-state incidence of all thyroid cancers. The authors also found that patients with private insurance, compared with no insurance, were more likely to receive more extensive surgical and adjuvant treatment.[27] Similarly, studies have found that

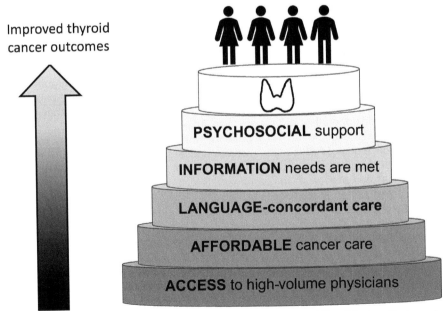

Improved thyroid cancer outcomes

PSYCHOSOCIAL support

INFORMATION needs are met

LANGUAGE-concordant care

AFFORDABLE cancer care

ACCESS to high-volume physicians

Fig. 1. Thyroid cancer patient outcomes are influenced by multilevel factors that can be visualized as a hierarchy of needs. To achieve improved thyroid cancer outcomes, it is necessary to fulfill the more critically important needs at the bottom of the hierarchy before moving on to the more advanced needs higher up in the hierarchy.

low socioeconomic status is associated with more advanced thyroid cancer and lower rates of adjuvant RAI therapy.[4,28] Hospital characteristics also have an impact, likely reflecting the health insurance and socioeconomic status of each hospital's patient population as well as resource availability.[14,29] In a retrospective cohort study, Lim and colleagues[29] found that patients at a large public hospital were 3.4 times more likely to present with advanced differentiated thyroid cancer than patients at the adjacent university teaching hospital (Lim). Notably, 96% of the public hospital patients self-reported as non-White compared with 16% of the university hospital patients. Similarly, White and colleagues[30] showed that guidelines from the ATA and the National Comprehensive Cancer Network (NCCN) were more likely to be followed for patients who traveled to academic centers for their thyroid cancer care compared with those who received treatment at a local hospital.

Physician-level factors that impact thyroid cancer diagnosis and treatment include variable use of thyroid ultrasound, experience with treating thyroid cancer, communication styles, conscious and unconscious biases, and cultural competency. The incidence of thyroid cancer increased substantially between 1973 and 2014, driven principally by the increased detection of small papillary thyroid cancers in the setting of widespread thyroid ultrasound screening.[11,31,32] Although the incidence of thyroid cancer has increased among all races and ethnicities, the magnitude of the increase has been larger for non-Hispanic patients than for Hispanic patients. This difference may be attributable to the differential use of thyroid ultrasound by physicians.[33,34] In a diverse cohort of 602 physicians involved in the care of patients with thyroid cancer, Chen and colleagues[35] found that although most physicians reported ultrasound use for clinically supported reasons, a substantial number endorsed ultrasound use for clinically unsupported reasons of patient request (33%), abnormal thyroid function tests (28%), and positive thyroid antibodies (23%). Furthermore, physicians in private practice were more likely to schedule ultrasounds for abnormal thyroid function tests and positive thyroid antibodies compared with those in academic medical centers.[35] Differences also exist in physicians' use of thyroid ultrasound during the long-term surveillance of thyroid cancer. In a cross-sectional study of 320 physicians who reported involvement with differentiated thyroid cancer surveillance, Kovatch and colleagues[36] found that only 27% reported personally performing bedside ultrasonography, and 33% did not report high confidence in either their ability or a radiologist's ability to use ultrasonography to detect cancer recurrence. Variations in thyroid cancer treatment in the postoperative setting are also influenced by physician factors. In a population-based sample of 1319 patients with differentiated thyroid cancer in whom selective use of RAI is recommended and shared decision making is encouraged, Wallner and colleagues[37] found that receipt of RAI was associated with physician attitudes and propensity to recommend RAI.

Patient-level factors that influence thyroid cancer care include patients' understanding of the disease, level of acculturation, treatment preferences, illness perception, and physician trust. An accurate understanding of thyroid cancer is critically important and influences patients' attitude and behavior toward the disease. Unfortunately, patients with thyroid cancer have significant unmet information needs, and this is exacerbated by preference for thyroid cancer information in a non-English language.[38–41] In a population-based survey study, Chen and colleagues[41] found that Hispanic women with thyroid cancer were significantly more likely to report the ability to access thyroid cancer information "all of the time" if they preferred information in English compared with Spanish. Furthermore, patient preference has been found to impact the intensity of thyroid cancer surveillance. Evron and colleagues[42] revealed that patient preference for a more maximal versus minimal approach to medical care is independently associated with increased health care utilization in the postoperative surveillance of thyroid cancer.

DISPARITIES IN THE TREATMENT OF BENIGN THYROID DISEASE
Racial Differences in the Treatment of Graves Disease

Hyperthyroidism is present in about 1.2% of the US population, with Graves disease accounting for up to 80% of cases and being more common in Blacks compared with Whites.[43–45] McLeod et al found that compared with Whites, the incidence rate ratios (IRRs) for Graves disease was significantly higher in Blacks (IRR 1.92 for Black women, and IRR 2.53 for Black men).[45] Independent of treatment modality, early and intensive control of hyperthyroidism in Graves disease is associated with decreased cardiovascular morbidity and all-cause mortality.[46–48] Treatment options for Graves disease include antithyroid drugs, RAI ablation, and thyroid surgery. Although the least used therapy in the United States, thyroid surgery is the most effective treatment for Graves disease and more likely to be used in the treatment of Black patients with Graves disease.[49–51] In a retrospective study of 427 patients with Graves disease, Elfenbein and colleagues[44] found that Black patients in the cohort underwent surgery 56% of the time as a first-line treatment compared with 28% of non-Black patients. In univariate analysis, surgical treatment (vs RAI) was found to be associated with Black race. In a study of 634 patients who were treated for Graves disease over a 10-year period at an urban county hospital, factors influencing the choice for surgical treatment of Graves disease were found to be patient preference and compressive symptoms.[52] Although thyroid surgery is the most efficacious treatment for Graves disease, there is variation in the incidence of postoperative complications that likely reflects differences in surgeons' experience and patient selection.[18,50] Among patients who underwent thyroid surgery for benign and malignant disease, Black patients were more likely to have neck hematoma and recurrent laryngeal nerve injury, unplanned hospitalization within 30 days after thyroidectomy, and negative voice outcomes compared with their White counterparts.[53–55]

Factors that Contribute to Disparities in Surgical Outcomes for Patients with Graves

The observed differences in surgical outcomes for Graves disease may arise partially due to differences in disease presentation and existing systemic disease of Black versus White patients undergoing thyroid surgery. In a study of 1189 patients with benign disease treated with thyroidectomy, Kuo and colleagues[56] found that Black (vs White) patients more commonly presented with compressive symptoms, larger thyroid glands, and after a longer disease duration. Interestingly, thyroid-associated ophthalmopathy, the most prevalent extrathyroidal manifestation of Graves disease, has not been found to be associated with race.[57] In addition, in a national database analysis of 1695 patients who had undergone thyroidectomy for Graves disease, Beck and colleagues[58] found that Black (vs Non-Hispanic White) patients were more likely to have an American Society of Anesthesiology (ASA) classification of physical health score of at least 3 and a higher rate of congestive heart failure. In univariate analysis, patients with an ASA score of at least 3 or with congestive heart failure were more likely to have complications.[58]

Ethnic Differences in the Treatment of Hypothyroidism

Hypothyroidism is present in 4.6% of the US population (0.3% clinical hypothyroidism and 4.3% subclinical hypothyroidism).[59,60] The standard of care for the treatment of hypothyroidism is levothyroxine, one of the most commonly prescribed drugs in the

United States with more than 11 million prescriptions filled in 2016.[61–63] However, disparities exist in the prescribing pattern for thyroid hormone replacement based on nonclinical factors. In a cohort of 1443 community participants in Baltimore, Mammen and colleagues[64] found that thyroid hormone initiation was more than twice as likely among White (vs Black) patients, and highest among women older than 80 years. Somwaru and colleagues[65] reported similar findings in their population-based longitudinal study of 5888 individuals aged 65 years and older, with those aged 85 years and older (vs 65–69 years) and White women more likely to be initiated on thyroid hormone replacement. To understand the clinical significance of disparities in thyroid hormone prescribing, Ettleson and colleagues[66] examined the sociodemographic characteristics between those with untreated and treated hypothyroidism using the National Health and Nutrition Examination Survey (NHANES), a nationally representative data set with available thyroid function data. Ettleson and colleagues[66] found that male gender, younger age, and lack of access to routine health care were associated with untreated hypothyroidism. Furthermore, Hispanic ethnicity was associated with inadequate treatment of hypothyroidism compared with non-Hispanic White.[66] More work is needed to understand why this disparity in treatment of hypothyroidism exists (eg, communication barriers, systemic barriers, etc) and its downstream implications (eg, coronary heart disease, heart failure, cognitive dysfunction, and pregnancy-related complications in those with untreated and undertreated hypothyroidism).

STRATEGIES TO ACHIEVE MORE EQUITABLE THYROID CARE

The causes of disparities in thyroid care are multifactorial and thus, innovative strategies that take an ecological approach to addressing racial disparities are needed to achieve equitable care for all patients with thyroid disease (**Table 1**). At the individual level, physicians need to have opportunities and protected time to obtain advanced training in thyroid ultrasonography, which is the cornerstone of long-term surveillance for thyroid cancer, and in effectively communicating with limited English proficient patients via trained medical interpreters.[67–70] In addition, the development of easily accessible multilingual and culturally sensitive information support tools and decision aids for thyroid disease will facilitate patients' understanding and involvement in the treatment decision making.[71,72] At the level of hospitals and health care systems, time and resources should be invested to (1) improve health care access for patients with limited English proficiency, a vulnerable and important population comprising more than 25 million individuals in the United States[73–76]; (2) provide opportunities for patients with thyroid cancer to meet with financial counselors given the substantial health care costs of thyroid cancer in the United States[77–80]; and (3) engage with the community to address social and environmental factors that impact the health of community members. In the realm of public policy, there needs to be increased access to high-volume surgeons, given findings from multiple studies that have demonstrated an association between higher-volume surgeons and improved patient outcomes.[7,8,17–19] To improve access, it is necessary to increase transparency on surgeons' performance of thyroid surgery (ie, volume per year and patient outcomes) and develop clinical practice guidelines with parameters on which patients would benefit from referral to a high-volume surgeon for thyroid surgery based on the extent of disease. In addition, the expansion of Medicaid or creation of an alternative mechanism to provide affordable health insurance to uninsured adults living in the United States will be essential to improving health care access.[81,82] Furthermore, even after the current coronavirus disease (COVID-19) pandemic ends, continued provider reimbursement for virtual visits, including those conducted by telephone and across state

Table 1
Strategies to address disparities in thyroid care

	Address System Factors	Address Physician Factors	Address Patient Factors
At the level of the individual			
Physician training and education on effective use of trained medical interpreters to provide care to limited English proficient patients	X	X	X
Continuing medical education courses in thyroid ultrasonography and effective shared decision making for physicians	X	X	X
Clinical practice guidelines on appropriate thyroid ultrasound use	X	X	
Easily accessible information support tools and decision aids for thyroid disease in patients' preferred language			X
At the level of hospitals and health care systems			
Financial investment to improve health care access for limited English proficient patients (ie, multilingual hospital signs/information, multilingual patient portal)	X	X	X
Use of nontraditional platforms for virtual visits (eg, FaceTime, telephone)	X		X
Availability of financial counselors to assist patients with thyroid cancer from the time of diagnosis	X		X
Community engagement to better understand and address the social and environmental factors that impact the health of its community members	X		X
Public policy			
Funding for disparities-focused research	X	X	X
Resource allocation to increase access to trained medical interpreters for limited English proficient patients, and to high-volume surgeons for all patients	X		X
Reimbursement by insurance companies for virtual visits and thyroid specialists across state lines	X		X
Expand Medicaid coverage or provide alternative affordable insurance options for uninsured adults	X		X

lines, will improve access to thyroid care for vulnerable patient populations living in underserved areas.[83] Continued funding for disparities-focused research, such as those available through the National Institutes of Health, American Cancer Society, the Association of American Medical Colleges, and the Centers for Medicare and Medicaid Services, is also essential to improve our understanding of disparities in thyroid care and provide actionable data that will yield more equitable care for all patients.[84–88]

SUMMARY

Given the high prevalence of thyroid disease in the United States and documented worse outcomes for racial and ethnic minorities, the endocrinology community faces an imperative to examine the factors contributing to such inequities and implement effective strategies to reduce disparities in thyroid care.[3] Current population-based data demonstrate that multiple factors contribute to disparities in the process and outcomes of thyroid care. These include socioeconomic status, health insurance status, and differential access to physicians and hospitals capable of providing the highest level of care. Continued funding for disparities-focused research and engagement of major stakeholders in the health care system are necessary to improve the health of vulnerable patient populations with thyroid disease. In addition, prioritizing the reduction of racial disparities in public policy and allocating resources to this effort will be essential.

CLINICS CARE POINTS

- Variation exists in the provision of guideline-concordant care for patients with thyroid cancer. Thus, it is important for all members of the thyroid cancer patient's treatment team to be familiar with and have access to the American Thyroid Association (ATA) and/or the National Comprehensive Cancer Network (NCCN) guidelines on treatment of thyroid cancer.

- Patients with thyroid cancer have significant unmet information needs. Because non–English-speaking patients with thyroid cancer may have greater unmet information needs that may impair shared decision making, physicians should use language interpreters liberally and have culturally and linguistically appropriate patient-centered literature available in various languages.

- To improve thyroid cancer care delivery and quality, clinics should have a list of endocrinologists, surgeons, and ultrasound radiologists on hand for all patients. The list of physicians should be available in several languages and include all the insurances accepted by each practitioner, as well as what languages they speak.

CONFLICT OF INTEREST STATEMENT

The authors have no conflicts of interest to disclose.

REFERENCES

1. Malone TE. Executive summary in report of the Secretary's Task force on Black and minority health, 1. Washington, D.C.: U.S. Department of Health and Human Services; 1985.
2. Smedley BD, Stith AY, Nelson AR, editors. Unequal treatment: confronting racial and ethnic disparities in healthcare. Washington, D.C.: The National Academes Press; 2003.
3. American Thyroid Association. General information/press room. Available at: https://www.thyroid.org/media-main/press-room/. Accessed July 1, 2021.
4. Harari A, Li N, Yeh MW. Racial and socioeconomic disparities in presentation and outcomes of well-differentiated thyroid cancer. J Clin Endocrinol Metab 2014; 99(1):133–41.
5. Golden SH, Brown A, Cauley JA, et al. Health disparities in endocrine disorders: biological, clinical, and nonclinical factors–an Endocrine Society scientific statement. J Clin Endocrinol Metab 2012;97(9):E1579–639.
6. Ramakrishnan K, Ahmad FZ. State of Asian Americans and Pacific Islanders Series: a multifaceted portrait of a growing population. Washington, DC: Center for American Progress; 2014.
7. Sosa JA, Mehta PJ, Wang TS, et al. Racial disparities in clinical and economic outcomes from thyroidectomy. Ann Surg 2007;246(6):1083–91.

8. Noureldine SI, Abbas A, Tufano RP, et al. The impact of surgical volume on racial disparity in thyroid and parathyroid surgery. Ann Surg Oncol 2014;21(8):2733–9.

9. Miller KD, Goding Sauer A, Ortiz AP, et al. Cancer Statistics for Hispanics/Latinos, 2018. CA Cancer J Clin 2018;68(6):425–45.

10. Torre LA, Sauer AM, Chen MS Jr, et al. Cancer statistics for Asian Americans, Native Hawaiians, and Pacific Islanders, 2016: Converging incidence in males and females. CA Cancer J Clin 2016;66(3):182–202.

11. National Cancer Institute. Cancer Stat Facts: thyroid cancer. Available at: https://seer.cancer.gov/statfacts/html/thyro.html. Accessed June 1, 2021.

12. Chen DW, Haymart MR. Disparities Research in Thyroid Cancer: Challenges and Strategies for Improvement. Thyroid 2020;30(9):1231–5.

13. Weeks KS, Kahl AR, Lynch CF, et al. Racial/ethnic differences in thyroid cancer incidence in the United States, 2007-2014. Cancer 2018;124(7):1483–91.

14. Zagzag J, Kenigsberg A, Patel KN, et al. Thyroid cancer is more likely to be detected incidentally on imaging in private hospital patients. J Surg Res 2017;215:239–44.

15. Hollenbeak CS, Wang L, Schneider P, et al. Outcomes of thyroid cancer in African Americans. Ethn Dis 2011;21(2):210–5.

16. Moten AS, Zhao H, Intenzo CM, et al. Disparity in the use of adjuvant radioactive iodine ablation among high-risk papillary thyroid cancer patients. Eur J Surg Oncol 2019;45(11):2090–5.

17. Al-Qurayshi Z, Randolph GW, Srivastav S, et al. Outcomes in endocrine cancer surgery are affected by racial, economic, and healthcare system demographics. Laryngoscope 2016;126(3):775–81.

18. Sosa JA, Bowman HM, Tielsch JM, et al. The importance of surgeon experience for clinical and economic outcomes from thyroidectomy. Ann Surg 1998;228(3):320–30.

19. Stavrakis AI, Ituarte PH, Ko CY, et al. Surgeon volume as a predictor of outcomes in inpatient and outpatient endocrine surgery. Surgery 2007;142(6):887–99.

20. Kovatch KJ, Reyes-Gastelum D, Hughes DT, et al. Assessment of Voice Outcomes Following Surgery for Thyroid Cancer. JAMA Otolaryngol Head Neck Surg 2019;145:823–9.

21. Shah SA, Adam MA, Thomas SM, et al. Racial Disparities in Differentiated Thyroid Cancer: Have We Bridged the Gap? Thyroid 2017;27(6):762–72.

22. Smallridge RC, Ain KB, Asa SL, et al. American Thyroid Association Anaplastic Thyroid Cancer Guidelines T. American Thyroid Association guidelines for management of patients with anaplastic thyroid cancer. Thyroid 2012;22(11):1104–39.

23. Roche AM, Fedewa SA, Shi LL, et al. Treatment and survival vary by race/ethnicity in patients with anaplastic thyroid cancer. Cancer 2018;124(8):1780–90.

24. Papaleontiou M, Reyes-Gastelum D, Gay BL, et al. Worry in Thyroid Cancer Survivors with a Favorable Prognosis. Thyroid 2019;29(8):1080–8.

25. Chen DW, Reyes-Gastelum D, Wallner LP, et al. Disparities in risk perception of thyroid cancer recurrence and death. Cancer 2020;126(7):1512–21.

26. Chen DW, Reyes-Gastelum D, Veenstra CM, et al. Financial Hardship Among Hispanic Women with Thyroid Cancer. Thyroid 2021;31(5):752–9.

27. Ullmann TM, Gray KD, Limberg J, et al. Insurance Status Is Associated with Extent of Treatment for Patients with Papillary Thyroid Carcinoma. Thyroid 2019;29(12):1784–91.

28. Zevallos JP, Xu L, Yiu Y. The impact of socioeconomic status on the use of adjuvant radioactive iodine for papillary thyroid cancer. Thyroid 2014;24(4):758–63.

29. Lim II, Hochman T, Blumberg SN, et al. Disparities in the initial presentation of differentiated thyroid cancer in a large public hospital and adjoining university teaching hospital. Thyroid 2012;22(3):269–74.

30. White MG, Applewhite MK, Kaplan EL, et al. A Tale of Two Cancers: Traveling to Treat Pancreatic and Thyroid Cancer. J Am Coll Surg 2017;225(1):125–136 e126.

31. Davies L, Welch HG. Increasing incidence of thyroid cancer in the United States, 1973-2002. JAMA 2006;295(18):2164–7.

32. Haymart MR, Banerjee M, Reyes-Gastelum D, et al. Thyroid Ultrasound and the Increase in Diagnosis of Low-Risk Thyroid Cancer. J Clin Endocrinol Metab 2019;104(3):785–92.

33. Magreni A, Bann DV, Schubart JR, et al. The effects of race and ethnicity on thyroid cancer incidence. JAMA Otolaryngol Head Neck Surg 2015;141(4):319–23.

34. Marcadis AR, Davies L, Marti JL, et al. Racial Disparities in Cancer Presentation and Outcomes: The Contribution of Overdiagnosis. JNCI Cancer Spectr 2020; 4(2):pkaa001.

35. Chen DW, Reyes-Gastelum D, Radhakrishnan A, et al. Physician-Reported Misuse of Thyroid Ultrasonography. JAMA Surg 2020;155:984–6.

36. Kovatch KJ, Reyes-Gastelum D, Sipos JA, et al. Physician Confidence in Neck Ultrasonography for Surveillance of Differentiated Thyroid Cancer Recurrence. JAMA Otolaryngol Head Neck Surg 2020;147(2):166–72.

37. Wallner LP, Reyes-Gastelum D, Hamilton AS, et al. Patient-Perceived Lack of Choice in Receipt of Radioactive Iodine for Treatment of Differentiated Thyroid Cancer. J Clin Oncol 2019;37(24):2152–61.

38. Sawka AM, Brierley JD, Tsang RW, et al. Unmet Information Needs of Low-Risk Thyroid Cancer Survivors. Thyroid 2016;26(3):474–5.

39. Morley S, Goldfarb M. Support needs and survivorship concerns of thyroid cancer patients. Thyroid 2015;25(6):649–56.

40. Husson O, Mols F, Oranje WA, et al. Unmet information needs and impact of cancer in (long-term) thyroid cancer survivors: results of the PROFILES registry. Psychooncology 2014;23(8):946–52.

41. Chen DW, Reyes-Gastelum D, Hawley ST, et al. Unmet Information Needs Among Hispanic Women with Thyroid Cancer. J Clin Endocrinol Metab 2021;106(7): e2680–7.

42. Evron JM, Reyes-Gastelum D, Banerjee M, et al. Role of Patient Maximizing-Minimizing Preferences in Thyroid Cancer Surveillance. J Clin Oncol 2019; 37(32):3042–9.

43. Ross DS, Burch HB, Cooper DS, et al. 2016 American Thyroid Association Guidelines for Diagnosis and Management of Hyperthyroidism and Other Causes of Thyrotoxicosis. Thyroid 2016;26(10):1343–421.

44. Elfenbein DM, Schneider DF, Havlena J, et al. Clinical and socioeconomic factors influence treatment decisions in Graves' disease. Ann Surg Oncol 2015;22(4): 1196–9.

45. McLeod DS, Caturegli P, Cooper DS, et al. Variation in rates of autoimmune thyroid disease by race/ethnicity in US military personnel. JAMA 2014;311(15): 1563–5.

46. Okosieme OE, Taylor PN, Evans C, et al. Primary therapy of Graves' disease and cardiovascular morbidity and mortality: a linked-record cohort study. Lancet Diabetes Endocrinol 2019;7(4):278–87.

47. Ryodi E, Metso S, Huhtala H, et al. Cardiovascular Morbidity and Mortality After Treatment of Hyperthyroidism with Either Radioactive Iodine or Thyroidectomy. Thyroid 2018;28(9):1111–20.

48. Lillevang-Johansen M, Abrahamsen B, Jorgensen HL, et al. Duration of Hyperthyroidism and Lack of Sufficient Treatment Are Associated with Increased Cardiovascular Risk. Thyroid 2019;29(3):332–40.

49. Brito JP, Payne S, Singh Ospina N, et al. Patterns of Use, Efficacy, and Safety of Treatment Options for Patients with Graves' Disease: A Nationwide Population-Based Study. Thyroid 2020;30(3):357–64.

50. Sundaresh V, Brito JP, Thapa P, et al. Comparative Effectiveness of Treatment Choices for Graves' Hyperthyroidism: A Historical Cohort Study. Thyroid 2017; 27(4):497–505.

51. Palit TK, Miller CC 3rd, Miltenburg DM. The efficacy of thyroidectomy for Graves' disease: A meta-analysis. J Surg Res 2000;90(2):161–5.

52. Jin J, Sandoval V, Lawless ME, et al. Disparity in the management of Graves' disease observed at an urban county hospital: a decade-long experience. Am J Surg 2012;204(2):199–202.

53. Maduka RC, Gibson CE, Chiu AS, et al. Racial disparities in surgical outcomes for benign thyroid disease. Am J Surg 2020;220(5):1219–24.

54. FitzGerald RA, Sehgal AR, Nichols JA, et al. Factors Predictive of Emergency Department Visits and Hospitalization Following Thyroidectomy and Parathyroidectomy. Ann Surg Oncol 2015;22(Suppl 3):S707–13.

55. Radowsky JS, Helou LB, Howard RS, et al. Racial disparities in voice outcomes after thyroid and parathyroid surgery. Surgery 2013;153(1):103–10.

56. Kuo LE, Simmons KD, Wachtel H, et al. Racial Disparities in Initial Presentation of Benign Thyroid Disease for Resection. Ann Surg Oncol 2016;23(8):2571–6.

57. Stein JD, Childers D, Gupta S, et al. Risk factors for developing thyroid-associated ophthalmopathy among individuals with Graves disease. JAMA Ophthalmol 2015;133(3):290–6.

58. Beck AC, Sugg SL, Weigel RJ, et al. Racial disparities in comorbid conditions among patients undergoing thyroidectomy for Graves' disease: An ACS-NSQIP analysis. Am J Surg 2021;221(1):106–10.

59. Hollowell JG, Staehling NW, Flanders WD, et al. Serum TSH, T(4), and thyroid antibodies in the United States population (1988 to 1994): National Health and Nutrition Examination Survey (NHANES III). J Clin Endocrinol Metab 2002;87(2): 489–99.

60. Canaris GJ, Manowitz NR, Mayor G, et al. The Colorado thyroid disease prevalence study. Arch Intern Med 2000;160(4):526–34.

61. Garber JR, Cobin RH, Gharib H, et al. American Thyroid Association Taskforce on Hypothyroidism in A. Clinical practice guidelines for hypothyroidism in adults: co-sponsored by the American Association of Clinical Endocrinologists and the American Thyroid Association. Endocr Pract 2012;18(6):988–1028.

62. Kantor ED, Rehm CD, Haas JS, et al. Trends in Prescription Drug Use Among Adults in the United States From 1999-2012. JAMA 2015;314(17):1818–31.

63. Ross JS, Rohde S, Sangaralingham L, et al. Generic and Brand-Name Thyroid Hormone Drug Use Among Commercially Insured and Medicare Beneficiaries, 2007 Through 2016. J Clin Endocrinol Metab 2019;104(6):2305–14.

64. Mammen JS, McGready J, Oxman R, et al. Thyroid Hormone Therapy and Risk of Thyrotoxicosis in Community-Resident Older Adults: Findings from the Baltimore Longitudinal Study of Aging. Thyroid 2015;25(9):979–86.

65. Somwaru LL, Arnold AM, Cappola AR. Predictors of thyroid hormone initiation in older adults: results from the cardiovascular health study. J Gerontol A Biol Sci Med Sci 2011;66(7):809–14.

66. Ettleson MD, Bianco AC, Zhu M, et al. Sociodemographic Disparities in the Treatment of Hypothyroidism: NHANES 2007-2012. J Endocr Soc 2021;5(7):bvab041.
67. Lubrano di Ciccone B, Brown RF, Gueguen JA, et al. Interviewing patients using interpreters in an oncology setting: initial evaluation of a communication skills module. Ann Oncol 2010;21(1):27–32.
68. Perez GK, Mutchler J, Yang MS, et al. Promoting quality care in patients with cancer with limited English proficiency: perspectives of medical interpreters. Psychooncology 2016;25(10):1241–5.
69. Gadon M, Balch GI, Jacobs EA. Caring for patients with limited English proficiency: the perspectives of small group practitioners. J Gen Intern Med 2007; 22(Suppl 2):341–6.
70. Wilson E, Chen AH, Grumbach K, et al. Effects of limited English proficiency and physician language on health care comprehension. J Gen Intern Med 2005;20(9): 800–6.
71. Sawka AM, Straus S, Rodin G, et al. Decision aid on radioactive iodine treatment for early stage papillary thyroid cancer: update to study protocol with follow-up extension. Trials 2015;16:302.
72. Pitt SC, Saucke MC. Novel Decision Support Interventions for Low-risk Thyroid Cancer. JAMA Otolaryngol Head Neck Surg 2020;146(11):1079–81.
73. Weiss L, Bauer T, Hill C, et al. Language as a barrier to health care for New York City children in immigrant families: Haitian, Russian and Latino perspectives. New York, NY: New York Academy of Medicine; 2006.
74. Ahn J, Abesamis-Mendoza N. Chinese American community health needs and resource assessment: an exploratory study of Chinese in NYC. New York, NY: NYU Center for the Study of Asian American Health; 2007.
75. Simon MA, Tom LS, Taylor S, et al. There's nothing you can do ... it's like that in Chinatown': Chinese immigrant women's perceptions of experiences in Chicago Chinatown healthcare settings. Ethn Health 2019;1–18.
76. United States Census Bureau. Detailed languages spoken at home and ability to speak English for the population 5 years and over: 2009-2013. Available at: https://www.census.gov/data/tables/2013/demo/2009-2013-lang-tables.html. Accessed June 1, 2021.
77. Lubitz CC, Kong CY, McMahon PM, et al. Annual financial impact of well-differentiated thyroid cancer care in the United States. Cancer 2014;120(9): 1345–52.
78. Ramsey S, Blough D, Kirchhoff A, et al. Washington State cancer patients found to be at greater risk for bankruptcy than people without a cancer diagnosis. Health Aff (Millwood) 2013;32(6):1143–52.
79. Barrows CE, Belle JM, Fleishman A, et al. Financial burden of thyroid cancer in the United States: An estimate of economic and psychological hardship among thyroid cancer survivors. Surgery 2020;167(2):378–84.
80. Kent EE, Forsythe LP, Yabroff KR, et al. Are survivors who report cancer-related financial problems more likely to forgo or delay medical care? Cancer 2013; 119(20):3710–7.
81. Garfield R, Orgera K. The coverage gap: uninsured poor adults in states that do not expand Medicaid. In: Kaiser Family Foundation. 2021. Available at: https://www.kff.org/medicaid/issue-brief/the-coverage-gap-uninsured-poor-adults-in-states-that-do-not-expand-medicaid/. Accessed June 29, 2021.
82. Finegold K, Conmy A, Chu RC, et al. Trends in the U.S. uninsured population, 2010-2020. Washington, DC: US Department of Health and Human Services; 2021.

83. Telehealth. Telehealth licensing requirements and interstate compacts. Available at: https://telehealth.hhs.gov/providers/policy-changes-during-the-covid-19-public-health-emergency/telehealth-licensing-requirements-and-interstate-compacts/#exceptions-for-interstate-telehealth-practice-and-liability-under-the-prep-act. Accessed June 29, 2021.
84. American Cancer Society. Cancer health disparities research. Available at: https://www.cancer.org/research/currently-funded-cancer-research/cancer-health-disparities-research.html. Accessed June 29, 2021.
85. Association of American Medical Colleges. Health equity grants and funding opportunities. Available at: https://www.aamc.org/what-we-do/mission-areas/medical-research/health-equity/funding-opportunities. Accessed June 29, 2021.
86. Centers for Medicare and Medicaid Services. Minority research grant program. Available at: https://www.cms.gov/About-CMS/Agency-Information/OMH/equity-initiatives/advancing-health-equity/minority-research-grant-program. Accessed June 29, 2021.
87. National Institutes of Health (NIH) Department of Health and Human Services. Funding Opportunity: NIMHD Health Disparities Research (R01). Available at: https://grants.nih.gov/grants/guide/rfa-files/rfa-md-12-001.html. Accessed September 1, 2021.
88. National Institutes of Health (NIH). National Institute on Minority Health and Health Disparities. Available at: https://www.nimhd.nih.gov/. Accessed September 1, 2021.

Role of Levothyroxine/ Liothyronine Combinations in Treating Hypothyroidism

Jacqueline Jonklaas, MD, PhD

KEYWORDS

- Hypothyroidism • Levothyroxine • Liothyronine • Combination therapy
- Patient-reported outcomes • Quality-of-life • Patient satisfaction • Risk-benefit ratio

KEY POINTS

- Most patients feel well while taking levothyroxine.
- Despite optimizing therapy based on biochemical parameters, about 10% to 15% of patients do not feel that their therapy has restored their quality of life.
- After other potential causes of decreased quality of life have been fully addressed, individual use of combination therapy with addition of liothyronine can be considered and continued as long as patient benefit is maintained and overtreatment is avoided.
- Prior trials of combination therapy were largely underpowered, did not target dissatisfied patients, were of short duration, and used once-daily liothyronine dosing, potentially contributing to lack of patient benefit.
- Sustained-release preparations have entered clinical trials, and future combination therapy trials that address some of the design limitations of prior trials and use a sustained-release liothyronine are anticipated.

TREATMENT WITH LEVOTHYROXINE

There is general agreement that levothyroxine (LT4) is the standard-of-care therapy for hypothyroidism.[1] When treated to consistently achieve a normal thyrotropin (TSH), most patients feel well while taking LT4. However, there is a subset of patients who do not feel fully restored to baseline health and who report reduced quality of life (QOL), although they are biochemically euthyroid. Thus, despite the success of LT4 therapy, the nuances and complexities of recapitulating the euthyroid state in those who have developed thyroid hormone deficiency have not yet been achieved for all patients. This has led to studies to try and understand the underpinnings of this reduced QOL and also to investigate whether alternative therapies for hypothyroidism might yield greater levels of satisfaction.

J. Jonklaas is supported by NIH grants R01DE025822 and UL1TR001409.
Division of Endocrinology, Georgetown University, Washington, DC 20007, USA
E-mail address: jonklaaj@georgetown.edu

Endocrinol Metab Clin N Am 51 (2022) 243–263
https://doi.org/10.1016/j.ecl.2021.12.003
endo.theclinics.com

Documentation of Residual Symptoms While Taking Levothyroxine

Questionnaires that assess QOL as judged by either general symptoms or thyroid-specific symptoms have shown differences between biochemically euthyroid patients and control individuals. One study from 2002 examined 397 patients receiving treatment for hypothyroidism and compared them with age- and sex-matched individuals without hypothyroidism, including an adjustment for other medical conditions, which were more frequent in the hypothyroid group. When well-being was assessed using the General Health Questionnaire (GHQ-12), 9% more patients were dissatisfied compared with controls. When the thyroid symptom questionnaire (TSQ) was used, approximately 14% more patients with hypothyroidism were dissatisfied compared with the control group.[2] Other cross-sectional studies (**Table 1**). Monotherapy with LT3 similarly showed worse scores in hypothyroid patients compared with control populations.[3–5]

Interpreting these types of studies is made challenging because findings are affected by the health of the control group and the possibility that recruitment methods may elicit more responses from individuals concerned about their health or who are dissatisfied with therapy. The results may also be affected by whether past or current QOL is being assessed and awareness of having a chronic condition. In a study of individuals with hyperthyroidism, QOL was assessed using a version of ThyPRO that assessed symptoms "at this moment" compared with symptoms assessed using the standard ThyPRO that retrospectively assesses symptoms over the last 4 weeks.[6] These individuals recalled worse QOL when it was recalled retrospectively, compared with when it was assessed in the current moment. An individual's perception of their health can be impacted by the knowledge that they have a chronic condition. In a cross-sectional population study, women had better self-reported health when they did not know of their diagnosis of hypothyroidism, and worse self-reported health when the diagnosis was known.[7]

More recent studies used e-mail, Web sites, and online forums to gather information. These data are even more subject to the limitation of the respondents being highly self-selected. An online survey of patients with hypothyroidism conducted by the American Thyroid Association evaluated the responses to questions about satisfaction with hypothyroidism therapy.[8] The entire group had a median score of 5 on a scale of 1 to 10. Areas identified as a source of the dissatisfaction were weight, fatigue/energy levels, mood, and memory in 69%, 77%, 48%, and 58%, respectively. A word cloud generated from questions/responses is shown in **Fig. 1**. In addition, those responding to the survey had a higher level of satisfaction with desiccated thyroid extract (DTE) than those receiving synthetic combination therapy with LT4 and liothyronine (LT3) or LT4 monotherapy.[8]

Potential Causes of Residual Symptoms During Levothyroxine Treatment

There are a host of potential explanations for why patients being treated with LT4 may have residual symptoms that overlap with symptoms of untreated hypothyroidism.[9,10]

Out of range or inappropriate thyrotropin values
Maintenance of a normal TSH cannot be presumed given the studies that show that as many as 40% of individuals receiving LT4 therapy may be either undertreated or overtreated.[11–13] With respect to studies showing TSH set points that are often patient-specific,[14,15] most studies do not show improvement in patients' symptoms with targeting specific TSH values within the normal range. For example, a recent trial randomly assigned patients to receive LT4 doses that targeted 3 different ranges of TSH values and showed that these different TSH values did not affect QOL, mood,

Table 1
Examples of cross-sectional studies showing reduced quality of life in patients with hypothyroidism and normal thyrotropin values

Study	QOL Assessments	How Recruited	Number of Hypothyroid	Score or % with Low Score for Hypothyroid	Number of Controls	Score or % with Low Score for Controls	Worse Score for Hypothyroid Group (%, P Value, or Rr)
Saravanan	GHQ-12 (poor score ≥3)	Questionnaire sent to patients and age- and sex-matched controls	381	34%	535	25%	9%
	TSQ (poor score ≥3)		389	49%	534	35%	14%
Wekking	SCL-90 (higher score = worse)	Invited by letter to participate in in-person testing, compared with standard reference values	140	155	745	118	$P = .001$
	RAND-36 mental health score		140	65	745	77	$P = .001$
	RAND-36 vitality score (energy and fatigue)		140	43	745	67	$P = .001$
Van de Ven	Self-reported fatigue	Survey participants invited by letter to participate in in-person testing, compared with controls	221	53%	5439	34%	Relative risk = 1.3
	RAND-36 vitality		221	61	5439	66	Regression coefficient = −2.9
	SFQ (shortened fatigue questionnaire)		221	13.7	5439	11.1	Regression coefficient = 1.4
Wouters	Physical functioning (<85%)	Female participants in Lifelines Cohort study	321	35.6%	1581	27.4%	$P = .003$
	Vitality (<55%)		321	30.8%	1581	18.1%	$P < .001$
	Mental health (<72%)		321	30.5%	1581	20.5%	$P < .001$
	Social functioning (<75%)		321	25.1%	1581	17.4%	$P < .001$
	Bodily pain (<67.4%)		321	23.8%	1581	15.4%	$P < .001$
	General health (<65%)		321	37.5%	1581	25.8%	$P < .001$

Data from Refs.[2-5]

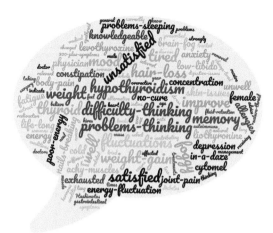

Fig. 1. Word cloud based on questions and answers to an American Thyroid Association survey about hypothyroidism. (*Data from* Peterson SJ, Cappola AR, Castro MR, Dayan CM, Farwell AP, Hennessey JV, Kopp PA, Ross DS, Samuels MH, Sawka AM, Taylor PN, Jonklaas J, Bianco AC. An Online Survey of Hypothyroid Patients Demonstrates Prominent Dissatisfaction. Thyroid. 2018;28(6):707-721.)

or cognition.[16] A prior randomized controlled study in which hypothyroid participants received each of 3 doses of LT4 for 8-week periods, with different mean TSH values of 0.3, 1.0, and 2.8 mIU/L being achieved, found that the different time periods were not associated with any differences in well-being, hypothyroid symptoms, QOL, or cognitive function.[17]

Thyroid peroxidase antibodies, coexistent conditions, or comorbidities

QOL is affected by many factors that impact the patient's perception of an illness and its treatment.[18] Assuming a normal TSH value, other factors to be considered as potentially negatively affecting QOL in patients being treated for hypothyroidism may include autoimmunity, symptoms that actually stem from coexistent conditions or comorbidities, a negative impact of awareness of having a chronic condition, or "tissue hypothyroidism"[9] (**Box 1**).

It is important to understand whether causes other than inadequately treated hypothyroidism are the underlying cause of patients' symptoms.[9,19] Alternate conditions that may be amenable to treatment, but require different therapy other than thyroid hormone, may be overlooked to the patient's detriment. It is possible that patients who take LT4 as their only medication (and their physicians) may have a tendency to preferentially attribute symptoms to hypothyroidism. This attribution could be either correct or incorrect. In addition, both patients and physicians may have unrealistic expectations for the outcome of hypothyroidism therapy.[20,21] Potentially beneficial activities, such as exercise, relaxation, and adequate sleep, may be underemphasized.

Existence of hypothyroidism at a "tissue level"

The tissue hypothyroidism hypothesis likely originated from a series of animal studies (**Box 2**) that measured tissue concentrations of thyroid hormones, including triiodothyronine (T3). In a classic study, it was determined that intravenous infusion of LT4 in thyroidectomized rats did not simultaneously normalize all the thyroid-related parameters studied.[22] Doses of LT4 that resulted in normal T3 concentrations in various tissues resulted in supraphysiologic serum concentrations of thyroxine (T4) and T3 and

---

Box 1
Potential causes of residual symptoms in patients with normal thyrotropin values

- TSH not at target (not within reference range, not at patient's set point)
- Negative effect of autoimmunity on quality of life (symptoms from another autoimmune disease, direct effect of thyroid peroxidase antibodies)
- Symptoms caused by accompanying conditions or comorbidities (comorbidity partially or entirely causal)
- Incorrect attribution and unrealistic expectations (hypothyroid symptoms anticipated based on diagnosis; symptoms actually due to lifestyle issues and normal aging)
- Awareness of chronic condition (burden from a chronic disease or reliance on a medication)
- Tissue hypothyroidism (low T3 levels at tissue or cellular level)
- LT4 does not recapitulate normal thyroid physiology (eg, T3 levels too low, free T4 levels too high)
- Genetic conditions causing impaired conversion of T4 to T3
- Genetic conditions causing impaired thyroid hormone entry into cells

---

suppressed serum TSH. Further studies from the same group using combined infusions of LT4 and LT3 in rats showed that all parameters could be normalized simultaneously with a dose of 0.9 μg/100 g body weight LT4 and 0.15 μg/100 g body weight LT3 per day.[23] A more recent animal study also showed similar findings.[24] Continuous-release pellets of LT4 and LT3 delivering "sustained-release" therapy normalized serum T4 and T3 concentrations, whereas intermittent daily doses of LT4 and LT3 did not.[24]

Lower triiodothyronine levels and elevated thyroxine/triiodothyronine ratios

LT4 monotherapy provides steady serum concentrations of T3 over a 24-hour period.[25] However, the resultant T4/T3 ratio is higher,[21] and conversely, the FT3/FT4 is lower[26] than that seen with native thyroid functioning. Several studies have examined the T3 levels achieved during LT4 monotherapy.[21] In a study that used patients as their own controls by studying the same patient before and after thyroidectomy, T3 levels were reasonably well maintained.[27] However, taking available studies together shows that T3 levels are lower in a proportion of LT4-treated patients[1,21] and may even be below the T3 reference range in some studies.[26] In a small

---

Box 2
Differences between rodent and human thyroid physiology

- Rat thyroid physiology and human thyroid physiology differ in several respects.
- The molar ratio of T3:T4 secreted by the thyroid gland is greater in the rat.
- The proportion of thyroid hormones bound to transport proteins is greater in the rat.
- The role of the type 2 deiodinase pathway is more developed in humans.
- Even with species differences, rodent studies suggest that local production of T3 is regulated in a tissue-specific manner.
- Rodent studies also suggest that specific tissues may have differential dependence on circulating T3 levels based on their deiodinase activity and different patterns of deiodinase inactivation.

---

study of thyroidectomized patients, lower T3 levels during LT4 monotherapy were associated with the presence of being either homozygous (13% of the group) or heterozygous for the Thr92Ala polymorphism of the type 2 deiodinase.[28] If replicated, these data could indicate that type 2 deiodinase polymorphisms may, in fact, affect circulating T3 levels in those who are athyreotic and dependent on LT4 therapy.

Type 2 deiodinase and thyroid hormone transporter polymorphisms

Data are available documenting the effect of type 2 deiodinase polymorphism status on either a patient's response to LT4 therapy or their preference for combined LT4/LT3 therapy.[21] One study by Panicker et al performed an analysis of retrospective type 2 deiodinase genotyping and the QOL data from the study of combination therapy by Saravanan and colleagues.[29] Thr92Ala polymorphism genotyping was performed, and participant scores on the GHQ-12 were analyzed according to their polymorphism status, both at baseline and when taking their assigned LT4 or LT4/LT3. Ala/Ala homozygotes had worse GHQ-12 scores while taking LT4.[29] In addition, they also had a better response to combination therapy compared with LT4 monotherapy based on their GHQ-12 scores.[29] Responses were not secondary to different TSH values, as median TSH values were not different over the course of study between patients with the same genotype receiving either combination therapy or monotherapy. As cautioned by the investigators, the study was underpowered, with a risk of a type 1 statistical error.

Two studies have reported lack of association between scores of QOL and cognition in LT4-treated patients according to their Thr92Ala genotype,[5,30] thus not confirming the findings of Panicker and colleagues regarding response to LT4 monotherapy. Two further genotyping studies have examined patients participating in the combination therapy trial conducted by Appelhof and colleagues.[31] One study examined the hypothesis that 2 type 2 deiodinase polymorphisms (ORFa-Gly3Asp and Thr92Ala) were associated with either response to LT4 monotherapy or preference for combination therapy. Neither polymorphism was associated with well-being, neurocognitive function, or preference for combination therapy.[32] The other study examined the hypothesis that OATP1C1 polymorphisms were associated with response to therapy. Two of the polymorphisms (OATP1C1-intron3C > T and the OATP1C1-C3035T) were associated with fatigue and depression that was worse in the wild types than in the homozygotes. There was no association with neurocognitive functioning or preference for combination therapy.[33] On the other hand, one small study,[34] that conducted retrospective genotyping of participants from a prospective combination therapy study,[35] found that patients with both the Thr92Ala polymorphism and a thyroid hormone transporter (MTC10) polymorphism preferred combination therapy.[34] As all these studies are retrospective and underpowered, the field will be greatly advanced when the results from a prospective, adequately powered study become available. This should answer the question of whether therapy for hypothyroidism should be informed by type 2 deiodinase or thyroid hormone transporter polymorphism genotypes.

THERAPY OTHER THAN LEVOTHYROXINE
Combination Therapy with Levothyroxine and Liothyronine or Liothyronine Therapy

Combination therapy with both LT4 and LT3 is frequently considered based on the findings that LT4 monotherapy results in a relatively lower serum T3 concentration and may be accompanied by some patient dissatisfaction with this therapy.[1,9,21] During endogenous thyroid functioning in humans, the molar ratio of T4:T3 is approximately 14:1 to 15:1.[1] If one of the goals of combination therapy is to strive for a similar ratio, this would be best achieved using small doses of synthetic LT3 with subsequent adjustments as necessary. Even though patients may express preference for DTE, its high T3 content makes it difficult to provide physiologic ratios with this product. Monotherapy with LT3 has not been well studied[36,37] (**Box 3, Table 2**).

Synthetic combination therapy
Excluding studies examining DTE alone,[38] patients with central hypothyroidism, only biochemical parameters, and patients who were not individually randomized, 15 randomized trials have been performed that examined the impact of synthetic combination therapy on patients with hypothyroidism.[1,21,31,35,39–51] The design of these studies was different with respect to the outcomes studied, the use of cross-over or parallel groups, blinding methodology, and the ratio of T4 to T3 used. However, autoimmune hypothyroidism was the prevailing diagnosis in most studies. The most recent study randomized patients to one of 3 treatment arms, with subsequent crossover to LT4, LT4/LT3, and DTE.[51] With the exception of 5 studies,[35,39,43,46,47] a benefit of LT4/LT3 combination therapy compared with LT4 monotherapy was not demonstrated (**Fig. 2**; see **Table 3**). Moreover, the heterogeneity of the trials with respect to causes of hypothyroidism, dosing regimens, outcome measures, duration of treatment, and TSH and T3 levels achieved in the combination therapy groups has made it challenging to draw conclusions in meta-analyses. Guidelines and recent reviews have stressed the need for larger, better-designed studies of longer duration that address some of the prior shortcomings[1,21,52] (**Table 4**).

Quality of life, neurocognitive function, and patient preference in combination therapy trials
Health-related QOL or mood was studied in 14 trials, with heterogeneous results[1,21,51] (see **Fig. 2** and **Table 3**). Superiority of combination therapy on multiple measures was demonstrated in 2 trials conducted by Bunevicius and colleagues[39] and Nygaard and colleagues.[35] These trials included patients with thyroid cancer and low TSH values[39] and used a large single dose of LT3 (20 µg)[35] respectively. Superiority of combination therapy on a minority of assessments was seen in 2 further trials.[46,47] In one of these trials, the benefit seen at 3 months was no longer detected at 12 months.[46] The latter is

---

Box 3
Considerations about liothyronine monotherapy

- LT3 is well absorbed in the gastrointestinal tract.
- LT3 is available in 3 dosages of 5, 25, and 50 µg.
- LT3 has a short half-life of slight less than 24 hours.
- Peak serum T3 levels are attained within 4 hours of administration.
- T3 peaks can be associated with symptoms such as anxiety, tremors, and palpitations.
- Would need to take LT3 multiple times a day to maintain a reasonably stable serum TSH.
- Would need to take LT3 multiple times a day to avoid T3 peaks and troughs.
- Approximately 150 µg LT4 is equivalent to 50 µg LT3.
- Preference for LT3 alone compared with LT4 alone has not been reported.
- Currently LT3 monotherapy is not recommended owing to uncertainty about benefits, difficulty with titration, lack of experience regarding parameters to monitor therapy, and concern about T3 thyrotoxicosis.

Table 2
Clinical trials of liothyronine monotherapy

Parameter	LT4 Monotherapy	LT3 Monotherapy
Frequency of administration	Three times daily	Three times daily
Dosage equivalence (3:1 ratio)	115 μg	40 μg
TSH value achieved (mIU/L)	1.2	1.4
Duration of trial	30 d	30 d
Weight	Comparator	3% decrease
Total cholesterol	Comparator	10.9% decrease
LDL-cholesterol	Comparator	13.3% decrease
Apolipoprotein B	Comparator	18.3% decrease
Sex hormone binding globulin	Comparator	22% increase

Data from Refs.[36,37]

the only combination therapy trial of 12 months' duration, with the next longest trials being 4 months and 6 months long. The remaining 10 trials did not show improved QOL with combination therapy for the whole group that was studied. With the most recent trial,[51] when a subgroup analysis was performed for those most symptomatic while taking LT4, there was significant improvement in QOL. In examining those who scored worst while taking LT4 as assessed by the TSQ-36, GHQ-12, and the Beck Depression Inventory (BDI), these individuals had significant improvement in these indices when switched to LT4/LT3.

Neurocognitive functioning was studied in 11 trials, again with heterogeneous results[1,21,51] (see **Fig. 2** and **Table 3**). Combination therapy was judged to be superior based on multiple measures in 1 trial.[39] Combination therapy was also found to be superior based on a minority of measures in another trial.[43] The remaining 9 trials did not

Studies showing improvement in QOL/mood or neurocognitive measures with LT4/LT3 compared with LT4

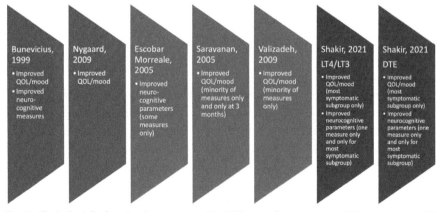

Fig. 2. Clinical trials showing improvement in QOL/mood or neurocognitive measures with combination therapy with LT4/LT3, compared with LT4 monotherapy. (*Data from* Refs.[35,39,43,46,47,51]).

Table 3
Selected characteristics of clinical trials of showing benefits of combination therapy (italics = desiccated thyroid extract) compared with LT4 monotherapy

Authors	LT3 Dosing Frequency	Approximate microgram Ratio of T4:T3	Serum T3 or FT3 Higher in T4/T3 Arm?	Trial Duration	Neuro-Cognitive Measures	QOL, Mood, Measures	Genotyping Done/Effect of Thr92Ala?
Bunevicius et al,[39] 1999	Once daily	10:1	Yes	5 wk	↑ Combo	↑ Combo	No
Escobar-Morreale et al,[43] 2005	Once daily	15:1 or 12:1	No	8 wk	↑ Combo (some parameters only)	No diff	No
Nygaard et al,[35] 2009	Once daily	4:1	Yes (FT3 index)	12 wk	n/a	↑ Combo	Retrospective, Yes
Saravanan et al,[46] 2005	Once daily	8:1	No	12 mo	n/a	↑ Combo (3 mo only) (minority of measures)	Retrospective, Yes
Shakir et al,[51] 2021	Once daily	9.5:1	Yes	22 wk	No diff (except in 1 domain in subgroup analysis of those with worst scores on LT4)	No diff (except in subgroup analysis of those with worst scores on LT4)	Prospective, No
Shakir et al,[51] 2021	*Once daily*	*4:1*	*Yes*	*22 wk*	*No diff (except in 1 domain in subgroup analysis of those with worst scores on LT4)*	*No diff (except in subgroup analysis of those with worst scores on LT4)*	*Prospective, No*
Valizadeh et al,[47] 2009	Twice daily	4:1	Yes	4mo	n/a	↑ Combo (minority of measures)	No

Data from Refs.[35,39,43,46,47,51]

Table 4
Consensus areas about future combination therapy trials

Characteristics Needed for Future Trials	Comments	Degree of Consensus (%)
Study Outcome		
Patient-reported outcome with content and validity for thyroid-related QOL, also with responsiveness to change should be used		100
ThyPRO 39 favored as a primary endpoint		100
Patient preference favored as a secondary trial outcome		100
Future studies should be powered for an effect size of at least 0.5, and preferably 0.3		100
Participant inclusion		
Following exclusion of other causes of symptoms, patients who do not report relief of their symptoms with LT4 therapy should specifically be recruited for future trials		75
A thyroid-related QOL questionnaire should be used to assess baseline satisfaction for the purpose of participant inclusion in the trial	Examples of potential inclusion criteria: (i) a score >4 in the 12-question TSQ, (ii) an overall health-related QOL score using the ThyPRO-39 composite score of >32	100
Participants should have a normal TSH while being treated with at least 1.2 µg/kg/d LT4		100
Patients with low serum T3 levels while taking LT4 monotherapy should be specifically recruited to any new trials		50
Results should be stratification according to baseline T3 levels or trough T3 levels		50
Trial design		
Should be a randomized, placebo-controlled, double-blind parallel design trial		100
A trial should be a year in duration	Concern about participant retention and the potential for participants to discontinue the trial in order to request LT3 from their health care provider	80
Trial should be "pragmatic" and include participants with comorbidities as long as they are managed to achieve stability	In order to ensure that trial results are representative and can be generalized to the hypothyroid population as a whole	90

(continued on next page)

| **Table 4** *(continued)* | | |
Characteristics Needed for Future Trials	Comments	Degree of Consensus (%)
A future combination therapy trial should include 3 arms (LT4, LT4/LT3, DTE)	Important because of the considerable patient interest in this product	67
Future trials should be adequately powered to study the effects of polymorphisms in the type 2 deiodinase and thyroid hormone transporters (MCT8, MCT10, OATP1C1)	Unless future prospective trials are large and well-funded, they are likely to remain underpowered	100
T3 administration		
A sustained-release T3 preparation is the preferred product for future trials	Two products have completed phase 1 and phase 2 clinical trials in humans	100
Twice-daily administration of LT3 should be used in a physiologic ratio (if sustained-release T3 is not available)	Has only been used in 4 previous trials	100

Adapted with permission from Jonklaas J, Bianco AC, Cappola AR, Celi FS, Fliers E, Heuer H, McAninch EA, Moeller LC, Nygaard B, Sawka AM, Watt T, Dayan CM. Evidence-Based Use of Levothyroxine/Liothyronine Combinations in Treating Hypothyroidism: A Consensus Document. Thyroid 2021;31(2):156-182 (Published by Mary Anne Liebert Inc, New Rochelle, NY), and Eur Thyroid J. 2021 Mar;10(1):10-38 (Published by S. Karger AG, Basel).

show a benefit of combination therapy on neurocognitive functioning.[1,21] The most recent trial showed significant improvement in 1 domain of the Wechsler memory scale-Version IV (visual memory index [VMI]) with synthetic combination therapy, but only for the subgroup of participants who scored worst on this test while taking LT4.[51]

Patient preference for therapy has been studied in 5 blinded 2-arm cross-over design trials and 2 blinded, parallel design trials.[1,21] With respect to the cross-over design trials, the combination therapy was preferred in 4 trials, which, when combined, included a total of 128 patients.[35,39,40,43] Another trial of 101 patients did not demonstrate a preference for combination therapy.[44] Of the 2 parallel design trials, patients reported a preference for combination therapy in 1 trial of 130 patients,[31] with no preference for combination therapy reported in another trial of 573 patients.[46] Akirov and colleagues[53] recently conducted a meta-analysis of preference data from the combination therapy trials in which they examined preference as a binomial distribution of choices (preference for combination therapy vs no preference for combination therapy). The preference rate was found to be no different from chance at 46.2%, although preference was associated with the magnitude of the LT3 dose.[53]

Combination therapy with desiccated thyroid extract
Combination therapy can also be provided by using DTE. Unlike synthetic combination therapy, the ratio of T4:T3 cannot be adjusted, unless LT4 therapy is added to lower the relative amount of T3. The T4/T3 ratio of DTE is approximately 4:1. Two trials of DTE have been reported.[38,51] The earlier trial of DTE randomized patients to either

LT4 or DTE and then switched participants to the other therapy with 16 weeks of therapy for each arm.[38] During the DTE treatment arm, patients had significantly higher serum levels of T3 and lower levels of FT4. Multiple different QOL parameters were assessed during the trial and did not differ between the 2 groups. However, 49% of patients preferred the DTE, compared with 19% preferring LT4 and 33% having no preference.[38] There was also no routine documentation of the daily excursions in T3 concentrations that were associated with DTE use. Only 2 patients had serum T3 levels measured on 1 occasion 3 hours after taking the thyroid extract.[38] The T3 concentration in these patients increased from 129 to 175 ng/dL and from 138 to 169 ng/dL, thus not providing data to counter the older studies showing hypertriiodothyroninemia 2 to 5 hours after DTE use. The clinical consequences of such serum T3 excursions are unknown, but these high T3 levels may be of particular concern in patients receiving suppressive therapy for thyroid cancer using a thyroid extract, or in frail or older populations. In the second trial of DTE,[51] similar to the situation seen with synthetic combination therapy in this trial, DTE resulted in improvement over LT4 when examining those who scored worst on assessments made while they were taking LT4. Significant improvements were seen in TSQ-36, GHQ-12, BDI, and VMI. There is continued patient interest in DTE as a "natural" form of combination therapy.[8] This would not be anticipated based on the negative results of the earlier randomized controlled trial of DTE,[38] but is in keeping with the subgroup analysis in the later trial.[51]

Risks of Combination Therapy

The risks of combination therapy have not been fully explored, as most studies of combination therapy have been of relatively short duration. Potential risks include iatrogenic hyperthyroidism in the form of T3 thyrotoxicosis, cardiac arrhythmias, and decrement in bone mineral density. The participants in most studies have consisted of relatively healthy middle-aged women, so the risks in men, in those with comorbidities, and in older or frail populations have not been studied. Most clinical trials of combination therapy have maintained normal TSH values in the study participants. However, it would be predicted that use of combination therapy in the clinical setting would likely be associated with some overtreatment. Based on a study of thyroid function tests in those who were 65 years and older and were taking thyroid hormone, overreplacement occurs at least as often in those taking combination therapy.[13] For those taking LT4, 37.5% had low TSH values, compared with those taking combination therapy in whom 42.5% had low TSH values.

Combination therapy should not be undertaken in pregnant women for fear of insufficient thyroid hormone reaching fetal tissues. Data about risk of LT3 in the general population have been inferred from observational studies. Comparison of 400 LT3 users with those who only used LT4 (n = 33,995) found no increase in atrial fibrillation or fractures with LT3 use over a 17-year period. There was, however, increased use of antipsychotic medications associated with LT3 use, with an adjusted hazard ratio of 2.26 (confidence interval, 1.64–3.11) for being prescribed an antipsychotic medication if LT3 was used.[54] There was also a trend for increased use of antidepressants, and a trend toward an increased hazard ratio for breast cancer.[54] A registry study from Sweden conducted over an 8.1-year period did not replicate the trend for breast cancer risk. LT3 users (n = 11,147) were compared with LT4 users (n = 575,461), and no increased incidence or mortality from breast cancer or other cancers was identified.[55]

Initiation and Monitoring of Combination Therapy

If synthetic combination therapy is chosen, the ratio of T4 to T3 and the frequency of the LT3 administration (daily, twice daily, 3 times daily) need to be selected. DTE is not recommended by clinical practice guidelines,[1,10,56] but if this was chosen, this would constitute fixed dose combination therapy with a T4/T3 ratio of approximately 4.2:1, with T3 being given once daily. The LT4/LT3 equivalence ratio has been shown as approximately 3:1 based on a pharmacodynamic study.[37] If a patient is being converted from LT4 monotherapy to combination therapy with the same dose being maintained, there would need to be a reduction in the LT4 dose according to the 3:1 conversion factor, depending on the LT3 dose being added. Dosage guidance for converting a patient who is not doing well while taking LT4 from LT4 monotherapy to combination therapy has been published.[56] In addition to consideration of dosage, the other consideration is frequency of LT3 administration. Endogenous fluctuations in FT3 are small and showed an excursion of approximately 0.6 pmol/L (0.39 pg/mL) in one study in which 24-hour blood sampling was conducted.[57] If steady serum levels of T3 are physiologic and desirable, multiple small doses of LT3 (eg, 2 μg 4 times daily or 2–3 μg 3 times a day) would be needed. Currently, LT3 is available as 5-μg, 25-μg, and 50-μg tablets, so these examples use small doses of LT3 that are not available as single tablets. In addition, there is agreement that expecting patients to be able to adhere to dosing of LT3 given more than twice daily is not realistic for a chronic therapy.[21,56] Alternatively, a sustained-release T3 preparation would be needed.

Monitoring of patient QOL during combination therapy is important because unresolved symptoms are what typically lead a patient to request such therapy. Symptoms can be assessed using validated QOL questionnaires. Because changes in thyroid symptoms might not be as apparent in general QOL questionnaires, it is important that standardized and/or validated thyroid-related QOL questionnaires be used. Examples of such questionnaires include ThyPRO, Chronic Thyroid Questionnaire, and Underactive-Thyroid-Dependent Quality of Life Questionnaire[58–60] (reviewed in Refs.[1,21]). However, such questionnaires have been used primarily in the research setting, rather than in a routine clinical setting, so more experience with this approach would be helpful.

It is not clear what biochemical parameters are most reflective of thyroid status when monitoring patients receiving combination therapy. Given the peaks and troughs of serum T3 levels, serum TSH may be harder to interpret as a marker of euthyroidism in a patient receiving combination therapy, compared with patients receiving traditional monotherapy.[21] Potential monitoring parameters, in addition to serum TSH, include FT4, T3, FT3, and the FT4/FT3 ratio.[21] The concept of using serum T3 as a therapeutic target has been quite controversial.[1,61] An additional concern exists if serum FT3 is being monitored, as assays for FT3 may be less accurate, in part because of the low concentrations of hormone being measured. The FT3/FT4 ratio has been proposed as an estimate of deiodinase activity during LT4 monotherapy.[62] It is possible that an FT3/FT4 ratio would reflect a combination of peripheral conversion plus the exogenous LT3 being supplied during combination therapy. However, even if the FT4/FT3 or FT3/FT4 ratio is a meaningful target, the desired target value has not been defined.[21] Any monitoring strategy that includes a combination of several laboratory analytes would entail additional phlebotomy and costs for the patient, in addition to any extra costs of the LT3 therapy itself.

Another consideration is the timing of testing and whether a peak or trough thyroid hormone level is being captured. Depending on the timing of T3 administration with respect to phlebotomy, high serum T3 levels may be encountered. Two trials of synthetic combination therapy documented postdosing T3 concentrations in a small subset of 10 to 12 patients.[25,42] In one study, patients were taking 10 μg LT3 once daily. A 42% increase in serum FT3 concentration was seen within 4 hours after the administration of 10 μg LT3.[25] Three of the 10 patients had serum T3 levels that were above the upper limit of the laboratory reference range for part of the day. In the other study, in which 5% of the patient's dose of LT4 was replaced by a single dose of LT3 that was prepared in house, there was a 54% increase in FT3 concentrations approximately 2 hours after LT3 administration.[42]

Attention to the timing of phlebotomy is particularly important if LT3 is given as a larger dose once daily, rather than in divided doses. Serum T3 and FT3 levels peak approximately 2.5 hours after LT3 administration.[25,42,63–65] A trough serum T3 level is both lower and more predictable than a postdose T3 level, as illustrated in 3 studies of once-daily LT3 dosing.[25,42,63] The 24-hour profile of serum TSH concentrations following once-daily LT4/LT3 administration appears to show more fluctuation than serum TSH levels following daily LT4 administration.[25] In patients receiving combination therapy, the TSH nadir was at 6 hours following LT4/LT3 dosing, before returning to the predosing value about 10 hours later.[25] If a trough T3 concentration, and its accompanying TSH level, was chosen for monitoring because of greater standardization of analyte values, phlebotomy in the early morning before any of that day's LT3 administration might be particularly useful.

Physician Practice Patterns for Prescribing of Triiodothyronine-containing Products

Surveys of physicians' prescribing practices demonstrate that despite the lack of conclusive data showing superiority of T3-containing therapies, physicians will prescribe combination therapy for their patients (**Box 4**; **Fig. 3**).[66–68] About a third of Polish endocrinologists responding to a survey expressed willingness to prescribe combination therapy for hypothyroid patients with unresolved symptoms despite a normal TSH. Nevertheless, the physicians attributed the symptoms to the burden of chronic disease, psychosocial factors, comorbidities, and unrealistic expectations, among other causes.[69]

Sustained-Release Triiodothyronine

The goal of a sustained-release T3 preparation that would avoid fluctuating serum T3 levels has been pursued for some years. T3 sulfate is a metabolite of T4 and T3 that does not itself have biological activity,[70] but has been shown to be converted to T3 and to lower TSH levels in thyroidectomized rats.[71] T3 sulfate has been reported to have a sustained-release profile, as initially demonstrated in patients who had been withdrawn from thyroid hormone. In such hypothyroid patients, administration of a single dose of T3 sulfate resulted in steady serum T3 levels for about 48 hours.[72]

Box 4
Survey of physicians regarding their T3-prescribing patterns (see Fig. 3)

- A survey of members of the American Thyroid Association described an index patient who was biochemically and clinically euthyroid while taking LT4 and queried the respondents regarding their choice of therapy.

- For this index patient, 98% of physicians continued current LT4 therapy.

- Modified patient scenarios incorporated other patient characteristics, and physicians then opted to increase LT4 dose or prescribe LT4/LT3 therapy (see **Fig. 3**).

- Physicians practicing in North America were more likely to prescribe T3-containing therapies than physicians practicing outside of North America.

- There was a trend for prescribing of T3 regimens to increase over time.

Data from Refs.[66–68]

Odds ratio of prescribing LT3 therapy over LT4 therapy

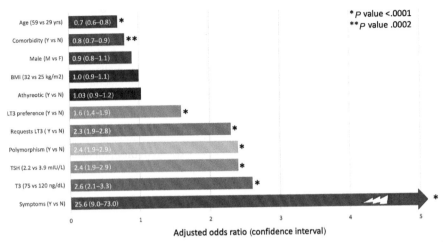

Fig. 3. Likelihood of prescribing LT3-containing therapy rather than LT4 therapy for several patient scenarios. BMI, body mass index; F, female; M, male; N, no; Y, yes. (*Data from* Jonklaas J, Tefera E, Shara N. Physician Choice of Hypothyroidism Therapy: Influence of Patient Characteristics. Thyroid. 2018;28(11):1416-1424.)

Subsequently, the same investigators conducted a phase 2 study,[73] in which they replaced 25 μg LT4 with 40 μg T3 sulfate in thyroidectomized patients and found that this lowered serum TSH and FT4 concentrations and produced a ratio of FT4/FT3 that was similar to the ratio seen in individuals with native euthyroidism.[26,27]

Efforts to attain delayed absorption of LT3 from the gastrointestinal tract or other depots so that a sustained-release profile is achieved have been pursued.[74] Recently, a zinc coordinated form of LT3 (poly-zinc-liothyronine) was administered as capsules to hypothyroid rats in a pharmacokinetic study.[75] The poly-zinc-liothyronine produced a lower serum T3 peak and exhibited a longer time period over which the T3 concentrations remained at a plateau, compared with LT3. Chronic poly-zinc-liothyronine administration lowered serum TSH, lowered body weight, decreased cholesterol levels, and stimulated T3-response genes in a similar manner to LT3.[75] Recently, a phase 1 single-dose, double-blind placebo-controlled trial of poly-zinc-liothyronine was completed in 12 healthy volunteers.[76] The poly-zinc-liothyronine reached a lower maximum serum T3 concentration than the LT3 and exhibited 6-hour and 12-hour plateaus. The area under the curve was greater for the poly-zinc-liothyronine at the 12- to 24-hour and 24- to 48-hour periods. Whether this profile will translate into improved stability of serum T3 levels and more satisfactory therapy for patients will be determined in future clinical trials.

SUMMARY

Although LT4 provides life-restoring therapy for most patients with hypothyroidism, perhaps as best shown in animal studies, LT4 does not recapitulate all aspects of normal thyroid physiology. The search for "physiologic" replacement therapy affords exciting opportunities for gaining understanding that may enable us to optimize thyroid hormone replacement therapy for as many patients as possible. Better understanding of deiodinase and thyroid hormone transporter polymorphisms may ultimately enable us to provide therapy tailored to individual patients. In addition to understanding the genetic underpinning of thyroid hormone delivery to tissues, additional goals include developing more physiologic, sustained-release combination thyroid hormone therapies, and ensuring adequate thyroid hormone levels in all tissues. It is exciting with regard to T3 preparations that products that have some sustained-release features have concluded phase 1 and 2 trials.[73,75] Other active areas of research are investigating the regeneration of functional thyroid follicles from embryonic or pluripotent stem cells in animal models. Such cells, once differentiated into thyroid follicular cells, have been shown to be capable of forming 3-dimensional follicles, expressing thyroid-specific genes, responding to TSH stimulation, actively transporting iodine, and expressing thyroglobulin.[77,78] Stem cells also seem to be involved in regenerating thyroid cells after experimentally induced thyroid damage in mouse models.[79] Should such successes be extended to humans, this would enable further studies to advance our understanding of thyroid physiology, pathophysiology, and disease, perhaps including how to prevent autoimmune damage to thyroid tissue. Ultimately, it could also pave the way for regenerating the full hormonal profile of a normally functioning thyroid gland and thereby restoring euthyroidism in its entirety for those affected by this life-long disease.[80]

CLINICS CARE POINTS

- For hypothyroid patients not restored to baseline health with levothyroxine, causes arising from coexistent medical conditions, stressors, lifestyle, and psychosocial factors should be addressed.

- If addressing such factors does not improve quality of life, and biochemical euthyroidism has been successfully maintained, there may be benefit to use of combination therapy with levothyroxine and liothyronine.

- It is important that any trial of combination therapy only be continued as long as a patient benefit is being experienced.

- Monitoring for adverse effects, particularly in older or frail individuals, is necessary, and combination therapy should not be used during pregnancy.

- Once they have completed clinical trials, sustained-release liothyronine preparations may become available as improved therapies for patients with hypothyroidism.

DISCLOSURE

J. Jonklaas has nothing to disclose.

REFERENCES

1. Jonklaas J, Bianco AC, Bauer AJ, et al. Guidelines for the treatment of hypothyroidism: prepared by the American Thyroid Association Task Force on thyroid hormone replacement. Thyroid 2014;24(12):1670–751.
2. Saravanan P, Chau WF, Roberts N, et al. Psychological well-being in patients on 'adequate' doses of l-thyroxine: results of a large, controlled community-based questionnaire study. Clin Endocrinol (Oxf) 2002;57(5):577–85.
3. Wekking EM, Appelhof BC, Fliers E, et al. Cognitive functioning and well-being in euthyroid patients on thyroxine replacement therapy for primary hypothyroidism. Eur J Endocrinol 2005;153(6):747–53.

4. van de Ven AC, Netea-Maier RT, de Vegt F, et al. Is there a relationship between fatigue perception and the serum levels of thyrotropin and free thyroxine in euthyroid subjects? Thyroid 2012;22(12):1236–43.

5. Wouters HJ, van Loon HC, van der Klauw MM, et al. No effect of the Thr92Ala polymorphism of deiodinase-2 on thyroid hormone parameters, health-related quality of life, and cognitive functioning in a large population-based cohort study. Thyroid 2017;27(2):147–55.

6. Boesen VB, Feldt-Rasmussen U, Bjorner JB, et al. How should thyroid-related quality of life be assessed? Recalled patient-reported outcomes compared to here-and-now measures. Thyroid 2018;28(12):1561–70.

7. Jørgensen P, Langhammer A, Krokstad S, et al. Diagnostic labelling influences self-rated health. A prospective cohort study: the HUNT Study, Norway. Fam Pract 2015;32(5):492–9.

8. Peterson SJ, Cappola AR, Castro MR, et al. An online survey of hypothyroid patients demonstrates prominent dissatisfaction. Thyroid 2018;28(6):707–21.

9. Jonklaas J. Persistent hypothyroid symptoms in a patient with a normal thyroid stimulating hormone level. Curr Opin Endocrinol Diabetes Obes 2017;24(5): 356–63.

10. Okosieme O, Gilbert J, Abraham P, et al. Management of primary hypothyroidism: statement by the British Thyroid Association Executive Committee. Clin Endocrinol (Oxf) 2016;84(6):799–808.

11. Thayakaran R, Adderley NJ, Sainsbury C, et al. Thyroid replacement therapy, thyroid stimulating hormone concentrations, and long term health outcomes in patients with hypothyroidism: longitudinal study. BMJ 2019;366:l4892.

12. Okosieme OE, Belludi G, Spittle K, et al. Adequacy of thyroid hormone replacement in a general population. QJM 2011;104(5):395–401.

13. Somwaru LL, Arnold AM, Joshi N, et al. High frequency of and factors associated with thyroid hormone over-replacement and under-replacement in men and women aged 65 and over. J Clin Endocrinol Metab 2009;94(4):1342–5.

14. Hoermann R, Midgley JEM, Larisch R, et al. Functional and symptomatic individuality in the response to levothyroxine treatment. Front Endocrinol (Lausanne) 2019;10:664.

15. Hoermann R, Midgley JEM, Larisch R, et al. Recent advances in thyroid hormone regulation: toward a new paradigm for optimal diagnosis and treatment. Front Endocrinol (Lausanne) 2017;8:364.

16. Samuels MH, Kolobova I, Niederhausen M, et al. Effects of altering levothyroxine (L-T4) doses on quality of life, mood, and cognition in L-T4 treated subjects. J Clin Endocrinol Metab 2018;103(5):1997–2008.

17. Walsh JP, Ward LC, Burke V, et al. Small changes in thyroxine dosage do not produce measurable changes in hypothyroid symptoms, well-being, or quality of life: results of a double-blind, randomized clinical trial. J Clin Endocrinol Metab 2006; 91(7):2624–30.

18. Deshpande PR, Rajan S, Sudeepthi BL, et al. Patient-reported outcomes: a new era in clinical research. Perspect Clin Res 2011;2(4):137–44.

19. Perros P, Van Der Feltz-Cornelis C, Papini E, et al. The enigma of persistent symptoms in hypothyroid patients treated with levothyroxine: a narrative review. Clin Endocrinol (Oxf) 2021. https://doi.org/10.1111/cen.14473.

20. Mitchell AL, Hegedüs L, Žarković M, et al. Patient satisfaction and quality of life in hypothyroidism: an online survey by the British Thyroid Foundation. Clin Endocrinol (Oxf) 2020;94(3):513–20.

21. Jonklaas J, Bianco AC, Cappola AR, et al. Evidence-based use of levothyroxine/liothyronine combinations in treating hypothyroidism: a consensus document. Thyroid 2021;31(2):156–82.
22. Escobar-Morreale HF, Obregón MJ, Escobar del Rey F, et al. Replacement therapy for hypothyroidism with thyroxine alone does not ensure euthyroidism in all tissues, as studied in thyroidectomized rats. J Clin Invest 1995;96(6):2828–38.
23. Escobar-Morreale HF, del Rey FE, Obregón MJ, et al. Only the combined treatment with thyroxine and triiodothyronine ensures euthyroidism in all tissues of the thyroidectomized rat. Endocrinology 1996;137(6):2490–502.
24. Werneck de Castro JP, Fonseca TL, Ueta CB, et al. Differences in hypothalamic type 2 deiodinase ubiquitination explain localized sensitivity to thyroxine. J Clin Invest 2015;125(2):769–81.
25. Saravanan P, Siddique H, Simmons DJ, et al. Twenty-four hour hormone profiles of TSH, free T3 and free T4 in hypothyroid patients on combined T3/T4 therapy. Exp Clin Endocrinol Diabetes 2007;115(4):261–7.
26. Gullo D, Latina A, Frasca F, et al. Levothyroxine monotherapy cannot guarantee euthyroidism in all athyreotic patients. PLoS One 2011;6(8):e22552.
27. Jonklaas J, Davidson B, Bhagat S, et al. Triiodothyronine levels in athyreotic individuals during levothyroxine therapy. JAMA 2008;299(7):769–77.
28. Castagna MG, Dentice M, Cantara S, et al. DIO2 Thr92Ala reduces deiodinase-2 activity and serum-T3 levels in thyroid-deficient patients. J Clin Endocrinol Metab 2017;102(5):1623–30.
29. Panicker V, Saravanan P, Vaidya B, et al. Common variation in the DIO2 gene predicts baseline psychological well-being and response to combination thyroxine plus triiodothyronine therapy in hypothyroid patients. J Clin Endocrinol Metab 2009;94(5):1623–9.
30. Young Cho Y, Jeong Kim H, Won Jang H, et al. The relationship of 19 functional polymorphisms in iodothyronine deiodinase and psychological well-being in hypothyroid patients. Endocrine 2017;57(1):115–24.
31. Appelhof BC, Fliers E, Wekking EM, et al. Combined therapy with levothyroxine and liothyronine in two ratios, compared with levothyroxine monotherapy in primary hypothyroidism: a double-blind, randomized, controlled clinical trial. J Clin Endocrinol Metab 2005;90(5):2666–74.
32. Appelhof BC, Peeters RP, Wiersinga WM, et al. Polymorphisms in type 2 deiodinase are not associated with well-being, neurocognitive functioning, and preference for combined thyroxine/3,5,3'-triiodothyronine therapy. J Clin Endocrinol Metab 2005;90(11):6296–9.
33. van der Deure WM, Appelhof BC, Peeters RP, et al. Polymorphisms in the brain-specific thyroid hormone transporter OATP1C1 are associated with fatigue and depression in hypothyroid patients. Clin Endocrinol (Oxf) 2008;69(5):804–11.
34. Carlé A, Faber J, Steffensen R, et al. Hypothyroid patients encoding combined MCT10 and DIO2 gene polymorphisms may prefer L-T3 + L-T4 combination treatment - data using a blind, randomized, clinical study. Eur Thyroid J 2017;6(3):143–51.
35. Nygaard B, Jensen EW, Kvetny J, et al. Effect of combination therapy with thyroxine (T4) and 3,5,3'-triiodothyronine versus T4 monotherapy in patients with hypothyroidism, a double-blind, randomised cross-over study. Eur J Endocrinol 2009;161(6):895–902.
36. Celi FS, Zemskova M, Linderman JD, et al. Metabolic effects of liothyronine therapy in hypothyroidism: a randomized, double-blind, crossover trial of liothyronine versus levothyroxine. J Clin Endocrinol Metab 2011;96(11):3466–74.

37. Celi FS, Zemskova M, Linderman JD, et al. The pharmacodynamic equivalence of levothyroxine and liothyronine: a randomized, double blind, cross-over study in thyroidectomized patients. Clin Endocrinol (Oxf) 2010;72(5):709–15.

38. Hoang TD, Olsen CH, Mai VQ, et al. Desiccated thyroid extract compared with levothyroxine in the treatment of hypothyroidism: a randomized, double-blind, crossover study. J Clin Endocrinol Metab 2013;98(5):1982–90.

39. Bunevicius R, Kazanavicius G, Zalinkevicius R, et al. Effects of thyroxine as compared with thyroxine plus triiodothyronine in patients with hypothyroidism. N Engl J Med 1999;340(6):424–9.

40. Bunevicius R, Jakuboniene N, Jakubonien N, et al. Thyroxine vs thyroxine plus triiodothyronine in treatment of hypothyroidism after thyroidectomy for Graves' disease. Endocrine 2002;18(2):129–33.

41. Clyde PW, Harari AE, Getka EJ, et al. Combined levothyroxine plus liothyronine compared with levothyroxine alone in primary hypothyroidism: a randomized controlled trial. JAMA 2003;290(22):2952–8.

42. Siegmund W, Spieker K, Weike AI, et al. Replacement therapy with levothyroxine plus triiodothyronine (bioavailable molar ratio 14:1) is not superior to thyroxine alone to improve well-being and cognitive performance in hypothyroidism. Clin Endocrinol (Oxf) 2004;60(6):750–7.

43. Escobar-Morreale HF, Botella-Carretero JI, Gómez-Bueno M, et al. Thyroid hormone replacement therapy in primary hypothyroidism: a randomized trial comparing L-thyroxine plus liothyronine with L-thyroxine alone. Ann Intern Med 2005;142(6):412–24.

44. Walsh JP, Shiels L, Lim EM, et al. Combined thyroxine/liothyronine treatment does not improve well-being, quality of life, or cognitive function compared to thyroxine alone: a randomized controlled trial in patients with primary hypothyroidism. J Clin Endocrinol Metab 2003;88(10):4543–50.

45. Fadeyev VV, Morgunova TB, Melnichenko GA, et al. Combined therapy with L-thyroxine and L-triiodothyronine compared to L-thyroxine alone in the treatment of primary hypothyroidism. Hormones (Athens) 2010;9(3):245–52.

46. Saravanan P, Simmons DJ, Greenwood R, et al. Partial substitution of thyroxine (T4) with tri-iodothyronine in patients on T4 replacement therapy: results of a large community-based randomized controlled trial. J Clin Endocrinol Metab 2005; 90(2):805–12.

47. Valizadeh M, Seyyed-Majidi MR, Hajibeigloo H, et al. Efficacy of combined levothyroxine and liothyronine as compared with levothyroxine monotherapy in primary hypothyroidism: a randomized controlled trial. Endocr Res 2009;34(3):80–9.

48. Rodriguez T, Lavis VR, Meininger JC, et al. Substitution of liothyronine at a 1:5 ratio for a portion of levothyroxine: effect on fatigue, symptoms of depression, and working memory versus treatment with levothyroxine alone. Endocr Pract 2005; 11(4):223–33.

49. Sawka AM, Gerstein HC, Marriott MJ, et al. Does a combination regimen of thyroxine (T4) and 3,5,3'-triiodothyronine improve depressive symptoms better than T4 alone in patients with hypothyroidism? Results of a double-blind, randomized, controlled trial. J Clin Endocrinol Metab 2003;88(10):4551–5.

50. Kaminski J, Miasaki FY, Paz-Filho G, et al. Treatment of hypothyroidism with levothyroxine plus liothyronine: a randomized, double-blind, crossover study. Arch Endocrinol Metab 2016;60(6):562–72.

51. Shakir MKM, Brooks DI, McAninch EA, et al. Comparative effectiveness of levothyroxine, desiccated thyroid extract, and levothyroxine+liothyronine in hypothyroidism. J Clin Endocrinol Metab 2021;106(11):e4400–13.

52. Jonklaas J, Cappola AR, Celi FS. Editorial: combination therapy for hypothyroidism: the journey from bench to bedside. Front Endocrinol (Lausanne) 2020; 11:422.

53. Akirov A, Fazelzad R, Ezzat S, et al. A systematic review and meta-analysis of patient preferences for combination thyroid hormone treatment for hypothyroidism. Front Endocrinol (Lausanne) 2019;10:477.

54. Leese GP, Soto-Pedre E, Donnelly LA. Liothyronine use in a 17 year observational population-based study - the tears study. Clin Endocrinol (Oxf) 2016;85(6): 918–25.

55. Planck T, Hedberg F, Calissendorff J, et al. Liothyronine use in hypothyroidism and its effects on cancer and mortality. Thyroid 2021;31(5):732–9.

56. Wiersinga WM, Duntas L, Fadeyev V, et al. 2012 ETA guidelines: the use of L-T4 + L-T3 in the treatment of hypothyroidism. Eur Thyroid J 2012;1(2):55–71.

57. Russell W, Harrison RF, Smith N, et al. Free triiodothyronine has a distinct circadian rhythm that is delayed but parallels thyrotropin levels. J Clin Endocrinol Metab 2008;93(6):2300–6.

58. Jaeschke R, Guyatt G, Cook D, et al. Spectrum of quality of life impairment in hypothyroidism. Qual Life Res 1994;3(5):323–7.

59. Watt T, Hegedüs L, Groenvold M, et al. Validity and reliability of the novel thyroid-specific quality of life questionnaire, ThyPRO. Eur J Endocrinol 2010;162(1): 161–7.

60. McMillan CV, Bradley C, Woodcock A, et al. Design of new questionnaires to measure quality of life and treatment satisfaction in hypothyroidism. Thyroid 2004;14(11):916–25.

61. Abdalla SM, Bianco AC. Defending plasma T3 is a biological priority. Clin Endocrinol (Oxf) 2014;81(5):633–41.

62. Hoermann R, Midgley JE, Larisch R, et al. Integration of peripheral and glandular regulation of triiodothyronine production by thyrotropin in untreated and thyroxine-treated subjects. Horm Metab Res 2015;47(9):674–80.

63. Jonklaas J, Burman KD. Daily administration of short-acting liothyronine is associated with significant triiodothyronine excursions and fails to alter thyroid-responsive parameters. Thyroid 2016;26(6):770–8.

64. Jonklaas J, Burman KD, Wang H, et al. Single dose T3 administration: kinetics and effects on biochemical and physiologic parameters. Ther Drug Monit 2015; 37(1):110–8.

65. Van Tassell B, Wohlford GF, Linderman JD, et al. Pharmacokinetics of L-triiodothyronine in patients undergoing thyroid hormone therapy withdrawal. Thyroid 2019; 29(10):1371–9.

66. Jonklaas J, Tefera E, Shara N. Physician choice of hypothyroidism therapy: influence of patient characteristics. Thyroid 2018;28(11):1416–24.

67. Jonklaas J, Tefera E, Shara N. Prescribing therapy for hypothyroidism: influence of physician characteristics. Thyroid 2019;29(1):44–52.

68. Jonklaas J, Tefera E, Shara N. Short-term time trends in prescribing therapy for hypothyroidism: results of a survey of American Thyroid Association Members. Front Endocrinol (Lausanne) 2019;10:31.

69. Bednarczuk T, Attanasio R, Hegedüs L, et al. Use of thyroid hormones in hypothyroid and euthyroid patients: a THESIS* questionnaire survey of Polish physicians. *THESIS: treatment of hypothyroidism in Europe by specialists: an international survey. Endokrynol Pol 2021;72(4):357–65.

70. Spaulding SW, Smith TJ, Hinkle PM, et al. Studies on the biological activity of triiodothyronine sulfate. J Clin Endocrinol Metab 1992;74(5):1062–7.

71. Santini F, Hurd RE, Lee B, et al. Thyromimetic effects of 3,5,3'-triiodothyronine sulfate in hypothyroid rats. Endocrinology 1993;133(1):105–10.

72. Santini F, Giannetti M, Ricco I, et al. Steady-state serum T3 concentrations for 48 hours following the oral administration of a single dose of 3,5,3'-triiodothyronine sulfate (T3S). Endocr Pract 2014;20(7):680–9.

73. Santini F, Ceccarini G, Pelosini C, et al. Treatment of hypothyroid patients with L-thyroxine (L-T4) plus triiodothyronine sulfate (T3S). A phase II, open-label, single center, parallel groups study on therapeutic efficacy and tolerability. Front Endocrinol (Lausanne) 2019;10:826.

74. Idrees T, Price JD, Piccariello T, et al. Sustained Release T3 therapy: animal models and translational applications. Front Endocrinol (Lausanne) 2019;10:544.

75. Da Conceição RR, Fernandes GW, Fonseca TL, et al. Metal coordinated poly-zinc-liothyronine provides stable circulating triiodothyronine levels in hypothyroid rats. Thyroid 2018;28(11):1425–33.

76. Dumitresecu A, Hanlon E, Arosemena M, et al. Extended absorption of liothyronine from ploy-zinc-liothyronine (PZL) in humans. medRxiv 2021. https://doi.org/10.1101/2021.06.14.21258437.

77. Ma R, Morshed SA, Latif R, et al. Thyroid cell differentiation from murine induced pluripotent stem cells. Front Endocrinol (Lausanne) 2015;6:56.

78. Antonica F, Kasprzyk DF, Opitz R, et al. Generation of functional thyroid from embryonic stem cells. Nature 2012;491(7422):66–71.

79. Ma R, Morshed SA, Latif R, et al. A stem cell surge during thyroid regeneration. Front Endocrinol (Lausanne) 2020;11:606269.

80. Hollenberg AN, Choi J, Serra M, et al. Regenerative therapy for hypothyroidism: mechanisms and possibilities. Mol Cell Endocrinol 2017;445:35–41.

Thyroid Dysfunction from Treatments for Solid Organ Cancers

Anupam Kotwal, MD[a],
Donald S.A. McLeod, MBBS (Hon I), FRACP, MPH, PhD[b,c],*

KEYWORDS

- Immune checkpoint inhibitors • Kinase inhibitors • Hypothyroidism
- Hyperthyroidism • Thyrotoxicosis • Thyroid function tests
- Iodine-131-metaiodobenzylguanidine • Malignancy

KEY POINTS

- Immune checkpoint inhibitors frequently cause thyroiditis mostly as hypothyroidism, either at presentation or preceded by a thyrotoxic phase.
- Thyroiditis from immune checkpoint inhibitors appears to be T lymphocyte mediated but requires further investigation.
- Kinase inhibitors may cause direct thyroid dysfunction from vascular injury or increase in levothyroxine metabolism.
- The high prevalence of thyroid dysfunction after I-131-metaiodobenzylguanidine despite iodine prophylaxis highlights the need for better risk prediction and prophylactic regimens.
- There appears to be a survival advantage of thyroid dysfunction from immune checkpoint and kinase inhibitors that supports their role as a potential marker for therapeutic efficacy against the malignancy.

INTRODUCTION

In recent years, cancer care has been transformed by immune-based and targeted treatments. Although these novel therapies have proved efficacious against various

[a] Division of Diabetes, Endocrinology and Metabolism, Department of Internal Medicine, University of Nebraska Medical Center, 984120 Nebraska Medical Center, Omaha, NE 68198, USA; [b] Department of Endocrinology and Diabetes, Royal Brisbane and Women's Hospital, Butterfield Street, Herston, Queensland 4029, Australia; [c] Population Health Department, QIMR Berghofer Medical Research Institute, Locked Bag 2000, Royal Brisbane Hospital, Queensland 4029, Australia
* Corresponding author. Department of Endocrinology and Diabetes, Royal Brisbane and Women's Hospital, Butterfield Street, Herston, Queensland 4029, Australia
E-mail address: donald.mcleod@qimrberghofer.edu.au
Twitter: @DrAKotwal (A.K.)

Endocrinol Metab Clin N Am 51 (2022) 265–286
https://doi.org/10.1016/j.ecl.2021.12.006
0889-8529/22/© 2021 Elsevier Inc. All rights reserved.

solid organ malignancies, they also cause multiple adverse effects, including thyroid dysfunction. In this review, the authors consider pertinent studies of treatments for solid organ cancers that affect the thyroid, focusing on immune checkpoint inhibitors (ICIs), kinase inhibitors (KIs), and radioactive iodine-conjugated treatment. They discuss the mechanisms causing thyroid dysfunction, provide a framework for their diagnosis and management, and explore the association with survival. Understanding the effects caused by targeted cancer therapies may yield insight into other thyroid disease processes and identify patients that have robust antitumor response from these therapies.

IMMUNE CHECKPOINT INHIBITORS

ICIs are monoclonal antibodies directed against immune checkpoints that otherwise promote self-tolerance and dampen immune responses. These therapies, with Food and Drug Administration (FDA) -approved targets of cytotoxic T-lymphocyte antigen-4 (CTLA-4) (ipilimumab, tremelimumab [not FDA approved]), programmed cell death protein-1 (PD-1) (pembrolizumab, nivolumab, cemipilimab), and programmed cell death protein-ligand 1 (PD-L1) (atezolizumab, avelumab, durvalumab), unshackle cytotoxic T cells. This restores and recruits host antitumor immunity, leading to potent T-cell activation, proliferation, and tumor cell destruction (**Fig. 1**).[1,2] However, these treatments also lead to a plethora of immune-related adverse events (irAEs), including endocrine disorders, such as thyroiditis,[3–11] hypophysitis,[12–14] diabetes mellitus,[15–17] and rarely, adrenalitis[18–20] and hypoparathyroidism.[21,22] Among endocrine irAEs, thyroid dysfunction is the most common.[3–11,13,23]

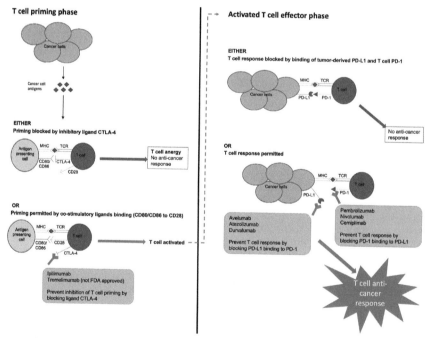

Fig. 1. Schematic for mechanism of ICIs. MHC, major histocompatibility complex; TCR, T-cell receptor.

Cumulative Incidence of Immune Checkpoint Inhibitor-Induced Thyroid Dysfunction

Two meta-analyses of ICI clinical trials[13,24] (**Table 1**) demonstrate that PD-1 and PD-L1 inhibitors cause more frequent thyroid dysfunction than CTLA-4 inhibitors. Observational cohort studies from major medical centers confirm a similar overall pattern.[3–11] These find that thyroid effects are more frequent with PD-1/PD-L1 inhibitors either alone or in combination with a CTLA-4 inhibitor (8%–60%), compared with CTLA-4 inhibitor alone (0%–6%; see **Table 1**).[3,4,6,7,9–11,23–29] The higher prevalence of thyroid disease seen in most cohort studies as compared with clinical trials is due to several factors. Thyroid dysfunction was not the focus of the trials and the follow-up of cohort studies is longer in most cases. While different phases of the same thyroid dysfunction (ie, thyrotoxic then hypothyroid phases of a thyroiditis) may have been captured as separate adverse events in trials, many cohort studies recorded subclinical thyroid dysfunction (normal thyroid hormone with abnormal thyroid-stimulating hormone [TSH]), whereas overt thyroid dysfunction was mostly recorded in clinical trials.

Potential Predictors for Immune Checkpoint Inhibitor-Induced Thyroid Dysfunction

Although autoimmune thyroid disease occurs more frequently in women,[30] ICI-induced thyroid dysfunction does not appear to have sex predisposition,[3,5] suggesting it to be a distinct entity. Its higher occurrence in older individuals reflects the age distribution of those receiving ICI therapy.[5] Diffuse thyroidal fluorodeoxyglucose (FDG) uptake on PET scan usually occurs before or concurrently with thyroid hormone dysfunction.[5,23] Higher baseline TSH level in the upper normal range may be another predictor for thyroid irAE, as some studies demonstrated levels greater than 1.67 mIU/L,[28,31] 1.72 mIU/L,[32] or 2.19 mIU/L[33] to be associated with thyroid irAE development. The severity of hypothyroidism has also been shown to correlate with the initial severity of thyrotoxicosis, which is in line with the underlying thyroiditis cause.[5,9]

As for autoantibodies against thyroid antigens thyroid peroxidase (TPOAb) and thyroglobulin (TgAb), 22% to 80% patients have positive autoantibodies at the time of thyroid irAE;[5–7,11,34] this is a lower percentage than for Hashimoto thyroiditis (which has greater than 90% TPOAb positivity),[35] but more than 10% to 18% reported in the general population.[35–37] Some studies have demonstrated TPOAb positivity to be associated with higher likelihood of developing overt as opposed to subclinical hypothyroidism,[5,26] hence may be helpful to guide therapy once thyroid irAE is identified. Although most studies measured thyroid autoantibodies only at the time of thyroid irAE, comprehensive autoantibody testing before ICI therapy was performed in a few prospective studies signaling their presence as a potential predictor of thyroid dysfunction.[11,28,32,34,38] For example, 2 studies demonstrated higher prevalence of positive TgAb and/or TPOAb at baseline in patients who developed destructive thyroiditis compared with those who did not (3/4 vs 3/62; $P = .002$;[34] and 13/22 vs 18/100; $P = .0002$,[38] respectively).

Pathogenesis of Immune Checkpoint Inhibitor-Induced Thyroid Dysfunction

The natural history of thyroid irAEs suggests a process of destructive thyroiditis, as most cases present with thyrotoxicosis progressing to normalization of thyroid function or hypothyroidism, or as hypothyroidism, in which case the initial mild thyrotoxic phase may have been missed.[3–11,13,23,24] The diffusely increased thyroid FDG uptake,[3,5,6] low radioactive iodine uptake, and ultrasound features[3] also support this cause. Microscopically, thyroid glands from 2 patients that developed thyroiditis

Table 1
Occurrence of thyroid immune-related adverse events in a meta-analysis, clinical trials, and observational cohort studies

Immune Checkpoint Inhibitor	Thyrotoxicosis Cumulative Incidence (95% CI) in Clinical Trials	Hypothyroidism Cumulative Incidence (95% CI) in Clinical Trials	Cumulative Incidence of Thyroid Dysfunction in Cohort Studies, %
CTLA-4 inhibitors[3,13,24,140]			
Studies assessing multiple CLTA-4 inhibitors	1.7% (0.8 - 3.8)[13]	3.8% (1.9 - 7.8)[13]	0-6[3,140]
Ipilimumab	1.4% (0.8-2.4)[24]	3.8% (2.6-5.5)[24]	
Tremelimumab	Up to 5.2%[24]	Up to 5.2%[24]	
PD-1 inhibitors[3,6,11,13,24,26,59]			
Studies assessing multiple PD-1 inhibitors	3.2% (1.7-5.7)[13]	7.0% (3.9-12.3)[13]	8-23[3,6,11,26,59]
Pembrolizumab	3.7% (2.8-4.7)[24]	8.5% (7.5-9.7)[24]	
Nivolumab	2.8 (2.1-3.8)[24]	8.0% (6.4-9.8)[24]	
Cemiplimab	Not reported/analyzed	Not reported/analyzed	
PD-L1 inhibitors[3,5,13,24]			
Studies assessing multiple PD-L1 inhibitors	0.6% (0.2-1.8)[13]	3.9% (1.7-8.4)[13]	10-25[3,5]
Atezolizumab	Not reported	6.0% (4.2-8.4)[24]	
Avelumab	2.3% (0.6-8.6)[24]	5.5% (3.5-8.7)[24]	
Durvalumab	Not reported	4.7% (2.5-8.8)[24]	
CTLA-4 and PD-1 inhibitor combination[3,4,13,24,29,141]			
Studies assessing multiple combination treatments	8.0% (4.1-15.3)[13]	13.2% (6.9-23.8)[13]	9-60[3,4,29,141]
Ipilimumab + Nivolumab	9.4% (7.1-12.3)[24]	16.4% (11.7-22.5)[24]	
Ipilimumab + Pembrolizumab	10.4% (6.6-16.1)[24]	15.1% (10.6-21.8)[24]	
Durvalumab + Tremelimumab	Not reported	10.2% (5.6-17.9)[24]	

contained abundant necrotic cells along with a rich infiltration of lymphocytes and his-tiocytic cells,[27,39] supporting the thyroiditis cause.

The underlying mechanism behind thyroid irAEs remains under investigation. Single nucleotide polymorphisms of immune checkpoint CTLA-4 are associated with autoim-mune thyroid disease, including Hashimoto thyroiditis and Graves disease.[40,41] Thy-roid dysfunction occurs less frequently with CTLA-4 inhibitors than with PD-1/PD-L1 inhibitors,[3,13] which raises the possibility of different causal pathways than classic autoimmune thyroid disease. Notably, the expression of PD-L1 was demonstrated on thyroid follicular cells,[25] suggesting a plausible mechanism for thyroid dysfunction from PD-1/PD-L1 inhibitors. Using flow cytometry, the authors' group demonstrated predominantly $CD8^+PD1^+$ and $CD4^-CD8^-$ T lymphocytes infiltrating the thyroid gland of patients with PD-1/PD-L1 inhibitor–induced thyroiditis, highlighting the role of these T-cell subsets in the pathogenesis.[42]

Mouse models are also beginning to yield insights into the molecular mechanisms of ICI-induced thyroiditis. In 1 model, PD-1 antibody administration after immunization with TgAb induced thyroiditis dependent on a subset of cytotoxic $CD4^+$ T cells expressing interferon-gamma and granzyme B.[43] In another model assessing combi-nation ICI treatment, ICI effects on $Foxp3^+$ regulatory T cells appeared to facilitate autoimmunity.[44] These studies suggest a role of $CD4^+$ T cells and regulatory T cells as the shared link between ICI-induced antitumor immunity and lowering of tolerance to self-antigen. A newly described model suggests distinct histologic, sonographic, and hormonal patterns of thyroiditis between PD-1 and CTLA-4 blockade.[45] In addi-tion, cytokine signatures differed between ICIs, most notably an increase in interleukin-6 production in PD-1 inhibitor-induced thyroiditis.[45]

Presentation of Immune Checkpoint Inhibitor-Induced Thyroid Dysfunction

Thyroid dysfunction occurs most frequently within the first 1 to 4 months following ICI initiation, with median time to onset being 6 to 10 weeks for thyrotoxicosis and 8 to 16 weeks for hypothyroidism, but it can occur as long as 2 years later.[3,5,6,46] It most commonly presents as thyrotoxicosis that usually progresses to normalization of thy-roid function or hypothyroidism, or as hypothyroidism, in which case the initial mild thyrotoxic phase may have been missed.[3,5–7,9,10,46] Owing to routine thyroid function screening in patients receiving ICIs, thyroid irAEs are usually readily identified. These are usually asymptomatic or have mild to moderate (according to standard clinical tri-als definitions for severity of adverse events) symptoms[5,6,9,10]; however, a few cases of thyroid storm[47] and severe hypothyroidism[48,49] have been reported. Compared with classical painless thyroiditis requiring 2 to 4 months to progress to hypothyroid-ism, the time for progression from thyrotoxicosis to hypothyroidism in thyroid irAEs is shorter (2–6 weeks).[3,5]

Other nonclassical presentations of thyroid irAEs have also been described. Wors-ening of preexisting hypothyroidism can occur owing to additional destructive thyroid-itis, but these cases are also at risk of thyrotoxicosis unless they already require full-replacement thyroid hormone doses.[5,6,9,10] Graves disease hyperthyroidism is extremely rare with ICIs but has been reported in some cases,[50–52] hence should be considered in the setting of persistent thyrotoxicosis with positive thyrotropin receptor autoantibody/thyroid stimulating immunoglobulin (TRAb/TSI) or with other features of Graves disease. Last, central hypothyroidism owing to hypophysitis should be consid-ered when patients manifest low or inappropriately normal TSH with low thyroxine (T4), after excluding nonthyroidal illness, hypothalamus-pituitary-adrenal axis suppression from high-dose glucocorticoids, and progression of thyroiditis from the phase of thyro-toxicosis to euthyroidism or hypothyroidism (**Fig. 2**).

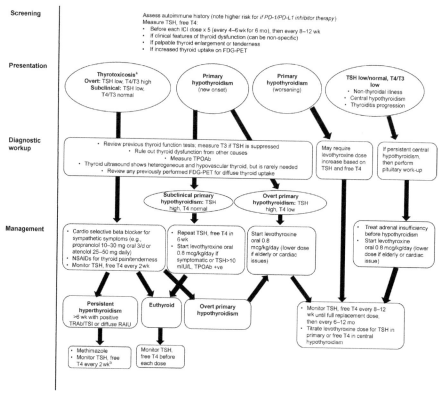

Fig. 2. A framework for the screening, diagnosis, and management of thyroid dysfunction from ICIs. [a]TSH may be normal initially due to rapid release of T4/T3. [b]This could progress to hypothyroidism. NSAIDs, nonsteroid anti-inflammatory drugs; RAIU, radioactive iodine uptake.

Screening and Diagnosis of Immune Checkpoint Inhibitor-Induced Thyroid Dysfunction

Society guidelines[53,54] and review articles[3,46,55] have provided recommendations for thyroid irAEs; however, a well-defined framework readily available for clinicians is still lacking. The authors have developed their approach based on those recommendations and their expertise in managing patients with thyroid irAEs. They recommend that TSH and free T4 levels be measured before each ICI infusion for at least 5 doses (which correspond to every 4–6 weeks for 6 months), then every 8 to 12 weeks, or when there is noted to be diffusely elevated FDG uptake on PET scan (see **Fig. 2**). The utility of measuring TPOAb/TgAb at baseline in addition to routine monitoring of thyroid function tests remains under investigation, but this could be considered if starting PD-1/PD-L1 inhibitor as their predictive role has been suggested.[11,26,28,34,38,56]

Once thyroid dysfunction occurs, it is essential to review the trend of thyroid function tests, rule out other causes, measure TPOAb/TgAb (to guide severity of thyroid dysfunction and influence management for subclinical hypothyroidism) and triiodothyronine (T3) level (if TSH is suppressed). Thyroid ultrasound usually demonstrates heterogeneous and hypovascular thyroid gland consistent with thyroiditis but is rarely needed for establishing the diagnosis. The frequent use of iodinated contrast for imaging in patients with cancer limits the utility of radioactive iodine uptake. If thyrotoxicosis is severe or persists greater than 6 weeks, then evaluation for Graves disease should be performed, including testing for TRAb or TSI (see **Fig. 2**).

Management of Immune Checkpoint Inhibitor-Induced Thyroid Dysfunction

The management of thyroid irAEs depends on the phase of thyroiditis in which the patient presents (see **Fig. 2**). Thyrotoxicosis can be managed symptomatically with beta-blockade and monitored for progression. If thyroid function normalizes, then it should be monitored, and if progression to overt hypothyroidism occurs, then thyroid hormone replacement with levothyroxine should be initiated, and for those with subclinical hypothyroidism if symptomatic or with serial serum TSH concentrations greater than 10 mIU/L. The authors support initiating levothyroxine dose of 0.8 µg/kg/d[3,55] as opposed to full dose of 1.6 µg/kg/d[53] because of risk of thyrotoxicosis in these patients who are usually elderly and have other comorbidities. If there is central hypothyroidism, it is essential to diagnose and treat adrenal insufficiency beforehand to prevent precipitation of adrenal crisis (see **Fig. 2**).

The discontinuation of ICI in the setting of thyroid disorders is not necessary except in cases of severe symptoms when the ICI may be temporarily held, and can be resumed once symptoms improve.[3,53,54] As for long-term thyroid function outcomes, overt hypothyroidism appears to be permanent, as the recovery of the thyroid gland has not been described.[3,55] However, subclinical mild thyroid dysfunction especially in the absence of TPOAb may resolve to normalization of thyroid function tests.[3,5,10]

Effect of Immune Checkpoint Inhibitor-Induced Thyroid Dysfunction on Cancer Outcomes

Multiple studies have demonstrated a strong and consistent association between thyroid irAEs and improved survival.[57] In a cohort of 91 PD-L1 inhibitor-treated patients at Mayo Clinic, median overall survival (OS) was not reached in those with thyroid irAEs, versus 9.8 months (95% confidence interval [CI], 6.3–12.9) in persistently euthyroid patients.[5] This survival benefit persisted after adjusting for age, sex, and cancer type, with patients who developed thyroid irAEs having a lower risk of mortality (hazard ratio, 0.49; 95% CI, 0.25–0.99; $P = .03$).[5] Additional retrospective[8,10,26,28,31,38,58] and a few prospective[11,59,60] studies have suggested similar 40% to 70% reductions in mortality risk for patients with cancer who developed thyroid irAEs.[57] Some studies demonstrated stronger survival benefit with overt and permanent as compared with subclinical and transient thyroid dysfunction, respectively.[10,23,28,60,61] These data suggest that not only the occurrence but also the severity and subtype of thyroid irAEs are important in the relationship with survival. In addition, a study demonstrated that TPOAb levels at baseline and their increase predict improved survival in PD-1 inhibitor-treated patients.[26] The authors postulate that the severity of autoimmunity parallels the degree of antitumor response.[57]

Despite the overall consistent evidence, some uncertainty about the relationship of thyroid irAEs with survival remains because a few studies have shown discordant observations. Two retrospective studies[62,63] of PD-1 inhibitors did not find improved OS with thyroid irAEs. In these studies, the limited mortality and lack of adjustment for confounding variables may explain the discordant observations. In addition, other noncausal explanations for the association between irAEs and survival need to be considered, such as the possibility for guarantee-time (lead-time, immortal-time) bias. However, thyroid irAEs develop early during ICI therapy[3,5,9,64] and most often before structural evidence of tumor response, and studies that addressed this bias also demonstrated a survival advantage of thyroid irAEs.[23,59,65]

KINASE INHIBITORS

KIs are antagonists of the cell surface receptor and intracellular kinase enzymes that play vital roles in cell signaling, growth, and proliferation. Most are orally administered small molecule inhibitors and are used against multiple cancer types. A critical component of kinases is an evolutionarily conserved ATP-binding pocket[66]; drugs binding these critical sites may therefore be poorly selective multi-KIs with both "on-target" and "off-target" kinase actions (although more specifically targeted KIs have now been developed). A further nuance is that "on-target" effects (for example, those directed at vascular growth factor pathways of tumors) may cause some adverse effects in noncancer tissues.[67] Thyroid function abnormalities are among the adverse effects reported with KIs and may be from a combination of on- and off-target drug actions.

Actions of Kinase Inhibitors on Peripheral Thyroid Hormone Metabolism

KIs are key treatment options for many patients with advanced thyroid cancers. Approved agents reporting thyroid-specific data include lenvatinib and sorafenib for radioactive iodine-refractory differentiated cancers, vandetanib and cabozantinib for medullary cancers, and most recently, selpercatinib and pralsetinib for *RET*-altered thyroid cancers (either differentiated or medullary). Because almost all such patients with thyroid cancer undergo thyroidectomy, alterations in thyroid hormone levels from KIs are caused by altered peripheral thyroid hormone metabolism.

Data from the key clinical trials assessing KIs in patients with thyroid cancer clearly demonstrate an effect on peripheral thyroid hormone metabolism (**Table 2**).[68–72] Although the definitions of reported effects varied between studies (so direct comparison of the severity of effects is not possible), the consistent outcome is an increase in serum TSH with potential for increased thyroid hormone requirements. For most patients, this corresponds to a relatively small increase in requirement for levothyroxine replacement, for example, approximately 10% mean increase has been reported for sorafenib.[73]

The mechanism for these peripheral thyroid hormone metabolism changes has been examined for sorafenib.[73] In a 26-week study including 21 athyreotic patients, levothyroxine requirements increased, serum-free thyroid hormone levels decreased,

---

Table 2
Kinase inhibitors approved for use in patients with thyroid cancer and effects on thyroid function in key trials leading to Food and Drug Administration approval

Kinase Inhibitor	Definition of Effect on Thyroid Function	Cumulative Incidence	Comparator, Cumulative Incidence
Lenvatinib[68]	Increase in serum TSH >0.5 mIU/L	57%	Placebo, 14%
Sorafenib[69]	Increase in serum TSH	33.3%	Placebo, 13.4%
Vandetanib[72]	Increase in thyroid hormone replacement	49%	Placebo, 17%
Cabozantinib[70]	Serum TSH above normal	57%	Placebo, 19%
Selpercatinib[71]	Hypothyroidism	15%	No comparator
Pralsetinib[142]	Change in thyroid hormone requirements	0% reported	No comparator

serum TSH concentration increased, and ratios of thyroid hormones and metabolites were altered consistent with an increase in type 3 iodothyronine deiodinase activity (serum T3/T4 and T3/reverse T3 ratios decreased by 18% and 22%, respectively).

Similar effects have also been reported for multiple other KIs in patients who were either athyreotic or with preexisting replaced hypothyroidism (who, like thyroidectomized patients could not enhance endogenous thyroid hormone secretion in the face of increased requirements). A well-studied example is imatinib. In an early report of 11 patients (8 after thyroidectomy and 3 without thyroid dysfunction), levothyroxine requirements increased, serum-free thyroid hormone levels decreased, and serum TSH concentration increased in all 8 thyroidectomized patients, but not in those with intact thyroid function.[74] In rat studies (using sunitinib), liver induction of type 3 iodothyronine deiodinase along with a reduction in type 1 iodothyronine deiodinase activity has been identified.[75] Although not reported for other tumor types, 1 cell-line study of gastrointestinal stromal tumors identified increased expression and activity of type 3 iodothyronine deiodinase when exposed to both imatinib and sunitinib,[76] which offers a further potential mechanism for KIs affecting thyroid hormone concentrations.

Despite an increase in type 3 iodothyronine deiodinase activity largely appearing to explain the thyroid function abnormalities seen in athyreotic patients exposed to multi-KIs, additional impacts on peripheral thyroid hormone transport and metabolism are possible. Two cell-line studies have shown that various KIs appear to also reduce thyroid hormone plasma membrane transport.[77,78] Computational protein modeling approaches have also postulated that KIs, specifically sunitinib and sorafenib, could bind retinoic acid receptors, which have important roles in complexing with thyroid hormone receptors.[79]

Direct Actions of Kinase Inhibitors on the Thyroid

Although peripheral effects of KIs on thyroid hormone metabolism may be important in nonthyroidectomized patients, less common but more profound effects can occur because of their direct action on the thyroid itself. How often KIs cause thyroid abnormalities likely varies with multiple factors. The most extensively studied KI causing thyroid dysfunction is sunitinib, approved for use in renal cell cancer, gastrointestinal stromal tumors, and pancreatic neuroendocrine tumors, although most multi-KIs used in cancer report some occurrence of thyroid dysfunction. Additional factors that influence the chance of thyroid dysfunction with sunitinib include the length of therapy (longer treatment time associated with higher prevalence)[80] and demographic characteristics of patients (more common in women).[79,81] **Table 3**[82–94] describes the cumulative incidence of thyroid dysfunction from KIs reported in nonthyroid cancer trials leading to FDA approval, noting that the exposure time to KIs in most was only a few months, hence likely underrepresenting the frequency of thyroid dysfunction.

Multiple lines of evidence suggest that destructive thyroiditis is the key process leading to KI-induced thyroid dysfunction. Transient thyrotoxicosis can be the first feature.[95,96] Hypothyroidism is the most common outcome, with or without prior thyrotoxicosis.[97] Thyroid autoantibodies can develop de novo after the cellular injury.[98] Although not universally reported, the vascularity of the gland is usually reduced on ultrasound after the thyroid injury.[99] The most common explanation for thyroiditis development is vascular injury, related to multi-KIs' effects on vascular growth factor signaling (such as VEGF-receptors [particularly VEGFR1 and VEGFR2] and PDGF-receptor).[100] This explanation is enticing, given that many multi-KIs that cause thyroid dysfunction have effects on receptors known to be crucial to angiogenesis and stabilizing vascular endothelium. However, other agents targeting VEGFR1

Table 3
Cumulative incidence of hypothyroidism from trials leading to Food and Drug Administration approval of multikinase inhibitors for their single-agent use in solid organ tumors

Kinase Inhibitor and Cancer	Cumulative Incidence of Hypothyroidism	Median Time on Treatment	Comparator, Cumulative Incidence of Hypothyroidism
Axitinib[82]			
Renal cell cancer[82]	19%	6.4 mo	Sorafenib, 8%
Cabozantinib[83,84,91]			
Renal cell cancer[83]	20%	7.6 mo	Everolimus, <1%
Hepatocellular cancer[84,91]	8%	3.8 mo	Placebo, <1%
Lenvatinib[85]			
Hepatocellular cancer[85]	16%	5.7 mo	Sorafenib, 2%
Pazopanib[86,87,92,143]			
Renal cell cancer[86]	7%	7.4 mo	Placebo, 0%
Renal cell cancer[143]	12%	8.0 mo	Sunitinib, 24%
Soft tissue sarcoma[87,92]	8%	4.1 mo	Placebo, 0%
Regorafenib[90,93]			
Colorectal cancer[90,93]	4.2%	2.8 mo	Placebo, 0.4%
Sorafenib[82,85]	Hypothyroidism not reported in initial sorafenib trials; reported as a comparator in Axitinib,[82] Lenvatinib,[85] and Tivozanib[82] trials		
Sunitinib[88,89,94,143]			
Gastrointestinal stromal tumors[88]	4%	1.9 mo	Placebo, 1%
Renal cell cancer[94,143]	16%	6 mo	Interferon-alpha, 1%
Pancreatic neuroendocrine tumors[89]	7%	4.3 mo	Placebo, 1%
Tivozanib[82]			
Renal cell cancer[82]	13%	6.6 mo	Sorafenib, 6%

and VEGFR2 signaling pathways (such as bevacizumab) are not known to cause thyroiditis; therefore, the importance of VEGFR is unclear.

An emerging treatment strategy for some cancers is a combination of KIs and ICIs. If KIs regularly induce thyroid injury (via vascular damage or other mechanisms) and expose antigens to an unrestrained immune system from ICI, high rates of thyroid dysfunction should ensue. Indeed, extremely high rates of hypothyroidism have been reported in the completed studies thus far (**Table 4**).[83,101–104]

Diagnosis and Management of Kinase Inhibitor-Induced Thyroid Dysfunction

In thyroidectomized patients or those already on thyroid hormone replacement commencing KI treatment, the authors recommend thyroid function testing before commencing treatment, every 4 weeks until levels/levothyroxine doses are stable or whenever KI dose adjustment has been made, and then every 3 to 6 months once stable.

In patients commencing KIs who are not known to have thyroid disease, baseline followed by regular thyroid function testing (no mandatory regimens, although testing

Table 4
Cumulative incidence of hypothyroidism from phase III trials of multikinase inhibitors combined with immune checkpoint inhibitors

Kinase Inhibitor + Immune Checkpoint Inhibitor	Cumulative Incidence of Hypothyroidism, %	Median Time on Treatment, mo	Comparator, Cumulative Incidence of Hypothyroidism
Axitinib + Avelumab[104]			
Renal cell cancer[104]	24.9	8.6	Sunitinib, 13.9%
Axitinib + Pembrolizumab[102]			
Renal cell cancer[102]	37	14.5	No comparator
Cabozantinib + Nivolumab[83]			
Renal cell cancer[83]	34.1	14.3	Sunitinib, 29.4%
Lenvatinib/Pembrolizumab[101,103]			
Endometrial cancer[101]	43.5	8.2	No comparator
Hepatocellular cancer[103]	47.2	17.0	Lenvatinib/everolimus, 26.8%; Sunitinib, 26.5%

every 2 months is reasonable) is recommended. When thyrotoxicosis is identified, symptomatic treatment with beta-blockade (expecting a transient thyrotoxic phase so long as TRAb/TSI is negative) and close monitoring for development of hypothyroidism are the gold-standard care. Levothyroxine replacement should be commenced when overt hypothyroidism occurs or if serial serum TSH concentrations are greater than 10 mIU/L.

Effect of Kinase Inhibitor-Induced Thyroid Dysfunction on Cancer Outcomes

If thyroid dysfunction from KIs is caused by actions on kinase-directed pathways that are also important in cancer growth, could thyroid side effects be a marker for better prognosis with KI treatment? Most evidence is supportive and has been accrued with sunitinib. Studies assessing sunitinib alone[105–111] or sunitinib with other agents[81,112–114] found that the occurrence of hypothyroidism with sunitinib treatment led to improved progression-free and/or overall survival, although this conclusion is not universal, as some studies did not show an association with improved survival.[115–117] In addition, studies assessing axitinib,[118] cabozantinib,[119] regorafenib,[60,110] and sorafenib[120] also support an improved prognosis in KI-treated patients who develop hypothyroidism. The only agent whereby evidence so far appears mixed is Lenvatinib.[121–124]

IODINE-131-LABELED METAIODOBENZYLGUANIDINE

Unbound radioactive iodine (I-131) is an important therapy for benign and malignant thyroid disease. It concentrates within thyroid tissue via the sodium-iodine symporter, followed by organification to TgAb. Trapped inside thyroid tissue, beta irradiation leads to DNA damage, causing the affected cells to undergo apoptosis, hence ablating the thyroid tissue. I-131 can also be bound to drugs to allow targeted uptake into other tissues. Metaiodobenzylguanidine (MIBG) resembles norepinephrine and enters cells through the norepinephrine transporter.[125] Tumors that may express sufficient norepinephrine transporters to allow therapeutic I-131-MIBG include pheochromocytomas/paragangliomas[126] and childhood neuroblastomas[127] (although

Table 5
Cumulative incidence of hypothyroidism from studies of radioactive iodine-131-metaiodobenzylguanidine treatment for neuroblastoma

Thyroid Prophylaxis with Each I-131-MIBG Treatment	Definition of Hypothyroidism	n	Treatment Details	Follow-Up Duration	Cumulative Incidence of Hypothyroidism
Lugol iodine for 5 d[132]	High TSH (minimum = 13.7 mIU/L)	16	Cumulative median activity 116 mCi	16 mo (median)	56.2%
Lugol iodine for 8 d[133]	Overt hypothyroidism	43	Cumulative median activity 160 MBq	Unclear[a]	35%
Potassium iodide for 5 d[134]	Hypothyroidism	55	Cumulative median 300 mCi	Unclear	19.6%
Potassium iodide for 14 d[135]	Permanent TSH elevation	42	Average 3.3 treatment courses (100–200 mCi each)	2.9 y (mean)	42.9%
Potassium iodide for 45 d, potassium perchlorate for 5 d[136]	Any onset or worsening of hypothyroidism	24	18.2 mCi/kg	3.5 mo	32%
Thyroxine, methimazole, potassium iodide until 28 d after last dose[137]	TSH >4.7 mIU/L	23	Average 2.3 treatment courses (100–200 mCi each)	19 mo (median)	17.4% within 5 y (5-y overall survival 38%)
Thyroxine, methimazole, potassium iodide until 28 d after last dose[138]	TSH >5 mIU/L or thyroxine use at last follow-up	24	Cumulative median activity 270 mCi	9 y (median)	37.5%

[a] Overt hypothyroidism occurred at a median of 12 mo; those with normal thyroid function were followed for a median of 45 mo.

occasional reports describe I-131-MIBG uptake into other tumor types, including medullary thyroid cancers[128] and gastroenteropancreatic neuroendocrine tumors,[125] the evidence for I-131-MIBG use in these settings is very weak).

Although most I-131 remains bound to MIBG, 3% to 5% dissociates and thus becomes available for thyroid uptake.[129] All patients receiving I-131-MIBG treatment should be prescribed prophylactic high-dose stable iodine treatment (eg, Lugol iodine or potassium iodide) commencing days before each treatment and continuing until I-131-MIBG is cleared. Varying protocols exist for both the dose of iodine and the time for which the prophylaxis continues.[129–131]

Given that patients with neuroblastoma are young children whose thyroids will be particularly sensitive to I-131 effects, most concern for thyroid complications of I-131-MIBG centers on this group. The late thyroid effects reported include hypothyroidism most commonly (**Table 5**),[132–138] thyroid nodules, and rarely, thyroid cancers.[139] Despite protocols for thyroid protection, all studies report high prevalence of hypothyroidism. In the short term, hypothyroidism rates are much lower after prophylactic regimens that include additional agents to Lugol iodine or potassium iodide.[135,137] However, in long-term survivors, hypothyroidism is extremely common.[138] Therefore, additional measures may be required in the future to prevent thyroid impacts from I-131-MIBG treatment in neuroblastoma patients.

SUMMARY

Thyroid dysfunction frequently occurs with all ICIs, but especially PD-1/PD-L1 inhibitors. It mostly presents as hypothyroidism, which may be preceded by a thyrotoxic phase. ICI-induced thyroid damage appears to be a T lymphocyte–mediated destructive thyroiditis, although underlying mechanisms are being investigated. KIs may cause direct thyroid dysfunction, potentially from vascular injury, or by alterations in thyroid hormone metabolism. The high prevalence of thyroid dysfunction after I-131-MIBG despite iodine prophylaxis highlights the need for better risk prediction and prophylactic regimens. Understanding the effects caused by cancer therapies may yield insight into other thyroid disease processes and identify patients that have robust antitumor response from these increasingly common targeted cancer therapies.

CLINICS CARE POINTS

- Monitor thyroid function in patients on immune checkpoint inhibitors and kinase inhibitors.
- Initiate levothyroxine at 0.8 μg/kg/d for overt hypothyroidism or symptomatic subclinical hypothyroidism with serum thyroid-stimulating hormone greater than 10 mIU/L.
- Manage thyrotoxicosis conservatively with beta-blockers unless it is persistent or severe, in which case evaluate for Graves disease.
- Evaluate and treat adrenal insufficiency before thyroid hormone replacement in the case of central hypothyroidism (low thyroid hormone, low or inappropriately normal thyroid-stimulating hormone).
- Provide iodine prophylaxis for patients receiving I-131-metaiodobenzylguanidine treatment and monitor thyroid function.

ACKNOWLEDGMENT

Don McLeod is supported by a Metro North Clinician Research Fellowship and a Queensland Advancing Clinical Research Fellowship.

DISCLOSURE

The authors have nothing to disclose.

REFERENCES

1. Pardoll DM. The blockade of immune checkpoints in cancer immunotherapy. Nat Rev Cancer 2012;12(4):252–64.
2. Anderson B, Morganstein DL. Endocrine toxicity of cancer immunotherapy: clinical challenges. Endocr Connect 2021;10(3):R116–24.
3. Chang LS, Barroso-Sousa R, Tolaney SM, et al. Endocrine toxicity of cancer immunotherapy targeting immune checkpoints. Endocr Rev 2019;40(1):17–65.
4. Morganstein DL, Lai Z, Spain L, et al. Thyroid abnormalities following the use of cytotoxic T-lymphocyte antigen-4 and programmed death receptor protein-1 inhibitors in the treatment of melanoma. Clin Endocrinol (Oxf) 2017;86(4):614–20.
5. Kotwal A, Kottschade L, Ryder M. PD-L1 inhibitor-induced thyroiditis is associated with better overall survival in cancer patients. Thyroid 2020;30(2):177–84.
6. Delivanis DA, Gustafson MP, Bornschlegl S, et al. Pembrolizumab-induced thyroiditis: comprehensive clinical review and insights into underlying involved mechanisms. J Clin Endocrinol Metab 2017;102(8):2770–80.
7. Iyer PC, Cabanillas ME, Waguespack SG, et al. Immune-related thyroiditis with immune checkpoint inhibitors. Thyroid 2018;28(10):1243–51.
8. Lui DTW, Lee CH, Tang V, et al. Thyroid immune-related adverse events in patients with cancer treated with anti-PD1/anti-CTLA4 immune checkpoint inhibitor combination: clinical course and outcomes. Endocr Pract 2021. https://doi.org/10.1016/j.eprac.2021.01.017.
9. Muir CA, Menzies AM, Clifton-Bligh R, et al. Thyroid toxicity following immune checkpoint inhibitor treatment in advanced cancer. Thyroid 2020;30(10):1458–69.
10. Muir CA, Clifton-Bligh RJ, Long GV, et al. Thyroid immune-related adverse events following immune checkpoint inhibitor treatment. J Clin Endocrinol Metab 2021. https://doi.org/10.1210/clinem/dgab263.
11. Osorio JC, Ni A, Chaft JE, et al. Antibody-mediated thyroid dysfunction during T-cell checkpoint blockade in patients with non-small-cell lung cancer. Ann Oncol 2017;28(3):583–9.
12. Faje A. Immunotherapy and hypophysitis: clinical presentation, treatment, and biologic insights. Pituitary 2016;19(1):82–92.
13. Barroso-Sousa R, Barry WT, Garrido-Castro AC, et al. Incidence of endocrine dysfunction following the use of different immune checkpoint inhibitor regimens: a systematic review and meta-analysis. JAMA Oncol 2018;4(2):173–82.
14. Kotwal A. Hypophysitis from immune checkpoint inhibitors: challenges in diagnosis and management. Curr Opin Endocrinol Diabetes Obes 2021;28(4):427–34.
15. Kotwal A, Haddox C, Block M, et al. Immune checkpoint inhibitors: an emerging cause of insulin-dependent diabetes. BMJ Open Diabetes Res Care 2019;7(1):e000591.
16. Stamatouli AM, Quandt Z, Perdigoto AL, et al. Collateral damage: insulin-dependent diabetes induced with checkpoint inhibitors. *Diabetes* Aug 2018;67(8):1471–80.
17. Quandt Z, Young A, Anderson M. Immune checkpoint inhibitor diabetes mellitus: a novel form of autoimmune diabetes. Clin Exp Immunol 2020;200(2):131–40.

18. Min L, Ibrahim N. Ipilimumab-induced autoimmune adrenalitis. *Lancet Diabetes Endocrinol* Nov 2013;1(3):e15.

19. Gaballa S, Hlaing KM, Mahler N, et al. A rare case of immune-mediated primary adrenal insufficiency with cytotoxic T-lymphocyte antigen-4 inhibitor ipilimumab in metastatic melanoma of lung and neck of unknown primary. Cureus 2020; 12(6):e8602.

20. Abdallah D, Johnson J, Goldner W, et al. Adrenal insufficiency from immune checkpoint inhibitors masquerading as sepsis. JCO Oncol Pract 2021;17(4): 212–4.

21. Piranavan P, Li Y, Brown E, et al. Immune checkpoint inhibitor-induced hypoparathyroidism associated with calcium-sensing receptor-activating autoantibodies. J Clin Endocrinol Metab 2019;104(2):550–6.

22. El Kawkgi OM, Li D, Kotwal A, et al. Hypoparathyroidism: an uncommon complication associated with immune checkpoint inhibitor therapy. Mayo Clinic Proc Innov Qual Outcomes 2020;4(6):821–5.

23. Yamauchi I, Yasoda A, Matsumoto S, et al. Incidence, features, and prognosis of immune-related adverse events involving the thyroid gland induced by nivolumab. PLoS One 2019;14(5):e0216954.

24. de Filette J, Andreescu CE, Cools F, et al. A systematic review and meta-analysis of endocrine-related adverse events associated with immune checkpoint inhibitors. Horm Metab Res 2019;51(3):145–56.

25. Yamauchi I, Sakane Y, Fukuda Y, et al. Clinical features of nivolumab-induced thyroiditis: a case series study. *Thyroid* Jul 2017;27(7):894–901.

26. Basak EA, van der Meer JWM, Hurkmans DP, et al. Overt thyroid dysfunction and anti-thyroid antibodies predict response to anti-PD-1 immunotherapy in cancer patients. Thyroid 2020;30(7):966–73.

27. Imblum BA, Baloch ZW, Fraker D, et al. Pembrolizumab-induced thyroiditis. Endocr Pathol 2019;30(2):163–7.

28. Luongo C, Morra R, Gambale C, et al. Higher baseline TSH levels predict early hypothyroidism during cancer immunotherapy. J Endocrinol Invest 2021.

29. Lee H, Hodi FS, Giobbie-Hurder A, et al. Characterization of thyroid disorders in patients receiving immune checkpoint inhibition therapy. Cancer Immunol Res 2017;5(12):1133–40.

30. Antonelli A, Ferrari SM, Corrado A, et al. Autoimmune thyroid disorders. Autoimmun Rev 2015;14(2):174–80.

31. Zhou Y, Xia R, Xiao H, et al. Thyroid function abnormality induced by PD-1 inhibitors have a positive impact on survival in patients with non-small cell lung cancer. Int Immunopharmacol 2021;91:107296.

32. Brilli L, Danielli R, Campanile M, et al. Baseline serum TSH levels predict the absence of thyroid dysfunction in cancer patients treated with immunotherapy. J Endocrinol Invest 2021;44(8):1719–26.

33. Pollack RM, Kagan M, Lotem M, et al. Baseline TSH level is associated with risk of anti–PD-1–induced thyroid dysfunction. Endocr Pract 2019;25(8):824–9. https://doi.org/10.4158/EP-2018-0472.

34. Kobayashi T, Iwama S, Yasuda Y, et al. Patients with antithyroid antibodies are prone to develop destructive thyroiditis by nivolumab: a prospective study. J Endocr Soc 2018;2(3):241–51.

35. Mariotti S, Caturegli P, Piccolo P, et al. Antithyroid peroxidase autoantibodies in thyroid diseases. J Clin Endocrinol Metab 1990;71(3):661–9.

36. Pedersen IB, Knudsen N, Jørgensen T, et al. Thyroid peroxidase and thyroglobulin autoantibodies in a large survey of populations with mild and moderate iodine deficiency. Clin Endocrinol (Oxf) 2003;58(1):36–42.

37. Hollowell JG, Staehling NW, Flanders WD, et al. Serum TSH, T(4), and thyroid antibodies in the United States population (1988 to 1994): National Health and Nutrition Examination Survey (NHANES III). J Clin Endocrinol Metab 2002; 87(2):489–99.

38. Sakakida T, Ishikawa T, Uchino J, et al. Clinical features of immune-related thyroid dysfunction and its association with outcomes in patients with advanced malignancies treated by PD-1 blockade. Oncol Lett 2019;18(2):2140–7.

39. Angell TE, Min L, Wieczorek TJ, et al. Unique cytologic features of thyroiditis caused by immune checkpoint inhibitor therapy for malignant melanoma. Genes Dis 2018;5(1):46–8.

40. Yanagawa T, Hidaka Y, Guimaraes V, et al. CTLA-4 gene polymorphism associated with Graves' disease in a Caucasian population. J Clin Endocrinol Metab 1995;80(1):41–5.

41. Kotsa K, Watson PF, Weetman AP. A CTLA-4 gene polymorphism is associated with both Graves disease and autoimmune hypothyroidism. Clin Endocrinol (Oxf) 1997;46(5):551–4.

42. Kotwal A, Gustafson MP, Bornschlegl S, et al. Immune checkpoint inhibitor-induced thyroiditis is associated with increased intrathyroidal T lymphocyte subpopulations. Thyroid 2020;30(10):1440–50.

43. Yasuda Y, Iwama S, Sugiyama D, et al. CD4$^+$ T cells are essential for the development of destructive thyroiditis induced by anti–PD-1 antibody in thyroglobulin-immunized mice. Sci Translational Med 2021;13(593):eabb7495.

44. Liu J, Blake SJ, Harjunpää H, et al. Assessing immune-related adverse events of efficacious combination immunotherapies in preclinical models of cancer. Cancer Res 2016;76(18):5288–301.

45. Ippolito S, Di Dalmazi G, Pani F, et al. Distinct cytokine signatures in thyroiditis induced by PD-1 or CTLA-4 blockade: insights from a new mouse model. Thyroid 2021. https://doi.org/10.1089/thy.2021.0165.

46. Wright JJ, Powers AC, Johnson DB. Endocrine toxicities of immune checkpoint inhibitors. Nat Rev Endocrinol 2021. https://doi.org/10.1038/s41574-021-00484-3.

47. McMillen B, Dhillon MS, Yong-Yow S. A rare case of thyroid storm. BMJ Case Rep 2016. https://doi.org/10.1136/bcr-2016-214603.

48. Min L, Hodi FS. Anti-PD1 following ipilimumab for mucosal melanoma: durable tumor response associated with severe hypothyroidism and rhabdomyolysis. Cancer Immunol Res 2014;2(1):15–8.

49. Khan U, Rizvi H, Sano D, et al. Nivolumab induced myxedema crisis. J Immunother Cancer 2017;5:13.

50. Gan EH, Mitchell AL, Plummer R, et al. Tremelimumab-induced Graves hyperthyroidism. Eur Thyroid J 2017;6(3):167–70.

51. Azmat U, Liebner D, Joehlin-Price A, et al. Treatment of ipilimumab induced Graves' disease in a patient with metastatic melanoma. Case Rep Endocrinol 2016;2016:2087525.

52. Peiffert M, Cugnet-Anceau C, Dalle S, et al. Graves' disease during immune checkpoint inhibitor therapy (a case series and literature review). Cancers (Basel) 2021;(8):13. https://doi.org/10.3390/cancers13081944.

53. Thompson JA, Schneider BJ, Brahmer J, et al. NCCN guidelines insights: management of immunotherapy-related toxicities, version 1.2020. J Natl Compr Canc Netw 2020;18(3):230–41.

54. Brahmer JR, Lacchetti C, Schneider BJ, et al. Management of immune-related adverse events in patients treated with immune checkpoint inhibitor therapy: American Society of Clinical Oncology Clinical Practice Guideline. J Clin Oncol 2018;36(17):1714–68.

55. Barroso-Sousa R, Ott PA, Hodi FS, et al. Endocrine dysfunction induced by immune checkpoint inhibitors: practical recommendations for diagnosis and clinical management. Cancer Mar 15 2018;124(6):1111–21.

56. Brilli L, Calabrò L, Campanile M, et al. Permanent diabetes insipidus in a patient with mesothelioma treated with immunotherapy. Arch Endocrinol Metab 2020; 64(4):483–6.

57. Kotwal A, Ryder M. Survival benefit of endocrine dysfunction following immune checkpoint inhibitors for nonthyroidal cancers. Curr Opin Endocrinol Diabetes Obes 2021. https://doi.org/10.1097/med.0000000000000664.

58. Lima Ferreira J, Costa C, Marques B, et al. Improved survival in patients with thyroid function test abnormalities secondary to immune-checkpoint inhibitors. Cancer Immunol Immunother 2021;70(2):299–309.

59. Peiró I, Palmero R, Iglesias P, et al. Thyroid dysfunction induced by nivolumab: searching for disease patterns and outcomes. Endocrine 2019;64(3):605–13.

60. Kim HI, Kim M, Lee S-H, et al. Development of thyroid dysfunction is associated with clinical response to PD-1 blockade treatment in patients with advanced non-small cell lung cancer. OncoImmunology 2018;7(1):e1375642.

61. Inaba H, Ariyasu H, Iwakura H, et al. Distinct clinical features and prognosis between persistent and temporary thyroid dysfunctions by immune-checkpoint inhibitors. Endocr J 2021;68(2):231–41.

62. Sbardella E, Tenuta M, Sirgiovanni G, et al. Thyroid disorders in programmed death 1 inhibitor-treated patients: Is previous therapy with tyrosine kinase inhibitors a predisposing factor? Clin Endocrinol (Oxf) 2020;92(3):258–65.

63. Al Mushref M, Guido PA, Collichio FA, et al. Thyroid dysfunction, recovery, and prognosis in melanoma patients treated with immune checkpoint inhibitors: a retrospective review. Endocr Pract 2020;26(1):36–42.

64. Nguyen H, Shah K, Waguespack SG, et al. Immune checkpoint inhibitor related hypophysitis: diagnostic criteria and recovery patterns. Endocr Relat Cancer 2021. https://doi.org/10.1530/erc-20-0513.

65. Haratani K, Hayashi H, Chiba Y, et al. Association of immune-related adverse events with nivolumab efficacy in non-small-cell lung cancer. JAMA Oncol 2018;4(3):374–8.

66. Anastassiadis T, Deacon SW, Devarajan K, et al. Comprehensive assay of kinase catalytic activity reveals features of kinase inhibitor selectivity. Nat Biotechnol 2011;29(11):1039–45.

67. Shah RR, Morganroth J, Shah DR. Hepatotoxicity of tyrosine kinase inhibitors: clinical and regulatory perspectives. Drug Saf 2013;36(7):491–503.

68. Lenvatinib prescribing information. Available at: http://www.lenvima.com/pdfs/prescribing-information.pdf. Accessed July 13, 2021.

69. Brose MS, Nutting CM, Jarzab B, et al. Sorafenib in radioactive iodine-refractory, locally advanced or metastatic differentiated thyroid cancer: a randomised, double-blind, phase 3 trial. Lancet 2014;384(9940):319–28.

70. Elisei R, Schlumberger MJ, Müller SP, et al. Cabozantinib in progressive medullary thyroid cancer. J Clin Oncol 2013;31(29):3639–46.

71. Wirth LJ, Sherman E, Robinson B, et al. Efficacy of selpercatinib in RET-altered thyroid cancers. New Engl J Med 2020;383(9):825–35.
72. Wells SA Jr, Robinson BG, Gagel RF, et al. Vandetanib in patients with locally advanced or metastatic medullary thyroid cancer: a randomized, double-blind phase III trial. J Clin Oncol 2012;30(2):134–41.
73. Abdulrahman RM, Verloop H, Hoftijzer H, et al. Sorafenib-induced hypothyroidism is associated with increased type 3 deiodination. The J Clin Endocrinol Metab 2010;95(8):3758–62.
74. de Groot JW, Zonnenberg BA, Plukker JT, et al. Imatinib induces hypothyroidism in patients receiving levothyroxine. Clin Pharmacol Ther 2005;78(4):433–8.
75. Kappers MHW, van Esch JHM, Smedts FMM, et al. Sunitinib-induced hypothyroidism is due to induction of type 3 deiodinase activity and thyroidal capillary regression. The J Clin Endocrinol Metab 2011;96(10):3087–94.
76. Maynard MA, Marino-Enriquez A, Fletcher JA, et al. Thyroid hormone inactivation in gastrointestinal stromal tumors. New Engl J Med 2014;370(14):1327–34.
77. Braun D, Kim TD, le Coutre P, et al. Tyrosine kinase inhibitors noncompetitively inhibit MCT8-mediated iodothyronine transport. The J Clin Endocrinol Metab 2012;97(1):E100–5.
78. Beukhof CM, van Doorn L, Visser TJ, et al. Sorafenib-induced changes in thyroid hormone levels in patients treated for hepatocellular carcinoma. The J Clin Endocrinol Metab 2017;102(8):2922–9.
79. Shu M, Zai X, Zhang B, et al. Hypothyroidism side effect in patients treated with sunitinib or sorafenib: clinical and structural analyses. PLOS ONE 2016;11(1): e0147048.
80. Funakoshi T, Shimada YJ. Risk of hypothyroidism in patients with cancer treated with sunitinib: a systematic review and meta-analysis. Acta Oncol 2013;52(4): 691–702.
81. Lechner MG, Vyas CM, Hamnvik OR, et al. Risk factors for new hypothyroidism during tyrosine kinase inhibitor therapy in advanced nonthyroidal cancer patients. Thyroid 2018;28(4):437–44.
82. Rini BI, Escudier B, Tomczak P, et al. Comparative effectiveness of axitinib versus sorafenib in advanced renal cell carcinoma (AXIS): a randomised phase 3 trial. Lancet 2011;378(9807):1931–9.
83. Choueiri TK, Escudier B, Powles T, et al. Cabozantinib versus everolimus in advanced renal-cell carcinoma. New Engl J Med 2015;373(19):1814–23.
84. Abou-Alfa GK, Meyer T, Cheng A-L, et al. Cabozantinib in patients with advanced and progressing hepatocellular carcinoma. New Engl J Med 2018; 379(1):54–63.
85. Kudo M, Finn RS, Qin S, et al. Lenvatinib versus sorafenib in first-line treatment of patients with unresectable hepatocellular carcinoma: a randomised phase 3 non-inferiority trial. Lancet 2018;391(10126):1163–73.
86. Sternberg CN, Hawkins RE, Wagstaff J, et al. A randomised, double-blind phase III study of pazopanib in patients with advanced and/or metastatic renal cell carcinoma: Final overall survival results and safety update. Eur J Cancer 2013; 49(6):1287–96.
87. van der Graaf WTA, Blay J-Y, Chawla SP, et al. Pazopanib for metastatic soft-tissue sarcoma (PALETTE): a randomised, double-blind, placebo-controlled phase 3 trial. Lancet 2012;379(9829):1879–86.
88. Demetri GD, van Oosterom AT, Garrett CR, et al. Efficacy and safety of sunitinib in patients with advanced gastrointestinal stromal tumour after failure of imatinib: a randomised controlled trial. Lancet 2006;368(9544):1329–38.

89. Raymond E, Dahan L, Raoul J-L, et al. Sunitinib malate for the treatment of pancreatic neuroendocrine tumors. New Engl J Med 2011;364(6):501–13.
90. Grothey A, Cutsem EV, Sobrero A, et al. Regorafenib monotherapy for previously treated metastatic colorectal cancer (CORRECT): an international, multicentre, randomised, placebo-controlled, phase 3 trial. The Lancet 2013;381(9863): 303–12.
91. Cabozantinib prescribing information. Available at: https://www.cabometyx. com/downloads/CABOMETYXUSPI.pdf. Accessed July 13, 2021.
92. Pazopanib prescribing information. Available at: https://www.novartis.us/sites/ www.novartis.us/files/votrient.pdf. Accessed July 14, 2021.
93. Regorafenib prescribing information. Available at: http://labeling. bayerhealthcare.com/html/products/pi/Stivarga_PI.pdf. Accessed July 13, 2021.
94. Sunitinib prescribing information. Available at: https://labeling.pfizer.com/ ShowLabeling.aspx?id=607. Accessed July 13, 2021.
95. Faris JE, Moore AF, Daniels GH. Sunitinib (sutent)-induced thyrotoxicosis due to destructive thyroiditis: a case report. Thyroid 2007;17(11):1147–9.
96. Grossmann M, Premaratne E, Desai J, et al. Thyrotoxicosis during sunitinib treatment for renal cell carcinoma. Clin Endocrinol (Oxf) 2008;69(4):669–72.
97. Abdel-Rahman O, Fouad M. Risk of thyroid dysfunction in patients with solid tumors treated with VEGF receptor tyrosine kinase inhibitors: a critical literature review and meta analysis. *Expert Rev Anticancer Ther* Sep 2014;14(9):1063–73.
98. Pani F, Atzori F, Baghino G, et al. Thyroid dysfunction in patients with metastatic carcinoma treated with sunitinib: is thyroid autoimmunity involved? Thyroid 2015;25(11):1255–61.
99. Desai J, Yassa L, Marqusee E, et al. Hypothyroidism after sunitinib treatment for patients with gastrointestinal stromal tumors. *Ann Intern Med* Nov 7 2006;145(9): 660–4.
100. Makita N, Iiri T. Tyrosine kinase inhibitor-induced thyroid disorders: a review and hypothesis. Thyroid 2013;23(2):151–9.
101. Makker V, Taylor MH, Aghajanian C, et al. Lenvatinib plus pembrolizumab in patients with advanced endometrial cancer. J Clin Oncol 2020;38(26):2981–92.
102. Atkins MB, Plimack ER, Puzanov I, et al. Axitinib in combination with pembrolizumab in patients with advanced renal cell cancer: a non-randomised, open-label, dose-finding, and dose-expansion phase 1b trial. Lancet Oncol 2018;19(3): 405–15.
103. Motzer R, Alekseev B, Rha S-Y, et al. Lenvatinib plus pembrolizumab or everolimus for advanced renal cell carcinoma. New Engl J Med 2021;384(14): 1289–300.
104. Motzer RJ, Penkov K, Haanen J, et al. Avelumab plus axitinib versus sunitinib for advanced renal-cell carcinoma. New Engl J Med 2019;380(12):1103–15.
105. Baldazzi V, Tassi R, Lapini A, et al. The impact of sunitinib-induced hypothyroidism on progression-free survival of metastatic renal cancer patients: a prospective single-center study. Urol Oncol 2012;30(5):704–10.
106. KUST D, PRPIĆ M, MURGIĆ J, et al. Hypothyroidism as a predictive clinical marker of better treatment response to sunitinib therapy. Anticancer Res 2014;34(6):3177–84.
107. Akaza H, Naito S, Ueno N, et al. Real-world use of sunitinib in Japanese patients with advanced renal cell carcinoma: efficacy, safety and biomarker analyses in 1689 consecutive patients. Jpn J Clin Oncol 2015;45(6):576–83.

108. Bailey EB, Tantravahi SK, Poole A, et al. Correlation of degree of hypothyroidism with survival outcomes in patients with metastatic renal cell carcinoma receiving vascular endothelial growth factor receptor tyrosine kinase inhibitors. Clin Genitourinary Cancer 2015;13(3):e131–7.

109. Bozkurt O, Karaca H, Hacıbekiroglu I, et al. Is sunitinib-induced hypothyroidism a predictive clinical marker for better response in metastatic renal cell carcinoma patients? J Chemother 2016;28(3):230–4.

110. Pani F, Atzori F, Baghino G, et al. Hypothyroidism and thyroid autoimmunity as a prognostic biomarker of better response in metastatic cancer long-term survivors treated with sunitinib. Thyroid 2016;26(9):1336–7.

111. Vasileiadis T, Chrisofos M, Safioleas M, et al. Impact of sunitinib-induced hypothyroidism on survival of patients with metastatic renal cancer. BMC Cancer 2019;19(1):407.

112. Riesenbeck LM, Bierer S, Hoffmeister I, et al. Hypothyroidism correlates with a better prognosis in metastatic renal cancer patients treated with sorafenib or sunitinib. World J Urol 2011;29(6):807–13.

113. Schmidinger M, Vogl UM, Bojic M, et al. Hypothyroidism in patients with renal cell carcinoma: blessing or curse? Cancer 2011;117(3):534–44.

114. Iacovelli R, Verri E, Cossu Rocca M, et al. Prognostic role of the cumulative toxicity in patients affected by metastatic renal cells carcinoma and treated with first-line tyrosine kinase inhibitors. Anticancer Drugs 2017;28(2):206–12.

115. Sabatier R, Eymard JC, Walz J, et al. Could thyroid dysfunction influence outcome in sunitinib-treated metastatic renal cell carcinoma? Ann Oncol 2012; 23(3):714–21.

116. Miyake M, Kuwada M, Hori S, et al. The best objective response of target lesions and the incidence of treatment-related hypertension are associated with the survival of patients with metastatic renal cell carcinoma treated with sunitinib: a Japanese retrospective study. BMC Res Notes 2016;9(1):79.

117. Bolzacchini E, Pinotti G, Bertù L, et al. On-target toxicities predictive of survival in metastatic renal cell carcinoma (mRCC) treated with sunitinib: a multicenter retrospective study. Clin Genitourinary Cancer 2020;18(2):e145–56. https://doi.org/10.1016/j.clgc.2019.10.003.

118. Takada S, Hashishita H, Nagamori S, et al. Axitinib-induced hypothyroidism as a predictor of long-term survival in patients with metastatic renal cell carcinoma. Urol Int 2019;102(4):435–40.

119. Kucharz J, Dumnicka P, Kusnierz-Cabala B, et al. The correlation between the incidence of adverse events and progression-free survival in patients treated with cabozantinib for metastatic renal cell carcinoma (mRCC). Med Oncol 21 2019;36(2):19.

120. Chu Y-D, Lin K-H, Huang Y-H, et al. A novel thyroid function index associated with opposite therapeutic outcomes in advanced hepatocellular carcinoma patients receiving chemotherapy or sorafenib. Asia-Pacific J Clin Oncol 2018; 14(5):e341–51. https://doi.org/10.1111/ajco.12983.

121. Shomura M, Okabe H, Sato E, et al. Hypothyroidism is a predictive factor for better clinical outcomes in patients with advanced hepatocellular carcinoma undergoing lenvatinib therapy. Cancers (Basel) 2020;(11):12. https://doi.org/10.3390/cancers12113078.

122. Shimose S, Kawaguchi T, Tanaka M, et al. Lenvatinib prolongs the progression-free survival time of patients with intermediate-stage hepatocellular carcinoma refractory to transarterial chemoembolization: a multicenter cohort study using data mining analysis. Oncol Lett 2020;20(3):2257–65.

123. Ohki T, Sato K, Kondo M, et al. Impact of adverse events on the progression-free survival of patients with advanced hepatocellular carcinoma treated with lenvatinib: a multicenter retrospective study. Drugs Real World Outcomes 2020;7(2):141–9.

124. Koizumi Y, Hirooka M, Hiraoka A, et al. Lenvatinib-induced thyroid abnormalities in unresectable hepatocellular carcinoma. Endocr J 2019;66(9):787–92.

125. Pandit-Taskar N, Modak S. Norepinephrine transporter as a target for imaging and therapy. J Nucl Med 2017;58(Suppl 2):39s–53s.

126. Pryma DA, Chin BB, Noto RB, et al. Efficacy and safety of high-specific-activity (131)I-MIBG therapy in patients with advanced pheochromocytoma or paraganglioma. J Nucl Med 2019;60(5):623–30.

127. Streby KA, Shah N, Ranalli MA, et al. Nothing but NET: a review of norepinephrine transporter expression and efficacy of 131I-mIBG therapy. Pediatr Blood Cancer 2015;62(1):5–11.

128. Wells SA Jr, Asa SL, Dralle H, et al. Revised American Thyroid Association guidelines for the management of medullary thyroid carcinoma. *Thyroid* Jun 2015;25(6):567–610.

129. Agrawal A, Rangarajan V, Shah S, et al. MIBG (metaiodobenzylguanidine) theranostics in pediatric and adult malignancies. Br J Radiol 2018;91(1091):20180103.

130. Giammarile F, Chiti A, Lassmann M, et al, EANM. EANM procedure guidelines for 131I-meta-iodobenzylguanidine (131I-mIBG) therapy. Eur J Nucl Med Mol Imaging 2008;35(5):1039–47.

131. Kinuya S, Yoshinaga K, Higuchi T, et al. Draft guidelines regarding appropriate use of (131)I-MIBG radiotherapy for neuroendocrine tumors: Guideline Drafting Committee for Radiotherapy with (131)I-MIBG, Committee for Nuclear Oncology and Immunology, the Japanese Society of Nuclear Medicine. Ann Nucl Med 2015;29(6):543–52.

132. Garrido Magaña E, Silva Estrada JA, Nishimura Meguro E, et al. [Thyroid dysfunction due to 131I-metaiodobenzylguanidine in patients with neuroblastoma]. Rev Chil Pediatr 2020;91(3):379–84. Disfunción tiroidea por I131-Metayodo Benzilguanidina en pacientes con neuroblastoma.

133. Garaventa A, Bellagamba O, Lo Piccolo MS, et al. 131I-metaiodobenzylguanidine (131I-MIBG) therapy for residual neuroblastoma: a mono-institutional experience with 43 patients. Br J Cancer 1999;81(8):1378–84.

134. Ussowicz M, Wieczorek A, Dłużniewska A, et al. Factors modifying outcome after MIBG therapy in children with neuroblastoma-a national retrospective study. Front Oncol 2021;11:647361.

135. van Santen HM, de Kraker J, van Eck BL, et al. High incidence of thyroid dysfunction despite prophylaxis with potassium iodide during (131)I-meta-iodobenzylguanidine treatment in children with neuroblastoma. Cancer 2002;94(7):2081–9.

136. Quach A, Ji L, Mishra V, et al. Thyroid and hepatic function after high-dose 131 I-metaiodobenzylguanidine (131 I-MIBG) therapy for neuroblastoma. Pediatr Blood Cancer 2011;56(2):191–201.

137. van Santen HM, de Kraker J, van Eck BL, et al. Improved radiation protection of the thyroid gland with thyroxine, methimazole, and potassium iodide during diagnostic and therapeutic use of radiolabeled metaiodobenzylguanidine in children with neuroblastoma. Cancer 2003;98(2):389–96.

138. Clement SC, van Rijn RR, van Eck-Smit BL, et al. Long-term efficacy of current thyroid prophylaxis and future perspectives on thyroid protection during 131I-

metaiodobenzylguanidine treatment in children with neuroblastoma. Eur J Nucl Med Mol Imaging 2015;42(5):706–15.

139. van Santen HM, Tytgat GA, van de Wetering MD, et al. Differentiated thyroid carcinoma after 131I-MIBG treatment for neuroblastoma during childhood: description of the first two cases. Thyroid 2012;22(6):643–6.

140. Ryder M, Callahan M, Postow MA, et al. Endocrine-related adverse events following ipilimumab in patients with advanced melanoma: a comprehensive retrospective review from a single institution. Endocr Relat Cancer 2014;21(2): 371–81.

141. Scott ES, Long GV, Guminski A, et al. The spectrum, incidence, kinetics and management of endocrinopathies with immune checkpoint inhibitors for metastatic melanoma. Eur J Endocrinol 2018;178(2):173–80.

142. Subbiah V, Hu MI, Wirth LJ, et al. Pralsetinib for patients with advanced or metastatic RET-altered thyroid cancer (ARROW): a multi-cohort, open-label, registrational, phase 1/2 study. Lancet Diabetes Endocrinol 2021;9(8):491–501.

143. Motzer RJ, Hutson TE, Tomczak P, et al. Sunitinib versus interferon alfa in metastatic renal-cell carcinoma. New Engl J Med 2007;356(2):115–24.

2022 Update on Clinical Management of Graves Disease and Thyroid Eye Disease

Thanh D. Hoang, DO[a,b], Derek J. Stocker, MD[c,d],
Eva L. Chou, MD[e,f], Henry B. Burch, MD[g,h],*

KEYWORDS

- Hyperthyroidism • Graves disease • Thyroid eye disease • Antithyroid drugs
- Radioiodine therapy • Thyroidectomy

KEY POINTS

- Initial ATD dosing should be individualized based on thyroid hormone levels. PTU should be used only in the first trimester of pregnancy, thyroid storm, or when patients develop minor adverse reactions to MMI.

Continued

*The views expressed in this article are those of the authors and do not reflect the official policy of the Department of the Army, Department of the Navy, the Department of Defense, the National Institutes of Health, or the United States Government. Authors are military service members or employees of the US Government. This work was prepared as part of our official duties. Title 17 U.S C. 105 provides the "Copyright protection under this title is not available for any work of the United States Government." Title 17 U.S C. 101 defines a US Government work as a work prepared by a military service member or employee of the US Government as part of that person's official duties. We certify that all individuals who qualify as authors have been listed; each has participated in the conception and design of this work, the analysis of data (when applicable), the writing of the document, and/or the approval of the submission of this version; that the document represents valid work; that if we used information derived from another source, we obtained all necessary approvals to use it and made appropriate acknowledgments in the document; and that each takes public responsibility for it.

[a] Division of Diabetes, Endocrinology and Metabolism, Walter Reed National Military Medical Center, 8901 Wisconsin Avenue, Bethesda, MD 20819, USA; [b] Uniformed Services University of the Health Sciences, Bethesda, MD 20814, USA; [c] Department of Radiology, Nuclear Medicine Service, Walter Reed National Military Medical Center, 8901 Wisconsin Avenue, Bethesda, MD 20819, USA; [d] Departments of Internal Medicine, Pathology, and Radiologic Sciences Uniformed Services University of the Health Sciences, Bethesda, MD 20814, USA; [e] Department of Ophthalmology, Oculoplastic Service, Walter Reed National Military Medical Center, 8901 Wisconsin Avenue, Bethesda, MD 20819, USA; [f] Uniformed Services University of the Health Sciences, Bethesda, MD 20814, USA; [g] Division of Diabetes, Endocrinology and Metabolic Diseases, National Institute of Diabetes and Digestive and Kidney Diseases, National Institutes of Health, 6707 Democracy Boulevard, Room 6054, Bethesda, MD 20892-5460, USA; [h] Uniformed Services University of the Health Sciences, Bethesda, MD 20814, USA
* Corresponding author.
E-mail address: Henry.Burch@nih.gov

Endocrinol Metab Clin N Am 51 (2022) 287–304
https://doi.org/10.1016/j.ecl.2021.12.004
0889-8529/22/© 2021 Elsevier Inc. All rights reserved.

Continued

- Baseline complete blood count with differential and liver function profile should be obtained prior to starting ATDs. Regular clinical and biochemical evaluation of thyroid function is required in patients taking ATDs.
- RAI is an effective and safe GD therapy which should be administered with sufficient activity to render the patient hypothyroid (greater than 150 μCi/g (5.55 MBq/g)), either in a fixed or calculated dose. RAI should not be used in patients with moderate or severe TED.
- General treatment of patients with TED includes (a) reversal of hyperthyroidism, (b) monitoring for and prompt treatment of hypothyroidism, and (c) cessation of smoking, if applicable.
- Treatment of TED should be initiated immediately to target the active, inflammatory phase of the disease to decrease disease severity. Surgical treatment may be required urgently in the case of compressive optic neuropathy, globe subluxation, or corneal decompensation.

INTRODUCTION
Background

Although the basic treatment options for hyperthyroidism due to Graves disease (GD) have seemed immutable for more than three-quarters of a century, its management remains complex. The endocrinologist must consider a multitude of factors including patient preference, age and comorbidity, pregnancy, or pregnancy potential, the influence of social factors such as tobacco smoking and the likelihood of adherence to medical therapy, and comanagement of extrathyroidal manifestations such as orbitopathy. This article leverages a multidisciplinary team to synthesize a current understanding of the pathophysiology, contemporary understanding of benefits and risks of treatment, and factors influencing trends in management of GD, arriving at a pragmatic approach to effective therapy. In addition, with the rollout of promising new therapeutic opportunities for thyroid eye disease (TED), a timely review of the complex management of this disorder is provided.

Diagnosis and Initial Management of Graves Disease

Initial triage

Evaluation of a new patient with thyrotoxicosis requires immediate answers to key questions (**Box 1**). Acute complications requiring immediate intervention include ischemia, atrial fibrillation,[1] congestive heart failure, thromboembolism,[2] stroke,[3] psychosis,[4] periodic paralysis,[5] and thyroid storm.[6] Each requires specific intervention in addition to normalization of thyroid hormone levels.

Diagnostic evaluation

A diagnosis of GD can be made clinically in a patient with diffuse goiter, elevations in serum thyroxine (T_4), and a suppressed thyroid-stimulating hormone (TSH) value. If uncertainty remains after initial evaluation, the 2016 American Thyroid Association (ATA) Guidelines for Diagnosis and Management of Hyperthyroidism and Other Causes of Thyrotoxicosis suggest that any one or more of 3 methods may be used, including TSH-receptor (TSH-R) antibody (TRAb) testing, radioactive iodine uptake (RAIU), or demonstration of diffusely increased vascularity on Doppler flow ultrasonography.[7] Modern TRAb testing has high sensitivity and specificity for the diagnosis of GD, on the order of 97% and 99%, respectively.[8]

Table 1
Comparative adverse effects of methimazole and propylthiouracil

Adverse Side Effects	MMI	PTU	Mean Onset	Treatment
Pruritus or minor rash	6%	3%	18–22 d of treatment	Antihistamines, CS, ± stop ATD
Hepatotoxicity (cholestatic & hepatocellular)	0.4%	2.7%	28–90 d	Stop ATD
Liver failure	0.03%	0.05%	27–127 d	Stop ATD, supportive care
Agranulocytosis	0.1%–0.3%	0.1%–0.3%	30–90 d	Stop ATD, recommend GCSF, CS, supportive care
Vasculitis (p-ANCA positive)	≤0.1%	≤0.1%	Weeks to months	Stop ATD, CS
Drug-induced lupus	None	Case reports only	Weeks to months	Stop ATD, CS
Insulin autoimmune syndrome with symptomatic hypoglycaemia	6.3%	0%	30–60 d	Stop ATD, CS, diazoxide

Abbreviations: ATD, antithyroid drug; CS, corticosteroids; GCSF, granulocyte colony-stimulating factor; p-ANCA, perinuclear anti-neutrophil cytoplasmic antibodies.

Shared Decision Making in Graves Disease

Equipping a patient with an understanding of the benefits and risks associated with each of the treatment options for GD and taking into consideration their personal values are both critical. Patients are asked to choose between treatments that damage or remove the thyroid, on the one hand, and pharmacologic therapy with a low cure rate and a potential for serious adverse effects, on the other. Patients must be aware that medical therapy may be required chronically to sustain euthyroidism, and that serial laboratory testing and monitoring for adverse effects will be required. In addition, patients should be apprised of the risk of new or worsened orbitopathy after radioiodine therapy, and transient or permanent hypoparathyroidism or vocal cord dysfunction following thyroidectomy. Finally, patients should be familiar with the relative costs and cost-sharing associated with each of the 3 modalities. Detailed analyses of clinical factors and patient preferences favoring a specific treatment of hyperthyroidism in GD are available.[7,9] Clinical factors influencing choice of therapy are summarized in **Box 2**.

MEDICAL THERAPY WITH THIONAMIDES
Antithyroid Drug Dosing Principles

Antithyroid drugs (ATDs) are effective in controlling hyperthyroidism when given in proper doses with patient adherence. Methimazole (MMI) should be used in patients who choose ATD therapy for GD, except (1) during the first trimester of pregnancy when propylthiouracil (PTU) is preferred, (2) in the management of thyroid storm[6], and (3) in patients with minor adverse reactions to MMI who refuse radioactive iodine (RAI) therapy or surgery.[7]

Current practice guidelines suggest an initial MMI dosing of 5 to 10 mg daily if free T_4 is 1 to 1.5 times the upper limit of normal; 10 to 20 mg daily if free T_4 is 1.5 to 2 times the upper limit of normal; and 30 to 40 mg daily for free T_4 2 to 3 times the upper limit of

> **Box 1**
> **Triage in patients presenting with overt thyrotoxicosis**
>
> - Is the patient experiencing acute complications requiring urgent intervention, such as ischemia, atrial fibrillation, or impending thyroid storm?
> - What is the cause of the patient's thyrotoxicosis? Is GD apparent clinically?
> - What are the patient's comorbidities?
> - What initial testing is required?
> - What therapy should be instituted at the first encounter?

normal.[7] The minimal effective dose of MMI is recommended to minimize adverse effects. MMI can be given once a day compared with PTU, which has a shorter duration of action and is usually administered as 50 to 150 mg 3 times daily. A comparison of adverse effects from MMI and PTU (**Table 1**).

Chronic Antithyroid Drug Therapy

ATDs have historically been prescribed with the objective of permitting a remission from GD within a prescribed period, after which patients were considered treatment failures and approached with radioiodine (RAI) therapy or thyroidectomy. However, chronic low-dose ATD therapy seems to be a reliable alternative to ablative therapy.[10,11] Patients in the United States increasingly select ATD therapy.[12,13] Adverse effects occur less frequently on low maintenance doses of MMI,[14,15] and most cases of agranulocytosis and severe hepatotoxicity occur within the first 3 months of therapy.[11,16] A study of patients failing to remit after an initial course of ATDs who were then randomized to either continued ATD therapy or radioiodine found 10-year costs

> **Box 2**
> **Clinical factors that favor a particular treatment modality for hyperthyroidism in Graves disease***
>
> ATDs
> - Patients with high likelihood of remission (women, mild disease, small goiter, negative or low titers of thyrotropin receptor antibody)
> - Elderly or those with comorbidities and increased surgical risk or short life expectancy
> - Patients with moderate to severe active Graves ophthalmopathy
>
> Radioiodine
> - Contraindication to ATD use (severe adverse reactions, liver disease)
> - Women planning pregnancy more than 6 to 12 months following RAI
> - Patients with increased surgical risk (comorbidities, prior neck surgery, or radiation)
> - Lack of access to high-volume thyroid surgeon
>
> Surgery
> - Patients with symptomatic compression or large goiters
> - Patients with low RAIU
> - When concurrent indications for surgery (thyroid cancer, hyperparathyroidism, suspicious thyroid nodules)
> - Patients with moderate to severe active TED
> - Women planning pregnancy in less than 6 months who wish to avoid ATDs
>
> *Abbreviations:* ATD, antithyroid drug; RAI; radioactive iodine.
>
> *Data from Refs.[7,10]*

of management similar or slightly lower with chronic ATD therapy, and episodes of hypothyroidism occurred more frequently after RAI therapy than with chronic ATDs.[17] In another study, long-term ATDs in patients with GD treated up to 11 years and then followed for an average of 4.5 years after stopping ATDs found a remission rate of 63%.[18] A retrospective study of patients treated with either continued low-dose ATDs or radioiodine after an initial relapse following ATD therapy showed that ATD-treated patients had better preservation of euthyroidism, less weight gain, and less orbitopathy deterioration compared with those treated with radioiodine.[19] Conversely, chronic ATD therapy requires serial dose adjustment and monitoring for rare late-occurring adverse effects related to ATDs.[20]

Monitoring Patients Taking Antithyroid Drug Therapy

Pretreatment considerations
Before starting ATD therapy, a baseline complete blood cell count, including white blood cell count with differential, and a baseline liver function profile, including transaminases and bilirubin, should be obtained. Mild leukocytopenia is common in patients with GD before starting ATDs. Notably, 10% of African Americans have neutrophil counts less than 2000 normally. Mild transaminase elevation occurs frequently in thyrotoxicosis.[21] Patients should be counseled verbally and in writing regarding the potential side effects of ATD therapy.[7]

Monitoring therapy
Serum TSH, free T_4, and total or free T_3 levels should be obtained initially at 2- to 4-week intervals after starting ATDs, and the dosage should be adjusted accordingly. Serum TSH levels may remain low for months after initiating ATD therapy. Serum free T_4 levels may normalize despite persistent elevated total or free T_3 level; thus, serum total or free T_3 level should also be monitored.[7]

Once the patient is biochemically euthyroid, gradual lowering of the MMI dose is advised, with repeated laboratory testing in 4 to 6 weeks. Euthyroid levels should be achieved with minimal ATD therapy dosage, and repeat testing should be done at approximately 2 to 3 months or longer intervals for long-term therapy.

Patients should be advised regarding the potential adverse effects of ATDs. A differential white blood cell count should be obtained during febrile illness or pharyngitis in all patients taking ATDs. Liver function tests should be checked in patients taking ATDs who develop jaundice, pruritic rash, light-colored stool or dark urine, arthralgia, abdominal pain, anorexia, nausea, or fatigue. After discontinuation of ATDs, liver function tests should be monitored weekly until normalization occurs. Routine monitoring of complete blood cell count and liver function by endocrinologists is commonly performed,[13] although controversial.[7] ATDs should be discontinued if transaminase levels are more than 3 times the upper limit of normal or if the transaminitis worsens.[7]

RADIOIODINE THERAPY
Background and Mechanism

RAI has been a safe and effective treatment option for hyperthyroidism for more than 8 decades.[22] RAI is well-tolerated and has few associated adverse effects in treatment doses for GD.[7] RAI is a β-radiation emitter with a long physical half-life of just more than 8 days, which is rapidly concentrated by the thyroid after oral ingestion. The β-particle has a range in tissue of approximately 2 mm and induces DNA damage and eventual thyroid cell death, rendering most patients with GD hypothyroid over a period of 6 weeks to 6 months.

Preparation for Radioiodine Therapy

The ATA hyperthyroidism guidelines identify several contraindications to the use of RAI, including pregnancy, lactation, known or suspected coexistent thyroid cancer, inability to comply with radiation safety guidelines, and planned pregnancy within the subsequent 6 months.[7] Moderate to severe and sight-threatening TED is also considered a contraindication to RAI.[7,23,24] In this clinical setting, ATDs or thyroidectomy are favored, because these demonstrate no significant effect on the course of TED.[24,25]

Patients with active mild TED are candidates for oral glucocorticoid therapy (0.3–0.5 mg of prednisone per kg of body mass per day, started 1–3 days after RAI administration, tapered over 3 months).[7,23,26] Shorter courses at lower doses (0.2 mg per kg of body mass per day for 6 weeks) may be equally protective.[7,26] Prophylactic use of glucocorticoids in patients without preexisting orbitopathy remains controversial.[23]

The goal of RAI treatment in GD is to administer sufficient activity to render the patient hypothyroid.[7] This goal can be accomplished with the use of a fixed dose or calculating the activity based on goiter size and RAI uptake.[7,27] To achieve hypothyroidism, activity of greater than 150 µCi/g (5.55 MBq/g) should be administered.[7] The efficacy of RAI strongly depends on the activity administered, with success rates ranging from 61% with 5.4 mCi (200 MBq) to 86% with 15.7 mCi (580 MBq).[28] To avoid the necessity for retreatment, therapy with lower activities is generally not recommended.[7]

Radioactive Iodine Therapy Outcomes

ATDs have a treatment failure rate of approximately 50%, followed by 7% for RAI and less than 1% for thyroidectomy.[29,30] In a nationwide population-based study, patients undergoing thyroidectomy had the highest rate of complications, at 24%, mostly either transient or chronic hypoparathyroidism. Patients on ATD had a complication rate of 12%, followed by patients receiving RAI at 6%. New-onset TED occurred in 7% of patients on ATD and 6% of those receiving RAI.[29] Early and successful RAI treatment was associated with a 50% reduction in mortality compared with ATD treatment, but this advantage was lost when the RAI failed to resolve the hyperthyroidism.[31,32]

Specifically addressing TED outcomes, RAI therapy for GD is associated with new or worsened TED with an incidence of 10% to 39%,[7,25,33–35] and in approximately 5%, these changes persisted after 1 year, requiring additional treatment.[25,36] The mechanism of this association is incompletely understood, but it is postulated that RAI-induced leakage of thyroid antigen and increased production of TRAb, thyroid peroxidase, and thyroglobulin contributes to the development or worsening of TED.[34] The risk of worsening TED can be mitigated and almost eliminated in cases of mild disease with a short course of oral glucocorticoids and avoiding posttreatment hypothyroidism.[7,36]

Radioactive Iodine Usage Trends in the United States

RAI was favored by 60% in the United States in a 2011 survey of endocrinologists,[13] reduced from 69% in 1990. A 2020 analysis of private insurance claims in 4661 patients for GD showed that only 33% of this selected group received initial therapy with RAI, whereas another 8.9% received RAI after ATD failure.[29]

Radioactive Iodine and Cancer Controversy

The association of RAI use in hyperthyroidism with an increased cancer incidence remains controversial. RAI in patients with hyperthyroidism has been associated with increased,[37–39] similar,[40] and even decreased[41,42] rates of overall cancer mortality. Those studies that demonstrated increased rates have been criticized for failing to adjust for confounders such as smoking, obesity, alcohol intake, and thyroid status.[31,39,43] In a recent analysis of a multicenter cohort of patients with hyperthyroidism treated with ATDs, RAI, or surgery, there were no differences in solid cancer mortality among groups when controlling for confounders, but within the RAI subgroup there was a modest dose-dependent association between RAI and mortality.[44] Hyperthyroidism itself is associated with an increased cancer risk, making a lack of a hyperthyroid control group a challenge in interpreting cohort studies.[31,42,43] The risks of both cardiovascular and cancer mortality in patients with hyperthyroidism can primarily be attributed to thyroid hormone excess, leading some to conclude that even a marginal increased cancer mortality in RAI would be offset by improved hyperthyroidism control with RAI over ATD.[31]

THYROIDECTOMY
Overview

Surgery is recommended by fewer than 1% of thyroid experts for the initial management of GD.[13] Indications include large goiters with compressive symptoms, concurrent suspicious thyroid nodules or hyperparathyroidism requiring surgery, and patient preference.[7] Health disparities are evident in the selection of thyroidectomy to treat GD, with black Americans twice as likely in one study to undergo surgery than whites with GD,[45] and this surgery is more frequently performed by lower-volume surgeons than that seen in whites.[46]

Preparation for Thyroidectomy

Patients selecting thyroidectomy to treat GD should first be rendered euthyroid using ATDs[7]; this typically requires 1 to 3 months of ATDs before thyroidectomy. Rapid preoperative preparation is occasionally needed for patients requiring urgent surgery[47] or in patients with contraindications to ATDs. Safe and effective oral therapy with a combination of β-blockers (propranolol 40 mg every 8 hours), high-dose glucocorticoids (betamethasone 0.5 mg every 6 hours), and sodium iopanoate (500 mg every 6 hours) has been reported in a small number of patients requiring urgent surgery.[48] This regimen was given for 5 days with surgery performed on the sixth day. Dexamethasone and hydrocortisone decrease T_4-to-T_3 conversion and have an important role in this setting. A recent case series reported the combination of iodine, dexamethasone, and propranolol to rapidly restore euthyroidism before thyroidectomy in 10 patients with GD.[49] Emergent preparation for thyroid surgery at our center in patients unable to use ATDs[47] has involved the regimen in **Box 3**, typically given in the inpatient setting for 5 to 10 days before thyroidectomy, with rapid correction of thyrotoxicosis.

THYROID EYE DISEASE
Referral Guidance

TED is a debilitating autoimmune disease with an incidence of 1.9 cases per 10,000 population per year.[50] Although most frequently associated with hyperthyroidism secondary to GD, about 10% of patients with TED are euthyroid or hypothyroid. The mechanism of action is not completely understood but is characterized by the activation of orbital fibroblasts by TRAb binding, leading to the expression of extracellular matrix molecules and deposition of glycosaminoglycans, resulting in swelling, congestion, and connective tissue modeling. The overall result is extraocular muscle enlargement and orbital fat expansion. As discussed later, recent work has suggested a role for cross-linking of the insulinlike growth factor 1 (IGF-1) receptor with the TSH-R in orbital tissue.[51]

Control of thyroid function is crucial in all patients with TED; however, the course and severity does not always correlate with thyroid hormone levels. When assessing patients for TED activity, the 7-point Clinical Activity Score (CAS) is frequently used, in which one point is assigned for pain behind the eyes, pain with eye movement, eyelid swelling, eyelid edema, conjunctival redness, chemosis (scleral edema), or caruncle swelling, and a score of 3 or greater is considered active disease.[52] The EUGOGO (European Group of Graves' Orbitopathy) system is commonly used to describe TED severity as mild, moderate to severe, or sight threatening, whereas the VISA (Vision, Inflammation, Strabismus, and Appearance) system may be used to assess both TED activity and severity.[53] If a patient exhibits any significant signs of TED or is experiencing eye discomfort, referral to an ophthalmologist is indicated.

Thyroid Eye Disease Risk Factors

In contrast to GD for which women are at higher risk, the role of sex in TED is controversial. Recent studies do not find an obvious sex-related risk for TED, whereas earlier studies suggested a slightly increased risk for men. This variability might relate to changes in smoking trends over the years. The prevalence of TED is higher with aging (40–60 years), and peaks in the fifth and sixth decades of life.[54–57]

Identified risk factors for TED include smoking, sex, advanced age, genetics including HLA DRB3*0101/*0202 heterozygosity,[58] wider lateral wall orbital angle, high TRAb levels, high pretreatment levels of T_3 and T_4, uncontrolled hypothyroidism/hyperthyroidism, and RAI therapy. Smoking is the most important risk factor for TED with the risk proportional to the number of cigarettes smoked per day. Former smokers have lower risk than current smokers. Patients should be referred to smoking cessation programs. Recent data suggest that statin usage is correlated with a lower risk of orbitopathy in patients with GD.[59]

Eye Assessment

Formal ophthalmology assessment

TED is diagnosed when 2 of 3 findings occur together, including immune-related thyroid dysfunction, one or more ocular signs, or radiologic evidence of tendon-sparing fusiform enlargement of one or more extraocular muscles. The most common signs of TED are eyelid retraction (Dalrymple sign), lid lag of the upper eyelid on downgaze (von Graefe sign), and lid edema. TED is the most common cause of proptosis, both unilateral and bilateral, in adults. Other clinical features include lagophthalmos, exposure keratopathy, chemosis and conjunctival injection, restrictive extraocular motility, and compressive optic neuropathy. Patients with TED typically have symptoms of ocular surface discomfort, such as tearing, dry eyes, swelling of the lids, or redness

---

Box 3
Rapid preparation for thyroidectomy in patients unable to use antithyroid drugs

- Propranolol, 60 mg orally, twice daily
- Dexamethasone, 2 mg intravenously, 4 times daily
- Cholestyramine, 4 g orally, 4 times daily
- SSKI*, 2 drops orally, 3 times daily

*SSKI, supersaturated potassium iodide.

of the lids or conjunctiva. Compressive optic neuropathy, often heralded by dyschromatopsia, decreased vision, and/or visual field defects, is considered an ophthalmic emergency requiring immediate treatment.

At every ophthalmology visit, best-corrected visual acuity, color vision, extraocular motility, and intraocular pressure are measured, and a pupillary examination is performed to assess for relative afferent pupillary defect. An external examination is performed assessing standard lid measurements, exophthalmometry, and resistance to retropulsion. A slit lamp and dilated funduscopic examination are performed. Static perimetric visual field examination is required at baseline to assess for visual field deficits with interval repeat testing as indicated by disease activity and severity.

Imaging

The diagnosis of TED is usually made clinically.[60,61] In unusual or unilateral cases, orbital imaging can play an important role in establishing the diagnosis, providing a differential diagnosis for management, and assisting in clinical and surgical follow-up. MRI, computed tomography (CT), ultrasonography, color Doppler imaging, and octreotide scintigraphy can each play a role in TED diagnosis and management.[60,61] CT continues to play a key role in the diagnosis of TED due to its superior characterization of the bones and soft tissues and remains the preferred imaging modality for orbital decompression planning in patients requiring surgical management.[23,61] MRI is considered the preferred imaging modality for detecting disease activity, given its superior ability to characterize soft tissues, and is also considered by some to be the preferred choice for diagnosis of TED.[23] MRI does not subject the lens of the eye to ionizing radiation, an important benefit over CT.[60,61] As in GD treatment options, significant regional practice variation exists in the use of imaging in moderate TED, with providers in the European Union obtaining CT and MRI imaging more often than those in the United States.[62]

General Treatment Measures

General treatment of patients with TED includes (1) reversal of hyperthyroidism, (2) monitoring for and prompt treatment of hypothyroidism, and (3) cessation of smoking, if applicable. Clinicians should advise their patients with GD to stop smoking and refer them to a structured smoking cessation program. Because both first- and second-hand smoking increase TED risk, patients with exposure to secondhand smoke should be advised of its negative effects and avoidance of second-hand smoke.[63,64]

Local measures to improve symptoms may include eye shades, artificial tears, elevation of head during sleep, and avoidance of eye cosmetics. For mild, active TED, topical artificial tears in drop, gel, and ointment (1% methylcellulose drops and/or petrolatum jelly) are key to maintaining a healthy ocular surface. If there are signs of focal eye inflammation, topical glucocorticoid ophthalmic drops may reduce inflammation, but evidence supporting this practice is scarce. Topical cyclosporine has been shown to be beneficial in reducing ocular surface inflammation. Selenium supplementation has been shown to improve the course of mild TED in areas of relative selenium deficiency.[65] Eye patching or prisms can be useful to treat diplopia while waiting for eye muscle stability before strabismus surgery.

TED is a self-limiting disease, with patients progressing from the active to quiescent phase within 1 to 3 years with a 5% to 10% risk of future recurrence. Once TED is diagnosed, treatment should commence immediately to target the active, inflammatory phase of the disease and decrease disease severity that can be more recalcitrant to treatment in the chronic or fibrotic phase of the disease.

Medical Therapy for Thyroid Eye Disease

Glucocorticoids

Intravenous (IV) glucocorticoids (IVGC) are considered first-line therapy in patients with moderate to severe TED. The preferred regimen involves delivery of a 4.5 g dose of methylprednisolone over 12 weeks, typically given as 0.5 mg IV weekly for 6 weeks and then 0.25 g weekly for another 6 weeks.[66] For patients with diplopia due to extraocular muscle involvement, higher cumulative doses up to 7.5 g have been used with greater benefit,[67] but it is important that the total dose remain under 8 g, to avoid potentially severe toxicity.[68,69] Oral glucocorticoids are less effective and more poorly tolerated than IVGC.[66] Topical glucocorticoid drops and intraocular depot injections have not been shown to be efficacious when compared with systemic therapy, and intraocular injections are associated with potentially severe adverse effects, including blindness. Patients receiving glucocorticoids for TED require continuous surveillance for a host of adverse effects including hyperglycemia, hypertension, glaucoma, hip osteonecrosis, and psychosis.

Teprotumumab

Teprotumumab, an IGF-1 receptor inhibitor, was approved to treat TED by the US Food and Drug Administration in 2020, based on the results of two 24-week trials comparing teprotumumab with placebo in patients with active, moderate to severe orbitopathy.[70,71] In the first trial, improvement of CAS by 2 points or more *and* reduction in proptosis by greater than or equal to 2 mm, together, occurred in 69% of patients with teprotumumab versus 20% with placebo.[71] In the second trial, the primary outcome of proptosis improvement by greater than or equal to 2 mm occurred in 83% of patients treated with teprotumumab versus 10% with placebo,[70] whereas a secondary outcome of combined improvement in CAS and proptosis occurred in 78% with teprotumumab versus 7% with placebo.[70] Assessment of the durability of effect will require further long-term follow-up studies. Cost may play a key role in clinical decision making.

Teprotumumab is administered IV every 3 weeks (10 mg/kg first dose, then 20 mg/kg) for a total of 8 infusions. Common side effects include nausea, diarrhea, muscle spasms, hearing impairment, dysgeusia, headaches, dry skin, infusion reactions, alopecia, paresthesia, weight loss, and hyperglycemia. Other possible serious effects reported include optic neuropathy, encephalopathy, urinary retention, inflammatory bowel disease activation, and neurocognitive decline.[72] Teprotumumab is contraindicated in pregnancy and not approved for children younger than 18 years.

Selenium

Selenium may improve symptoms in patients with mild TED, especially in regions of selenium insufficiency. One study compared selenium (100 μg twice a day), pentoxifylline (600 mg twice a day), or placebo in 159 patients with mild TED from a region in which selenium levels are marginally decreased.[65] These patients had at least one sign of mild orbitopathy (chemosis, mild to moderate eyelid swelling, exophthalmos ≤22 mm) and disease duration of less than 18 months. After 6 months of treatment, selenium (but not pentoxifylline) was associated with an improved quality of life (both visual functioning and appearance scores), and less eye involvement and slowed the progression of TED. Evaluation at 12 months confirmed the results at 6 months. Neither placebo nor pentoxifylline improved quality-of-life measures.

It is uncertain whether selenium benefits individuals with mild TED who reside in selenium-sufficient regions such as the United States.

At present, the european thyroid association (ETA)/ EUGOGO recommends 6 months of selenium supplementation in patients with mild TED of short duration because it may improve eye manifestations and quality of life and prevent TED progression to severe forms.[73,74]

Mycophenolate mofetil

Mycophenolate mofetil is an immunosuppressive with relatively mild side effects, commonly used after organ transplantation. As a potent selective, noncompetitive, and reversible inhibitor of inosine-5'-monophosphate dehydrogenase, it inhibits T- and B-lymphocyte proliferation and reduces immunoglobulin production; it also suppresses dendritic cell maturation, reducing its ability for antigen presentation to T lymphocytes.[75,76] In a trial comparing mycophenolate mofetil 500 mg twice a day for 24 weeks with glucocorticoids 0.5 g IV daily for 3 days, followed by 60 mg oral daily for 8 weeks and then tapered in 174 Chinese patients with active moderate to severe TED, the overall result was better with mycophenolate at 24 weeks (91.3% vs 67.9%) with concurrent improvement in 3 or more features including CAS, diplopia, proptosis, visual acuity, soft tissue swelling, or diplopia.[77] Another randomized study of 164 patients with active moderate to severe TED treated with methylprednisolone alone versus methylprednisolone with mycophenolate showed no significant difference in the rate of response at 12 weeks or rate of relapse at 24 and 36 weeks; however, posthoc analysis showed that addition of mycophenolate to methylprednisolone improved response to therapy at 24 weeks in patients with active and moderate to severe TED.[78] A recent study found a favorable risk-benefit ratio for low-dose mycophenolate therapy in active moderate to severe TED.[79] The 2021 EUGOGO Clinical Practice Guidelines recommend combined use of IVGC and mycophenolate as first-line therapy for active moderate to severe TED.[74]

Tocilizumab

Tocilizumab is a humanized monoclonal antibody against the interleukin (IL)-6 receptor. Dosing is 8 mg/kg at 4 monthly infusions. This agent targets IL-6. A randomized trial of 32 patients with moderate to severe corticosteroid-resistant TED randomly assigned patients to tocilizumab (8 mg/kg) or placebo, administered IV at weeks 0, 4, 8, and 12. Tocilizumab therapy was associated with greater improvement in CAS at 16 weeks (93.3% vs 58.8%) and improved composite ophthalmic score at 16 weeks (73.3% vs 29.4%); however, no significant differences persisted between groups at 40 weeks.[80] Case reports and a small series of 9 patients (aged 40–84 years) with chronic, active, moderate to severe TED treated with subcutaneous tocilizumab after failing other interventions showed clinical improvement in CAS, with decreases in thyroid-stimulating immunoglobulins (TSI) also observed.[81,82] Optimal duration of treatment with tocilizumab remains undetermined.

Rituximab

Rituximab is a chimeric human and mouse monoclonal antibody against CD20 antigen on B cells. Rituximab decreases TRAb levels and depletes B cells in the thyroid and retro-orbital tissues.[83] For treatment of TED, 2 infusions of rituximab (1000 mg each and 2 weeks apart) have been used without immunosuppressive effects.

Two prospective studies using rituximab for TED produced conflicting results,[84,85] possibly related to shorter disease duration in the trial showing beneficial effects.[84] Both trials reported a high rate of adverse effects from rituximab (ie, optic neuropathy and infusion reactions). Meta-analyses suggest that IV rituximab has an acute and long-lasting beneficial effect on reducing both CAS and TRAb; however, the effect on proptosis is limited.[86–88] At present, the therapeutic role of rituximab remains uncertain.

Surgical Approach to Thyroid Eye Disease: What an Endocrinologist Needs to Know

Surgery for TED is typically performed either emergently, such as for optic neuropathy, globe subluxation, or corneal thinning/perforation due to exposure keratopathy, or for rehabilitation after the disease has run its active course.

Dysthyroid optic neuropathy (DON) occurring in the setting of TED is due to inflammation and congestion of the orbital apex, which compresses the blood supply of the optic nerve within the bony orbit. DON presents with insidious, progressive, typically bilateral (but asymmetric) vision loss; dyschromatopsia; and visual field deficits. DON is surgically treated with orbital decompression to relieve the pressure on the optic nerve and blood supply; this is often performed in combination with systemic IV corticosteroids. Orbital decompression is performed by removing bone, and sometimes orbital fat, to expand the boundaries of the orbit,[89] allowing for the enlarged retroocular tissue mass to decompress from its normal confined space. The most commonly decompressed walls of the orbit are the lateral, medial, and floor. Orbital roof decompressions are performed rarely, and always with the involvement of neurosurgeons. This surgery is performed under general anesthesia and, if done emergently, requires inpatient admission for close interval evaluation.

Globe subluxation occurs when the pressure inside the orbit due to tissue expansion leads to anterior displacement of the eye, usually when then equator of the globe protrudes beyond the retracted lids. This is a rare and dramatic orbital complication. Immediate treatment is vital, with digital or surgical repositioning of the globe.[90] If this fails, lateral tarsorrhaphy or orbital decompression is warranted to protect the exposed ocular surface.

If corneal integrity is threatened due to prolonged exposure from proptosis, eyelid retraction, lagophthalmos, or a poor Bell reflex, urgent surgery is also indicated. Corneal desiccation can lead to decreased vision, diminished barrier to infection, corneal thinning, and corneal perforation. If the cornea has perforated, it must be emergently repaired or patched to maintain the integrity of the globe. If the cornea is threatened, a surgical temporary tarsorrhaphy may be performed to close the lids partially or fully and decrease corneal exposure.

Nonemergent surgery for TED can be considered when the disease is in the quiescent phase and no reactivation is suspected. The surgery occurs in 3 phases—orbital decompression, strabismus surgery, and eyelid surgery—with the potential for more than one surgery per phase. Because orbital decompression can alter globe positioning, decrease eyelid retraction, and affect extraocular motility, it should precede any strabismus or eyelid surgeries.[91]

TED affects extraocular muscles through inflammation and fibrosis of the muscle belly, leading to diplopia through restriction of extraocular motility. Most patients with diplopia due to strabismus will not require surgery and can be managed with prism spectacles. Strabismus surgery is reserved for patients with intractable diplopia in primary gaze or with reading, abnormal head positioning due to compensation for diplopia, or cosmetically unacceptable globe position. Owing to the relationship of the vertical eye muscles with the eyelid, strabismus surgery should be performed before eyelid procedures.

Eyelid changes due to TED are common and include upper and lower eyelid retraction and eyelid fat compartment expansion. Eyelid retraction surgery is aimed at lowering the upper eyelid and raising the lower eyelid to correct the "thyroid stare" appearance. Eyelid contouring is targeted to restore the natural height and contour of the eyelid, including decreasing the fat compartment expansion and minimizing the temporal flare, which occur as part of the disease state. Eyelid surgery is typically the last step in the rehabilitation of the patient's appearance. The total time between onset of TED to the final eyelid surgery can span several years.

CLINICS CARE POINTS

- Assess new patients with hyperthyroidism for acute severe complications including cardiac ischemia, arrhythmia, congestive heart failure, and thyroid storm
- Shared decision making that includes the patient and family members should be maximized when selecting primary treatment of GD
- Liver-associated enzymes and a complete blood cell count should be obtained before starting ATDs
- Dosing with methimazole should be individualized and based on the severity of thyrotoxicosis
- Patients treated with ATDs should be repeatedly apprised of warning signs for agranulocytosis, hepatotoxicity, and vasculitis
- Radioiodine therapy should be avoided in patients with active moderate to severe TED
- Patients unable to take ATDs who are not candidates for radioiodine therapy may generally be prepared for surgery with combination therapy using corticosteroids, potassium iodide, beta-adrenergic blocking agents, and cholestyramine to normalize thyroid hormone levels preoperatively
- TED should be comanaged by endocrinologists and ophthalmologists with experience managing this disorder
- IVGCs should be considered primary initial therapy for active TED
- Teprotumumab should be considered in patients with moderate to severe TED with proptosis, but it should be acknowledged that the long-term durability of benefit and cost-effectiveness remain to be determined
- Surgical rehabilitation should be considered for stable TED and includes orbital decompression to reduce proptosis and congestion, strabismus surgery to improve ocular motility, and eyelid procedures to treat fibrosis-related eyelid retraction

DISCLOSURE

The authors have nothing to disclose.

REFERENCES

1. Frost L, Vestergaard P, Mosekilde L. Hyperthyroidism and risk of atrial fibrillation or flutter: a population-based study. Arch Intern Med 2004;164(15):1675–8.
2. Srisawat S, Sitasuwan T, Ungprasert P. Increased risk of venous thromboembolism among patients with hyperthyroidism: a systematic review and meta-analysis of cohort studies. Eur J Intern Med 2019;67:65–9.
3. Kim HJ, Kang T, Kang MJ, et al. Incidence and mortality of myocardial infarction and stroke in patients with hyperthyroidism: A Nationwide Cohort Study in Korea. Thyroid 2020;30(7):955–65.
4. Golub D, Rodack V. Antipsychotics in hyperthyroid-related psychosis: case report and systematic review. Neuro Endocrinol Lett 2018;39(1):65–74.
5. Rivas AM, Thavaraputta S, Orellana-Barrios MA, et al. Thyrotoxic periodic paralysis and complicated thyrotoxicosis, two presentations of hyperthyroidism with

notable differences in their clinical manifestations: an experience from a Tertiary Care Hospital in the United States. Endocr Pract 2020;26(7):699–706.

6. Warnock AL, Cooper DS, Burch HB. Life-threatening thyrotoxicosis. In: Matfin G, editor. Endocrine and metabolic medical emergencies: a clinician's guide. 2nd edition. John Wiley & Sons, Ltd.; 2018.

7. Ross DS, Burch HB, Cooper DS, et al. 2016 American Thyroid Association Guidelines for Diagnosis and Management of Hyperthyroidism and Other Causes of Thyrotoxicosis. Thyroid 2016;26(10):1343–421.

8. Kahaly GJ, Diana T, Olivo PD. TSH receptor antibodies: relevance & utility. Endocr Pract 2020;26(1):97–106.

9. Muldoon BT, Mai VQ, Burch HB. Management of Graves' disease: an overview and comparison of clinical practice guidelines with actual practice trends. Endocrinol Metab Clin North Am 2014;43(2):495–516.

10. Azizi F. Long-Term Treatment of Hyperthyroidism with Antithyroid Drugs: 35 Years of Personal Clinical Experience. Thyroid 2020;30(10):1451–7.

11. Burch HB, Cooper DS. ANNIVERSARY REVIEW: Antithyroid drug therapy: 70 years later. Eur J Endocrinol 2018;179(5):R261–74.

12. Brito JP, Schilz S, Singh Ospina N, et al. Antithyroid Drugs-The Most Common Treatment for Graves' Disease in the United States: A Nationwide Population-Based Study. Thyroid 2016;26(8):1144–5.

13. Burch HB, Burman KD, Cooper DS. A 2011 survey of clinical practice patterns in the management of Graves' disease. J Clin Endocrinol Metab 2012;97(12): 4549–58.

14. Reinwein D, Benker G, Lazarus JH, et al. A prospective randomized trial of antithyroid drug dose in Graves' disease therapy. European Multicenter Study Group on Antithyroid Drug Treatment. J Clin Endocrinol Metab 1993;76(6):1516–21.

15. Sato S, Noh JY, Sato S, et al. Comparison of efficacy and adverse effects between methimazole 15 mg+inorganic iodine 38 mg/day and methimazole 30 mg/day as initial therapy for Graves' disease patients with moderate to severe hyperthyroidism. Thyroid 2015;25(1):43–50.

16. Nakamura H, Miyauchi A, Miyawaki N, et al. Analysis of 754 cases of antithyroid drug-induced agranulocytosis over 30 years in Japan. J Clin Endocrinol Metab 2013;98(12):4776–83.

17. Azizi F, Ataie L, Hedayati M, et al. Effect of long-term continuous methimazole treatment of hyperthyroidism: comparison with radioiodine. Eur J Endocrinol 2005;152(5):695–701.

18. Elbers L, Mourits M, Wiersinga W. Outcome of very long-term treatment with antithyroid drugs in Graves' hyperthyroidism associated with Graves' orbitopathy. Thyroid 2011;21(3):279–83.

19. Villagelin D, Romaldini JH, Santos RB, et al. Outcomes in Relapsed Graves' Disease Patients Following Radioiodine or Prolonged Low Dose of Methimazole Treatment. Thyroid 2015;25(12):1282–90.

20. Laurberg P, Berman DC, Andersen S, et al. Sustained control of Graves' hyperthyroidism during long-term low-dose antithyroid drug therapy of patients with severe Graves' orbitopathy. Thyroid 2011;21(9):951–6.

21. Goichot B, Raverot V, Klein M, et al. Management of thyroid dysfunctions in the elderly. French Endocrine Society consensus 2019 guidelines. Short version. Ann Endocrinol (Paris) 2020;81(5):511–5.

22. Becker DV, Sawin CT. Radioiodine and thyroid disease: the beginning. Semin Nucl Med 1996;26(3):155–64.

23. Gontarz-Nowak K, Szychlińska M, Matuszewski W, et al. Current Knowledge on Graves' Orbitopathy. J Clin Med 2020;10(1):16.

24. Bahn Chair RS, Burch HB, Cooper DS, et al. Hyperthyroidism and other causes of thyrotoxicosis: management guidelines of the American Thyroid Association and American Association of Clinical Endocrinologists. Thyroid 2011;21(6):593–646.

25. Bartalena L, Marcocci C, Bogazzi F, et al. Relation between therapy for hyperthyroidism and the course of Graves' ophthalmopathy. N Engl J Med 1998; 338(2):73–8.

26. Bartalena L, Baldeschi L, Dickinson A, et al. Consensus statement of the European Group on Graves' orbitopathy (EUGOGO) on management of GO. Eur J Endocrinol 2008;158(3):273–85.

27. Ariamanesh S, Ayati N, Mazloum Khorasani Z, et al. Effect of Different 131I Dose Strategies for Treatment of Hyperthyroidism on Graves' Ophthalmopathy. Clin Nucl Med 2020;45(7):514–8.

28. Braga M, Walpert N, Burch HB, et al. The effect of methimazole on cure rates after radioiodine treatment for Graves' hyperthyroidism: a randomized clinical trial. Thyroid 2002;12(2):135–9.

29. Brito JP, Payne S, Singh Ospina N, et al. Patterns of use, efficacy, and safety of treatment options for patients with Graves' Disease: A Nationwide Population-Based Study. Thyroid 2020;30(3):357–64.

30. Sundaresh V, Brito JP, Thapa P, et al. Comparative effectiveness of treatment choices for Graves' Hyperthyroidism: a Historical Cohort Study. Thyroid 2017; 27(4):497–505.

31. Okosieme OE, Taylor PN, Dayan CM. Should radioiodine now be first line treatment for Graves' disease? Thyroid Res 2020;13:3.

32. Okosieme OE, Taylor PN, Evans C, et al. Primary therapy of Graves' disease and cardiovascular morbidity and mortality: a linked-record cohort study. Lancet Diabetes Endocrinol 2019;7(4):278–87.

33. Träisk F, Tallstedt L, Abraham-Nordling M, et al. Thyroid-associated ophthalmopathy after treatment for Graves' hyperthyroidism with antithyroid drugs or iodine-131. J Clin Endocrinol Metab 2009;94(10):3700–7.

34. Ponto KA, Zang S, Kahaly GJ. The tale of radioiodine and Graves' orbitopathy. Thyroid 2010;20(7):785–93.

35. Stan MN, Durski JM, Brito JP, et al. Cohort study on radioactive iodine-induced hypothyroidism: implications for Graves' ophthalmopathy and optimal timing for thyroid hormone assessment. Thyroid 2013;23(5):620–5.

36. Bartalena L, Marcocci C, Bogazzi F, et al. Use of corticosteroids to prevent progression of Graves' ophthalmopathy after radioiodine therapy for hyperthyroidism. N Engl J Med 1989;321(20):1349–52.

37. Hall P, Berg G, Bjelkengren G, et al. Cancer mortality after iodine-131 therapy for hyperthyroidism. Int J Cancer 1992;50(6):886–90.

38. Metso S, Auvinen A, Huhtala H, et al. Increased cancer incidence after radioiodine treatment for hyperthyroidism. Cancer 2007;109(10):1972–9.

39. Kitahara CM, Berrington de Gonzalez A, Bouville A, et al. Association of radioactive iodine treatment with cancer mortality in patients with hyperthyroidism. JAMA Intern Med 2019;179(8):1034–42.

40. Goldman MB, Maloof F, Monson RR, et al. Radioactive iodine therapy and breast cancer. A follow-up study of hyperthyroid women. Am J Epidemiol 1988;127(5): 969–80.

41. Franklyn JA, Maisonneuve P, Sheppard M, et al. Cancer incidence and mortality after radioiodine treatment for hyperthyroidism: a population-based cohort study. Lancet 1999;353(9170):2111–5.

42. Ron E, Doody MM, Becker DV, et al. Cancer mortality following treatment for adult hyperthyroidism. Cooperative Thyrotoxicosis Therapy Follow-up Study Group. Jama 1998;280(4):347–55.

43. Greenspan BS, Siegel JA, Hassan A, et al. There is no association of radioactive iodine treatment with cancer mortality in patients with hyperthyroidism. J Nucl Med 2019;60(11):1500–1.

44. Kitahara CM, Preston DL, Sosa JA, et al. Association of radioactive iodine, anti-thyroid drug, and surgical treatments with solid cancer mortality in patients with hyperthyroidism. JAMA Netw Open 2020;3(7):e209660.

45. Elfenbein DM, Schneider DF, Havlena J, et al. Clinical and socioeconomic factors influence treatment decisions in Graves' disease. Ann Surg Oncol 2015;22(4):1196–9.

46. Sosa JA, Mehta PJ, Wang TS, et al. Racial disparities in clinical and economic outcomes from thyroidectomy. Ann Surg 2007;246(6):1083–91.

47. Langley RW, Burch HB. Perioperative management of the thyrotoxic patient. Endocrinol Metab Clin North Am 2003;32(2):519–34.

48. Baeza A, Aguayo J, Barria M, et al. Rapid preoperative preparation in hyperthyroidism. Clin Endocrinol (Oxf) 1991;35(5):439–42.

49. Fischli S, Lucchini B, Müller W, et al. Rapid preoperative blockage of thyroid hormone production/secretion in patients with Graves' disease. Swiss Med Wkly 2016;146:w14243.

50. Smith TJ, Hegedüs L. Graves' Disease. N Engl J Med 2016;375(16):1552–65.

51. Smith TJ, Janssen J. Insulin-like growth factor-i receptor and thyroid-associated ophthalmopathy. Endocr Rev 2019;40(1):236–67.

52. Mourits MP, Prummel MF, Wiersinga WM, et al. Clinical activity score as a guide in the management of patients with Graves' ophthalmopathy. Clin Endocrinol (Oxf) 1997;47(1):9–14.

53. Barrio-Barrio J, Sabater AL, Bonet-Farriol E, et al. Graves' Ophthalmopathy: VISA versus EUGOGO Classification, Assessment, and Management. J Ophthalmol 2015;2015:249125.

54. Bartley GB. The epidemiologic characteristics and clinical course of ophthalmopathy associated with autoimmune thyroid disease in Olmsted County, Minnesota. Trans Am Ophthalmol Soc 1994;92:477–588.

55. Laurberg P, Berman DC, Bülow Pedersen I, et al. Incidence and clinical presentation of moderate to severe graves' orbitopathy in a Danish population before and after iodine fortification of salt. J Clin Endocrinol Metab 2012;97(7):2325–32.

56. Perros P, Crombie AL, Kendall-Taylor P. Natural history of thyroid associated ophthalmopathy. Clin Endocrinol (Oxf) 1995;42(1):45–50.

57. Tanda ML, Piantanida E, Liparulo L, et al. Prevalence and natural history of Graves' orbitopathy in a large series of patients with newly diagnosed graves' hyperthyroidism seen at a single center. J Clin Endocrinol Metab 2013;98(4):1443–9.

58. Lombardi A, Menconi F, Greenberg D, et al. Dissecting the Genetic Susceptibility to Graves' Disease in a Cohort of Patients of Italian Origin. Front Endocrinol (Lausanne) 2016;7:21.

59. Nilsson A, Tsoumani K, Planck T. Statins decrease the risk of orbitopathy in newly diagnosed patients with Graves Disease. J Clin Endocrinol Metab 2021;106(5):1325–32.

60. Müller-Forell W, Kahaly GJ. Neuroimaging of Graves' orbitopathy. Best Pract Res Clin Endocrinol Metab 2012;26(3):259–71.

61. Gonçalves AC, Gebrim EM, Monteiro ML. Imaging studies for diagnosing Graves' orbitopathy and dysthyroid optic neuropathy. Clinics (Sao Paulo) 2012;67(11): 1327–34.

62. Negro R, Attanasio R, Grimaldi F, et al. 2015 Italian Survey of Clinical Practice Patterns in the Management of Graves' Disease: Comparison with European and North American Surveys. Eur Thyroid J 2016;5(2):112–9.

63. Khong JJ, Finch S, De Silva C, et al. Risk Factors for Graves' Orbitopathy; the Australian Thyroid-Associated Orbitopathy Research (ATOR) Study. J Clin Endocrinol Metab 2016;101(7):2711–20.

64. Krassas GE, Perros P. Prevention of thyroid associated-ophthalmopathy in children and adults: current views and management of preventable risk factors. Pediatr Endocrinol Rev 2007;4(3):218–24.

65. Marcocci C, Kahaly GJ, Krassas GE, et al. Selenium and the course of mild Graves' orbitopathy. N Engl J Med 2011;364(20):1920–31.

66. Kahaly GJ, Pitz S, Hommel G, et al. Randomized, single blind trial of intravenous versus oral steroid monotherapy in Graves' orbitopathy. J Clin Endocrinol Metab 2005;90(9):5234–40.

67. Bartalena L, Krassas GE, Wiersinga W, et al. Efficacy and safety of three different cumulative doses of intravenous methylprednisolone for moderate to severe and active Graves' orbitopathy. J Clin Endocrinol Metab 2012;97(12):4454–63.

68. Weissel M, Hauff W. Fatal liver failure after high-dose glucocorticoid pulse therapy in a patient with severe thyroid eye disease. Thyroid 2000;10(6):521.

69. Marcocci C, Watt T, Altea MA, et al. Fatal and non-fatal adverse events of glucocorticoid therapy for Graves' orbitopathy: a questionnaire survey among members of the European Thyroid Association. Eur J Endocrinol 2012;166(2):247–53.

70. Douglas RS, Kahaly GJ, Patel A, et al. Teprotumumab for the Treatment of Active Thyroid Eye Disease. N Engl J Med 2020;382(4):341–52.

71. Smith TJ, Kahaly GJ, Ezra DG, et al. Teprotumumab for Thyroid-Associated Ophthalmopathy. N Engl J Med 2017;376(18):1748–61.

72. Hoang TD, Nguyen NT, Chou E, et al. Rapidly progressive cognitive decline associated with teprotumumab in thyroid eye disease. BMJ Case Rep 2021;14(5).

73. Bednarczuk T, Schomburg L. Challenges and perspectives of selenium supplementation in Graves' disease and orbitopathy. Hormones (Athens) 2020; 19(1):31–9.

74. Bartalena L, Kahaly GJ, Baldeschi L, et al. The 2021 European Group on Graves' orbitopathy (EUGOGO) clinical practice guidelines for the medical management of Graves' orbitopathy. Eur J Endocrinol 2021;185(4):G43–67.

75. Riedl M, Kuhn A, Krämer I, et al. Prospective, systematically recorded mycophenolate safety data in Graves' orbitopathy. J Endocrinol Invest 2016;39(6):687–94.

76. Villarroel MC, Hidalgo M, Jimeno A. Mycophenolate mofetil: an update. Drugs Today (Barc) 2009;45(7):521–32.

77. Ye X, Bo X, Hu X, et al. Efficacy and safety of mycophenolate mofetil in patients with active moderate-to-severe Graves' orbitopathy. Clin Endocrinol (Oxf) 2017; 86(2):247–55.

78. Kahaly GJ, Riedl M, Konig J, et al. Mycophenolate plus methylprednisolone versus methylprednisolone alone in active, moderate-to-severe Graves' orbitopathy (MINGO): a randomised, observer-masked, multicentre trial. Lancet Diabetes Endocrinol 2018;6(4):287–98.

79. Lee ACH, Riedl M, Frommer L, et al. Systemic safety analysis of mycophenolate in Graves' orbitopathy. J Endocrinol Invest 2020;43(6):767–77.

80. Perez-Moreiras JV, Gomez-Reino JJ, Maneiro JR, et al. Efficacy of tocilizumab in patients with moderate-to-severe corticosteroid-resistant graves orbitopathy: a randomized clinical trial. Am J Ophthalmol 2018;195:181–90.

81. Copperman T, Idowu OO, Kersten RC, et al. Subcutaneous tocilizumab for thyroid Eye Disease: Simplified Dosing and Delivery. Ophthalmic Plast Reconstr Surg 2019;35(3):e64–6.

82. Silkiss RZ, Paap MK, Roelofs KA, et al. Treatment of corticosteroid-resistant thyroid eye disease with subcutaneous tocilizumab. Can J Ophthalmol 2021;56(1): 66–70.

83. Salvi M, Vannucchi G, Campi I, et al. Rituximab treatment in a patient with severe thyroid-associated ophthalmopathy: effects on orbital lymphocytic infiltrates. Clin Immunol 2009;131(2):360–5.

84. Salvi M, Vannucchi G, Currò N, et al. Efficacy of B-cell targeted therapy with rituximab in patients with active moderate to severe Graves' orbitopathy: a randomized controlled study. J Clin Endocrinol Metab 2015;100(2):422–31.

85. Stan MN, Garrity JA, Carranza Leon BG, et al. Randomized controlled trial of rituximab in patients with Graves' orbitopathy. J Clin Endocrinol Metab 2015;100(2): 432–41.

86. Chen J, Chen G, Sun H. Intravenous rituximab therapy for active Graves' ophthalmopathy: a meta-analysis. Hormones (Athens) 2021;20(2):279–86.

87. Shen WC, Lee CH, Loh EW, et al. Efficacy and safety of rituximab for the treatment of Graves' Orbitopathy: a meta-analysis of randomized controlled trials. Pharmacotherapy 2018;38(5):503–10.

88. Wang C, Ning Q, Jin K, et al. Does rituximab improve clinical outcomes of patients with thyroid-associated ophthalmopathy? A systematic review and meta-analysis. BMC Ophthalmol 2018;18(1):46.

89. Jefferis JM, Jones RK, Currie ZI, et al. Orbital decompression for thyroid eye disease: methods, outcomes, and complications. Eye (Lond) 2018;32(3):626–36.

90. Tse DT. A simple maneuver to reposit a subluxed globe. Arch Ophthalmol 2000; 118(3):410–1.

91. Chang EL, Bernardino CR, Rubin PA. Normalization of upper eyelid height and contour after bony decompression in thyroid-related ophthalmopathy: a digital image analysis. Arch Ophthalmol 2004;122(12):1882–5.

The Future of Thyroid Nodule Risk Stratification

Nydia Burgos, MD[a], Naykky Singh Ospina, MD, MS[b], Jennifer A. Sipos, MD[c],*

KEYWORDS

- Thyroid nodules • Thyroid cancer • Artificial intelligence • Risk stratification

KEY POINTS

- Sonographic risk stratification of thyroid nodules is the first step to personalize the care of patients with thyroid nodules.
- Multiple systems are available for sonographic risk stratification of thyroid nodules, each associated with different advantages and limitations.
- The use of artificial intelligence to improve thyroid cancer risk estimation and assessment reproducibility is promising.
- Future studies using artificial intelligence should focus on improving patient outcomes and use rigorous scientific methods.

INTRODUCTION

Over the last 2 decades, the use of sonographic risk stratification systems (SRSS) has become an integral part in the evaluation of patients with thyroid nodules.[1–4] The aim of these systems is to standardize the evaluation of thyroid cancer risk according to ultrasound features, in order to individualize the management of patients with thyroid nodules.[1–3,5,6] Clinical evidence and practice guidelines further support the routine use of risk stratification, as it can decrease the number of unnecessary thyroid biopsies and improve reporting of thyroid cancer risk while avoiding missed diagnoses of clinically relevant thyroid cancer.[7–10]

More recently, artificial intelligence (AI) methodologies have been applied to improve thyroid cancer risk stratification and the care of patients with thyroid nodules with promising results.[11,12] This article aims to review ultrasound features, SRSS, and current clinical evidence incorporating AI in the diagnostic evaluation of patients with thyroid nodules.

---

[a] Division of Endocrinology, Diabetes and Metabolism, Department of Medicine, University of Puerto Rico, Medical Sciences Campus, Paseo Dr. Jose Celso Barbosa, San Juan 00921, Puerto Rico; [b] Division of Endocrinology, Diabetes and Metabolism, Department of Medicine, University of Florida, 1600 SW Archer Road, Gainesville, FL 32610, USA; [c] Division of Endocrinology, Diabetes and Metabolism, Department of Medicine, The Ohio State University Wexner Medical Center, 1581 Dodd Drive, Columbus, OH 43210, USA
* Corresponding author.
E-mail address: Jennifer.sipos@osumc.edu

Endocrinol Metab Clin N Am 51 (2022) 305–321
https://doi.org/10.1016/j.ecl.2021.12.002
0889-8529/21/© 2021 Elsevier Inc. All rights reserved.

ASSOCIATION OF THYROID NODULES, ULTRASOUND FEATURES, AND THYROID CANCER

Certain individual ultrasound features are specific for malignancy, while others are associated with benign histology.[1,2,13] Ultrasound features of benign and malignant nodules may overlap, limiting their diagnostic properties as a single rule-in or rule-out test for thyroid cancer diagnosis. However, they are extremely useful to stratify the risk for thyroid malignancy.[1,2,13] Suspicious features include microcalcifications, local invasion, taller-than-wide shape, irregular/infiltrative margins, and markedly reduced echogenicity. However, the absence of a halo, ill-defined margins, solid composition, and vascularity are less specific.[14–16] Cystic nodules and spongiform nodules have a high diagnostic odds ratio to predict benign nodules.[17] Although a solitary suspicious finding may be associated with variable rates of cancer, the accumulation of suspicious findings significantly increases the malignancy risk. Indeed, a retrospective study of 1658 thyroid nodules measuring at least 1 cm showed in a univariate analysis that there was a significant association of malignancy with a single suspicious ultrasound feature, and on multivariate analysis, the malignancy risk was further increased with an escalating number of high-risk sonographic features.[18]

Table 1 summarizes thyroid ultrasound features, their associated histologic findings, and diagnostic odds ratios to predict benign or malignant thyroid nodules.[2,13,15,19]

CONTEMPORARY THYROID ULTRASOUND RISK STRATIFICATION SYSTEMS - OVERVIEW

Numerous SRSS exist with the goal of standardizing the evaluation of patients with thyroid nodules.[1,3,20,21] Fundamentally, these systems aim to separate thyroid nodules according to thyroid cancer risk and propose a nodule size at which biopsy should be recommended, according to the estimated risk for thyroid cancer.[1,3,5,21]

Evaluation of individual thyroid ultrasound features provides insight into the nature of the underlying lesion and its estimated cancer risk. Moreover, the presence of ultrasound features suspicious for malignancy are rarely independent of each other.[15] For this reason, establishing sonographic patterns to aid the management of patients with thyroid nodules is based on the concept that sonographic features are present concurrently. Although pattern-based SRSS are associated with improved interobserver variability in assigning risk classification,[1] these systems[1,3,22] have the disadvantage that 5% to 17% of nodules are nonclassifiable.[23,24] Therefore, point-based systems, such as the American College of Radiology Thyroid Imaging Reporting & Data System (ACR TIRADS) have the advantage of being inclusive of all nodule types.[2] However, classification of nodules using the ACR TIRADS is limited by interobserver variability in assigning scores for each feature and can be time consuming in the setting of classifying multiple nodules.[2]

Table 2 summarizes contemporary thyroid nodule SRSS, their diagnostic performance, and clinical implications.[1–3,5,7,21,23,25,26]

CLINICAL BENEFITS OF THYROID NODULE RISK STRATIFICATION

The use of thyroid nodule SRSS has revolutionized the management of patients with thyroid nodules by improving the quality of thyroid ultrasound assessment and communication between clinicians, potentially decreasing the number of unnecessary biopsies, and using thyroid cancer risk to personalize patient care.

Table 1
Thyroid ultrasound features, definitions, and diagnostic odds ratio

US Feature	Definition	Descriptors	Histologic Background	Diagnostic Odds Ratio (DOR)[13]
Composition	Proportion of solid tissue and fluid in a nodule	Solid Predominantly solid Predominantly cystic Cystic	Hyperplastic nodules have abundant colloid, which appears cystic on sonography Neoplasms can undergo cystic degeneration and have cystic areas	Solid (DOR-M) (4.45, 2.63–7.5) Cystic (DOR-B) (6.78, 2.26–20.3) Spongiform (DOR-B) (12, 0.61–234.3)
Echogenicity	Brightness relative to normal thyroid parenchyma	Hyperechoic Isoechoic Hypoechoic Very hypoechoic	Classic PTC and MTC produce less acoustic interfaces than microfollicles and may appear hypoechoic	Hypoechoic (DOR-M) (4.5, 3.2–6.4) Isoechoic (DOR-B) (3.6, 2–6.3)
Borders	Interface between nodule and surrounding thyroid parenchyma	Smooth Ill-defined Irregular Infiltrative Extrathyroidal extension	Infiltrative or lobular borders may be concerning for invasive thyroid carcinoma Hyperplastic nodules may have ill-defined borders because of similar echogenicity to surrounding parenchyma, which may not be suspicious for malignancy	Infiltrative margins (DOR-M) (6.89, 3.35–14.1)
Shape	Evaluated in the axial plane by comparing the height (tallness) and width of a nodule measured parallel and perpendicular to the ultrasound beam	Taller-than-wide Wider-than-tall	Disproportionate growth in anteroposterior dimension is considered an aggressive growth pattern	Taller-than-wide (DOR-M) (11.14, 6.6–18.9)
Echogenic foci	Hyperechoic foci	Large comet tail artifacts Macrocalcifications Peripheral rim calcifications Punctate echogenic foci	Large comet tail artifacts are associated with colloid Punctuate echogenic foci have been associated with psammoma bodies, which may be associated with PTC	Internal microcalcifications (DOR-M) (6.78, 4.48–10.24)

DOR-M, diagnostic odds ratio to predict malignant nodules and DOR-B, diagnostic odds ratio to predict benign nodules, presented as estimate and 95% CI.
Abbreviations: MTC, medullary thyroid cancer; PTC, papillary thyroid cancer.

Table 2
Diagnostic performance of sonographic risk stratification systems

SRSS	System Type	Categories	Biopsy Cut-off	POM[5]	Unnecessary Biopsy rate[7] (95% CI)	Missed Malignancy rate[23]%	Sensitivity[25] (95% CI)	Specificity[25] (95% CI)	Likelihood Ratio for Positive Results (LR+)[25] (95% CI)	DOR[25] (95% CI)	Interobserver agreement[26]
ATA	Ultrasound pattern based	Benign	No FNA	0	51% (44–58)	4.1%	87% (75–94)	31% (24–40)	1.2 (1.0–1.4)	3.1 (1.3–7.1)	0.5 (0.4–0.6)
		Very low risk	>2 cm or no FNA	<3%							
		Low risk	1.5 cm	5%–10%							
		Intermediate risk	≥ 1 cm	10%–20%							
		High risk	≥ 1 cm	70%–90%							
ACR-TIRADS	Weighted point-based system	Benign (TIRADS-1)	No FNA	<2%	25% (22–29)	2.2%	74% (61–83)	64% (56–70)	1.9 (1.6–2.3)	4.9 (3.1–7.7)	0.5 (0.4–0.6)
		Not suspicious (TIRADS-2)	No FNA	<2%							
		Mildly suspicious (TIRADS-3)	≥ 2.5 cm	5%							
		Moderately suspicious (TIRADS-4)	≥ 1.5 cm	5%–20%							
		Highly suspicious (TIRADS-5)	≥ 1 cm	>20%							

Guideline	Method	Category	Size / FNA threshold	POM							
ETA	Ultrasound pattern based	EU-TIRADS 1 – normal	-	0	38% (16–66)	3.2%	54% (51–57)	53% (51–55)	1.4 (1.0–1.8)	2.2 (0.9–5.1)	0.6 (0.5–0.6)
		EU-TIRADS 2- benign	No FNA	0							
		EU-TIRADS 3- low risk	>2 cm	2%–4%							
		EU-TIRADS 4- intermediate risk	>1.5 cm	6%–17%							
		EU-TIRADS 5- high risk	>1 cm	26%–87%							
AACE/ACE/AME	Ultrasound pattern based	Low risk	>2 cm, increase in size, clinical features	1%	N/A	2.9%	74% (71–78)	53% (51–55)	1.5 (1.1–2.1)	3.1 (1.0–9.4)	0.4 (0.4–0.6)
		Intermediate risk	>2 cm	5%–15%							
		High risk	≥1 cm	50%–90%							
K-TIRADS	Ultrasound pattern based	K-TIRADS 1 – no nodule	NA	-	55% (42–67)	3.5%	86 (73–94)	28% (20–38)	1.2 (1.0–1.4)	2.5 (1.1–5.5)	0.5 (0.4–0.6)
		K-TIRADS 2 – benign	≥2 cm	<3%							
		K-TIRADS 3 – low suspicion	≥1.5 cm	3%–15%							
		K-TIRADS 4 – Intermediate suspicion	≥1 cm	15%–50%							
		K-TIRADS 5 – High suspicion	≥1 cm (>0.5 cm selective)	>60%							

Abbreviations: AACE, American Association of Clinical Endocrinologists; ACE, American College of Endocrinology; ACR, American College of Radiology; AME, Associazione Medici Endocrinologi (AME); ATA, American Thyroid Association; CI, confidence interval; DOR, diagnostic odds ratio; ETA, European Thyroid Association; EU-TIRADS, European Thyroid Imaging Reporting and Data System; FNA, fine needle aspiration; K-TIRADS, Korean Thyroid Imaging Reporting and Data System; LR; likelihood ratio; N/A, not available; POM, prevalence of malignancy; TIRADS, - Thyroid Imaging Reporting and Data System.

Although the details included in thyroid and neck ultrasound reports are variable, SRSS provide a means to standardize reporting and communication among clinicians. For example, a retrospective study of ultrasound reports of 478 thyroid nodules found that most reports did not include the size of the dominant nodule (71%) or comment on suspicious features (91%) or the presence of suspicious lymph nodes (83%), with 46% of the reports lacking a description of malignancy risk.[27] Multiple studies have shown a positive effect of implementation of thyroid nodule risk stratification in the quality of the ultrasound report, with increased inclusion of ultrasound features of interest, thyroid cancer risk, and suggestions of management strategies to address this risk.[10,28,29]

Moreover, better reporting of thyroid ultrasound features and cancer risk translates to improved clinical care. For example, observational data suggest that strict implementation of recommendations for thyroid biopsy according to the different SRSS can result in decreased rates of unnecessary biopsies.[5,7,23,30] However, most commonly, these studies consider nodules with benign cytology as unnecessary. This is a narrow definition, given that the necessity and appropriateness of a thyroid biopsy depend on additional factors beyond thyroid nodule risk and size.[5,6,31]

COMPARISONS OF CURRENT THYROID NODULE RISK STRATIFICATION SYSTEMS

Castellana and colleagues performed a systematic review and meta-analysis to compare 5 thyroid nodule SRSS and found that American Thyroid Association (ATA) guidelines had the highest pooled sensitivity, and ACR-TIRADS the highest pooled specificity.[25] Moreover, when performing a direct comparison analysis, the diagnostic odds ratio for selecting patients for thyroid biopsy was higher for ACR-TIRADS than for ATA (5.6 vs 2.9 $P=.002$) or Korean Society of Thyroid Radiology's Thyroid Imaging Reporting and Data System (K-TIRADS) (4.5 vs 2.5, $P=.002$). The review included 12 studies and 18,750 thyroid nodules.

Kim and colleagues performed a systematic review of 8 articles including 13,092 nodules and compared unnecessary biopsy rates among 4 thyroid nodule SRSS.[7] ACR-TIRADS had the lowest unnecessary biopsy rates (25%). However, low unnecessary biopsy rates may exist at the expense of higher missed malignancy rates.[5,32] ACR-TIRADS is associated with the higher proportion of malignant nodules that do not receive a recommendation for biopsy; however, for nodules that do not meet biopsy criteria but carry a relevant risk of malignancy, active surveillance instead of biopsy is recommended, potentially decreasing the risk of a significant adverse outcome.[33] Overall, SRSS improve the prediction of benign or malignant disease, with high-risk categories having a strong association with malignant or suspicious histology.[20,23,25,34]

SIZE THRESHOLD

Current guidelines offer variable size cutoffs according to risk stratification category, with a lower threshold for biopsy as the risk for thyroid cancer increases, although limited clinical evidence guides the selection of these thresholds.[1–3,21] In fact, the selection of size thresholds for thyroid nodule fine needle aspiration (FNA) has remained controversial given that the association of thyroid nodule size and malignancy risk is not linear (but could result in higher risk for false-negative cytology), and size only partly correlates with thyroid cancer prognosis.[5,35–38] Machens and colleagues reported increased cumulative risk for distant metastases from papillary thyroid cancer and follicular thyroid cancer above 2 cm.[39] Based on this, ACR-TIRADS selects a slightly higher threshold for biopsy in the lower risk categories of 2.5 cm, after considering the reported discrepancy of pathologic tumor size and estimated sonographic size.[2]

Ha and colleagues evaluated the effect of size thresholds using the current biopsy indications for ATA, K-TIRADS, and ACR-TIRADS, in 3323 consecutive thyroid nodules. Overall, the sensitivity for detecting malignancy was higher for ATA and K-TIRADS compared with ACR-TIRADS at 89.6% and 94.5%, versus 74.7%, respectively. ACR-TIRADS, on the other hand, was associated with higher specificity (67.3%) compared with ATA (33.2%) and K-TIRADS (26.4%). This improved specificity with ACR-TIRADS translated to the lowest rate of unnecessary FNA at 25.3%, in comparison with ATA (51.7%) and K-TIRADS (56.9%). However, if a higher threshold for thyroid biopsy of 1.5 cm for intermediate-risk thyroid nodules (instead of the existing 1 cm threshold) and of 2.5 cm for low suspicion thyroid nodules (as opposed to the existing 1.5 cm threshold) was used, the specificity and rates of unnecessary biopsies for this revised ATA system would be similar to those for ACR-TIRADS, highlighting the effects of size thresholds on the performance of these SRSS.[5,40,41]

LIMITATIONS OF THYROID NODULE RISK STRATIFICATION

The clinical evidence supporting the prevalence of malignancy associated with the different thyroid cancer risk categories is mostly derived from observational studies that are enriched with malignant cases, which can lead to overestimation of the diagnostic performance.[5,42] In addition, SRSS have been validated mostly among thyroid nodules potentially harboring PTC; however, the diagnostic performance for patients with medullary or follicular thyroid carcinoma might differ.[25,43] Another limitation when using risk stratification in practice is the inability to classify all nodules (when using a pattern-based system), with an unknown percentage of these nodules harboring malignancy.[34,43,44]

Structured evaluation and report of thyroid ultrasounds requires expertise and availability of clinical time, both potential barriers to implementation.[10] Similarly, reproducibility of ultrasound assessments is pivotal; yet most of the clinical evidence reporting moderate interobserver agreement is derived from small groups of expert thyroid examiners.[26,45–48]

Finally, another potential unintended consequence of the implementation of thyroid nodule risk stratification is the over-reliance on the radiology report and recommendations (of observation and/or biopsy) that may not take into consideration the clinical situation of the patient.[6]

CLINICAL FACTORS AND RISK STRATIFICATION

Because thyroid nodules are such a common clinical entity, individual risk stratification based on patient characteristics is an important component of the evaluation. Various clinical and demographic factors should be assessed to further refine the malignancy risk and aid in the next steps of clinical management.

Age at diagnosis of a nodule influences the risk that any nodule is cancerous; younger age is associated with an increased malignancy risk.[49,50] In a single-center study of 6391 adult patients with thyroid nodules, the risk of malignancy was highest (22.9%) in the group aged 20 to 30 years, and declined by 2.2% per year until the risk reached a plateau of 12.6% at age 60. It is important to note, however, that in spite of the overall lower likelihood of malignancy in the older patients, there was a greater risk of a more aggressive histologic phenotype when a cancer was identified.[49]

Sex also plays an important role in risk stratification of patients with thyroid nodules. Although not consistently reported,[51,52] a greater risk of malignancy in those with a thyroid nodule has been suggested in men.[53] In the largest reported experience with thyroid nodules, a single-study center of 20,001 consecutive thyroid nodules determined that the odds ratio for malignancy in men was 1.7 (1.5–1.9, confidence interval [CI], P<.0001), compared with women.[54]

Although the etiology of most thyroid malignancies is unclear, a small proportion of differentiated cancers may be attributable to an inherited condition. Because thyroid cancer may be seen in up to 10% to 15% of the population at autopsy,[55,56] the occurrence of 2 cases of thyroid cancer among first-degree relatives in most families is attributable to chance, rather than a genetic predisposition.[57] However, the identification of nonmedullary thyroid cancer in 3 or more first-degree relatives is associated with a 96% chance of an inherited condition.[57]

Exposure to radiation in childhood is a well-recognized cause of differentiated thyroid carcinoma, and the impact may be seen for decades after therapy.[58–60] Additionally, those patients exposed during childhood or adolescence to ionizing radiation from a nuclear fallout are at increased risk of malignancy.[61] Consequently, clinicians should consider these risk factors in the decision-making process of whether to perform FNA.[1]

Another important consideration in the evaluation of a patient with a thyroid nodule is the presence of comorbid conditions. It is well recognized that thyroid cancers are often associated with an indolent clinical course. If the patient has a low-risk thyroid nodule in the setting of another, more aggressive primary malignancy or uncontrolled chronic condition, consideration may be given to postponing the evaluation of an identified thyroid nodule. A recent study examined the likelihood of identification of a clinically significant thyroid cancer (defined as anaplastic, medullary, or poorly differentiated carcinoma, or the presence of distant metastases) in a cohort of 1129 patients over the age of 70 years. Only 17 (1.5%) significant risk thyroid cancers (SRTCs) were found among 2527 nodules, all of which were readily identifiable by initial imaging and cytology. During a median follow-up of 4 years, there were only 10 (0.9%) thyroid cancer deaths, all of which occurred in patients with SRTCs. Interestingly, they found that among all other patients, there were 160 deaths (14.4%), and there was a more than twofold increased risk of death among those with a separate nonthyroidal malignancy or coronary artery disease at the time of nodule evaluation. The authors concluded that the evaluation of thyroid nodules in patients over the age of 70 years without high-risk imaging or cytologic findings should be tempered in the setting of significant comorbid illness.[62]

ARTIFICIAL INTELLIGENCE AND THYROID NODULE RISK STRATIFICATION
Background and Definition of Artificial Intelligence

AI refers to the imitation of human abilities such as learning and problem solving by computer systems.[63–65] Although the idea of AI is not new, the application to enhance clinical care has expanded recently given the availability of computers that are fast and able to analyze large datasets.[65,66] Within AI, machine learning is the use of mathematical operations to solve problems and for systems to learn from the evaluation of data over time.[65,67] Machine learning algorithms can be classified according to how the data are provided and whether the outcome of interest is labeled during the development of the model.[65,67,68] Specifically, in thyroid nodule risk stratification, the use of images in which the ultrasound features of interest have been manually extracted by a human operator (eg, echogenicity or composition) is considered conventional machine learning. On the other hand, if thyroid nodule images are analyzed as raw data (pixels) by the computer model, this is considered deep learning. Similarly, if the nodule is labeled as thyroid cancer or a benign nodule during the model development, this is considered supervised machine learning, where the goal is for the system to learn to classify/predict the desired outcome (eg, malignancy). Alternatively, if the thyroid nodule is not labeled for the outcome of interest (thyroid cancer or benign), this is considered unsupervised learning, and the goal is the identification of new clusters/groups (**Fig. 1**).[67–69]

A particular modality of interest for imaging-based diagnosis is computer-aided diagnosis (CAD). These methods are based on machine learning models for the evaluation of images and can be used to complement and enhance the human operator assessment.[70] Augmented intelligence refers to AI models that seek to support human cognition, instead of replacing it. In addition, models of human in the loop refer to models in which the outputs from machine learning algorithms require review from human operators.[64]

Overview of How Artificial Intelligence can Improve Ultrasound Risk Stratification

Thyroid nodule risk stratification allows clinicians to estimate the risk for thyroid cancer and personalize the care of patients with thyroid nodules.[6,31] However, concerns in terms of thyroid nodule ultrasound feature assessment reproducibility, time requirement for these assessments, and overall precision of the current frameworks can limit the clinical benefits.[10,33,71] The use of AI can help resolve these concerns by improving frameworks for thyroid nodule risk stratification and increasing the automation of thyroid nodule risk stratification.[11,69,72] In addition, these systems can be used in areas in which experts in thyroid ultrasonography are not available, possibly improving the quality of care across different health care systems.[72]

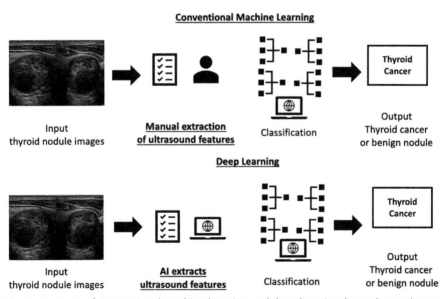

Fig. 1. Structure of conventional machine learning and deep learning (according to human or computer model extraction of the images or pixels) for thyroid nodule risk stratification. Supervised machine learning as during development classification/prediction of thyroid cancer/benign is provided to the model.

Improving frameworks for thyroid nodule risk stratification

The use of machine learning algorithms offers an opportunity to re-evaluate the weight of the ultrasound features that are currently used for thyroid cancer risk stratification and to increase the number of variables that are evaluated.[11]

For example, Zhang and colleagues aimed to develop a machine learning model for the diagnosis of thyroid nodules, based on the evaluation of 11 ultrasound features that were manually extracted and real-time elastography.[73] Their model was developed using a sample of 2064 nodules, with histologic diagnosis of thyroid cancer in 36%. The diagnostic properties were compared with a radiologist. The machine learning model was able to integrate information from the provided variables, with higher weight given to the presence of calcification, hypoechoic halo, and elastography.[73] In fact, the random forest algorithm had a higher area under the curve than the radiologist (AUC = 0.92 [95% CI 0.90-0.95] vs 0.83 [95% CI 0.82–0.85]).[73] Interestingly, size was included as a potential variable and was given lower importance by the machine-learning model, highlighting the need to understand potential biases in the datasets used to train machine-learning models and the importance of collaboration between expert clinicians and machine-learning data scientists. The evidence that links thyroid nodule size and malignancy risk is somewhat controversial, and instead, this variable may provide more prognostic information.[5,35,36,39,74]

Similarly, the study by Wildman-Tobriner and colleagues[75] aimed to optimize the diagnostic performance of ACR-TIRADS using AI. A dataset of 1425 biopsy-proven thyroid nodules (malignancy rate of 11%) was evaluated for the 5 ACR-TIRADS components, and a genetic AI algorithm was used to optimize the classification.[75] The optimized AI ACR-TIRADS, assigned new weights to 8 features, and for 6 features, the new system assigned 0 points. The optimized AI ACR- TIRADS had similar receiver operator curves and sensitivity, but higher specificity than the radiologists using the original ACR-TIRADS.[75]

Multiple additional studies have explored the use of AI to improve understanding of what ultrasound features are associated with thyroid cancer risk, what weight should be assigned to each of the features, and taking advantage of the ability of the algorithms to integrate variables in order to provide a more accurate and precise estimate of thyroid cancer.[11,12] Future studies should include large datasets of patients with thyroid nodules, with different risk for thyroid cancer and representative of the populations of interest, in order to take full advantage of AI methods and enhancing thyroid cancer risk estimation.

Increasing automation of thyroid nodule risk stratification

Another barrier to routine implementation of thyroid nodule risk stratification is the need for accurate and reproducible assessment of thyroid nodule features.[33,71] These assessments have shown that highly trained evaluators and time are important considerations that can affect reproducibility, given that ultrasound assessment is an operator-dependent task.[10,48] AI algorithms could help solve this clinical gap by supporting highly reproducible, fast ,and automated thyroid nodule risk stratification.

Xu and colleagues conducted a systematic review that included 19 studies (4781 nodules) assessing the diagnostic performance of machine-learning algorithms for the diagnosis of thyroid nodules.[76] Only the results from the external validation cohorts were included in the analysis. There were 6 studies that evaluated conventional machine learning and 13 that evaluated deep learning models. Overall, the studies were considered to be at moderate risk of bias, and the prevalence of thyroid cancer cases was high.[76] The conventional machine-learning models had a sensitivity of 0.86

(95% CI 0.79–0.92), specificity of 0.85 (95% CI 0.77–0.91), and diagnostic odds ratio (DOR) of 37.4 (95% CI 24.9–56.2). Models based on deep learning had a sensitivity of 0.89 (95% CI 0.81–0.93), specificity of 0.84 (95% CI 0.75–0.90), and DOR of 40.9 (95% CI 18.1–92.1). The performance of deep learning-based algorithms was comparable to the diagnostic performance of radiologists (DOR of 40.1 [95% CI 15.6–103.3] vs DOR of 44.9 [95% CI 30.7–65.6], respectively).[76] These findings are consistent with the systematic review by Chambara and colleagues, that evaluated 14 studies of CAD models for thyroid nodules, demonstrating comparable diagnostic performance of the AI models to human evaluators.[70] These reviews suggest good diagnostic performance of machine learning algorithms for the identification of thyroid cancer.[76]

The study by Li and colleagues was a large multicenter study conducted in China including greater than 300,000 images from 17,627 patients with thyroid cancer and 25,325 patients with benign thyroid nodules.[69] The area under the curve in each external validation site was 0.91 (95% CI 0.87–0.96) and 0.91 (95% CI 0.89–0.93). Moreover, the sensitivity of the machine-learning model was 84.3% versus 92.9% (P=.048) in 1 site and 84.7% versus 89% (P=.25), while the specificity was 86.9% versus 56.1% (P<.0001) and 87.8% versus 68.6% in the second site (P<.0001), when compared with radiologists.[69]

Thomas and colleagues developed a similarity algorithm for thyroid nodule risk stratification and used heat maps to attempt to explain the algorithm output. Heat-maps are visual representations that can help identify the areas (in an image in this case) that were used to support the output of the AI model.[77] Their development cohort included 2025 images from 482 patients, and the overall malignancy prevalence was 32%.[77] In this model, the physician is always in the loop as he or she selects the images of interest and is presented with the final output that he or she can accept or reject. The similarity model was used to classify test images and demonstrated an accuracy of 81.5%.[77] Interestingly, the heatmap was not able to completely explain the rationale for the model outputs.[77]

This body of evidence suggests that machine-learning algorithms can enhance thyroid nodule risk stratification by analyzing thyroid nodule images without the need for expert extraction of ultrasound features.

LESSONS LEARNED AND NEXT STEPS FOR THE USE OF ARTIFICIAL INTELLIGENCE FOR THYROID NODULE RISK STRATIFICATION

The ultimate goal of applying AI methods to improve thyroid nodule risk stratification is to improve the care of patients with thyroid nodules (**Fig. 2**). The preliminary evidence presented suggests reasonable diagnostic performance of machine-learning algorithms. However, a few concerns arise. Similar to the existent thyroid nodule diagnostic literature, the datasets that are used to train these models suffer from bias related to: high prevalence of thyroid cancer (improves diagnostic performance), over-representation of papillary thyroid cancer, variable gold standards, and inappropriate exclusions.[5,11,42] These biases cannot be completely overcome by large datasets or by advanced machine-learning algorithms and limit the validity and generalizability of findings.[78]

Several studies have focused on deep learning algorithms, but understanding of the features and/or rationale used by the algorithm to reach conclusions continues to be poorly understood for most models.[12] This black box and limited interpretability significantly hinder the reliability, trust, and adoption of these methods in practice.[79]

Similarly, as is the case for other areas of AI for diagnosis based on imaging, there is paucity of randomized, controlled trials focused not only on diagnostic performance,

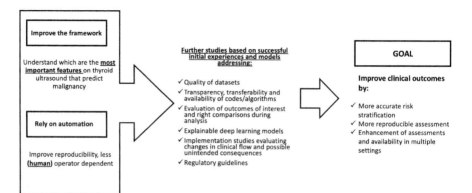

Fig. 2. Potential applications of AI to improve thyroid nodule risk stratifications, areas that need to be addressed in future studies in order to achieve the goal of improved clinical outcomes.

but also of effects on clinical care and outcomes (ie, increased reproducibility, accuracy/discussion of thyroid cancer risk, and unnecessary biopsies). Although most models have focused on providing a dichotomous answer of benign/malignant classification for thyroid nodules, models that provide an estimate of thyroid cancer risk can also assist and support personalization of care for patients with thyroid nodules.[79] Moreover, the possible unintended consequences of implementation of these models in clinical practice have rarely been assessed (ie, clinician/patient distrust and legal implications).[64,68]

SUMMARY

Ultrasound risk stratification is an essential tool in the management of patients with thyroid nodules. The application of AI to thyroid nodule risk stratification can help improve the diagnostic accuracy of current SRSS and the reproducibility of assessments. The results of preliminary studies using AI to enhance thyroid nodule risk stratification are promising, supporting the need for future research that moves from diagnostic performance to effects on clinical outcomes.

CLINICS CARE POINTS

- The use of risk stratification systems in the evaluation of thyroid nodules can lead to a decrease of unnecessary thyroid biopsies without missed diagnosis of clinically relevant thyroid cancer.
- Reproducible and accurate risk stratification of thyroid nodules can be time consuming and requires expertise, which represents potential limitations for widespread implementation.
- Deep learning models for thyroid nodule risk stratification have shown good diagnostic properties for thyroid cancer; yet their impact on patient care requires further evaluation.

DISCLOSURE

The authors have nothing to disclose.

REFERENCES

1. Haugen BR, Alexander EK, Bible KC, et al. 2015 American Thyroid Association Management guidelines for adult patients with thyroid nodules and differentiated thyroid cancer: The American Thyroid Association Guidelines Task Force on Thyroid Nodules and Differentiated Thyroid Cancer. Thyroid 2016. https://doi.org/10.1089/thy.2015.0020.
2. Tessler FN, Middleton WD, Grant EG, et al. ACR thyroid imaging, reporting and data system (TI-RADS): white paper of the ACR TI-RADS Committee. J Am Coll Radiol 2017;14(5):587–95.
3. Pearce SHS, Brabant G, Duntas LH, et al. 2013 ETA guideline: management of subclinical hypothyroidism. Eur Thyroid J 2014;2:215–28.
4. Tessler FN, Middleton WD, Hoang JK. Commentary on a direct comparison of the ATA and TI-RADS ultrasound scoring systems. Endocr Pract 2019;25(5):503–5.
5. Singh Ospina N, Iñiguez-Ariza NM, Castro MR. Thyroid nodules: diagnostic evaluation based on thyroid cancer risk assessment. BMJ 2020;368. https://doi.org/10.1136/bmj.l6670.
6. Ospina NS, Genere N, Hoang JK, et al. ACR TI-RADS Recommendations: a call to contextualize radiologists' recommendations for thyroid nodules with the clinical scenario. J Am Coll Radiol 2021. https://doi.org/10.1016/j.jacr.2021.04.019.
7. Kim PH, Suh CH, Baek JH, et al. Unnecessary thyroid nodule biopsy rates under four ultrasound risk stratification systems: a systematic review and meta-analysis. Eur Radiol 2021. https://doi.org/10.1007/s00330-020-07384-6.
8. Zhang Q, Ma J, Sun W, et al. Comparison of diagnostic performance between the American college of radiology thyroid imaging reporting and data system and American thyroid association guidelines: a systematic review. Endocr Pract 2020;26(5):552–63.
9. Li W, Wang Y, Wen J, et al. Diagnostic performance of American college of radiology TI-RADS: a systematic review and meta-analysis. Am J Roentgenol 2021;216(1):38–47.
10. Hamour AF, Yang W, Lee JJW, et al. Association of the Implementation of a Standardized Thyroid Ultrasonography Reporting Program with Documentation of Nodule Characteristics. JAMA Otolaryngol Head Neck Surg 2021;147(4):343–9.
11. Li LR, Du B, Liu HQ, et al. Artificial intelligence for personalized medicine in thyroid cancer: current status and future perspectives. Front Oncol 2021;10. https://doi.org/10.3389/fonc.2020.604051.
12. Thomas J, Ledger GA, Mamillapalli CK. Use of artificial intelligence and machine learning for estimating malignancy risk of thyroid nodules. Curr Opin Endocrinol Diabetes Obes 2020;27(5):345–50.
13. Brito JP, Gionfriddo MR, Al Nofal A, et al. The accuracy of thyroid nodule ultrasound to predict thyroid cancer: systematic review and meta-analysis. J Clin Endocrinol Metab 2014;99(4):1253–63.
14. Wienke JR, Chong WK, Fielding JR, et al. Sonographic features of benign thyroid nodules. J Ultrasound Med 2003;22(10):1027–31.
15. Moon W-J, Lee YH, Kim J, et al. Benign and malignant thyroid purpose : methods : results : conclusion. Radiology 2008;247(3):762–70.
16. Hoang JK, Wai KL, Lee M, et al. US features of thyroid malignancy: Pearls and pitfalls. Radiographics 2007;27(3):847–60.
17. Kim DW, Lee EJ, In HS, et al. Sonographic differentiation of partially cystic thyroid nodules: A prospective study. AJNR Am J Neuroradiol 2010;31(10):1961–6.

18. Kwak JY, Han KH, Yoon JH, et al. Thyroid imaging reporting and data system for us features of nodules: a step in establishing better stratification of cancer risk. Radiology 2011;260(3):892–9.

19. Mandel SJ, Langer JE. Ultrasound of thyroid nodules. Thyroid Parathyr Ultrasound Ultrasound-Guided FNA 2018;189–223.

20. Trimboli P, Durante C. Ultrasound risk stratification systems for thyroid nodule: between lights and shadows, we are moving towards a new era. Endocrine 2020; 69(1):20–3.

21. Gharib H, Papini E, Garber JR, et al. American Association of Clinical Endocrinologists, American College of Endocrinology, and Associazione Medici Endocrinologi medical guidelines for clinical practice for the diagnosis and management of thyroid nodules - 2016 update. Endocr Pract 2016;22(May):1–60.

22. Yi KH. The revised 2016 Korean Thyroid Association guidelines for thyroid nodules and cancers: differences from the 2015 American Thyroid Association guidelines. Endocrinol Metab 2016;31(3):373–8.

23. Grani G, Lamartina L, Ascoli V, et al. Reducing the number of unnecessary thyroid biopsies while improving diagnostic accuracy: toward the "right" TIRADS. J Clin Endocrinol Metab 2019;104(1):95–102.

24. Lauria Pantano A, Maddaloni E, Briganti SI, et al. Differences between ATA, AACE/ACE/AME and ACR TI-RADS ultrasound classifications performance in identifying cytological high-risk thyroid nodules. Eur J Endocrinol 2018;178(6): 595–603.

25. Castellana M, Castellana C, Treglia G, et al. Performance of five ultrasound risk stratification systems in selecting thyroid nodules for FNA. J Clin Endocrinol Metab 2020;105(5):1–32.

26. Grani G, Lamartina L, Cantisani V, et al. Interobserver agreement of various thyroid imaging reporting and data systems. Endocr Connect 2018;7(1):1–7.

27. Karkada M, Costa AF, Imran SA, et al. Incomplete thyroid ultrasound reports for patients with thyroid nodules: Implications regarding risk assessment and management. Am J Roentgenol 2018;211(6):1348–53.

28. Griffin AS, Mitsky J, Rawal U, et al. Improved quality of thyroid ultrasound reports after implementation of the ACR thyroid imaging reporting and data system nodule lexicon and risk stratification system. J Am Coll Radiol 2018;15(5):743–8.

29. Ghazizadeh S, Kelly TL, Khajanchee YS, et al. Standardization of thyroid ultrasound reporting in the community setting decreases biopsy rates. Clin Endocrinol (Oxf) 2021;94(6):1035–42.

30. Persichetti A, Di Stasio E, Guglielmi R, et al. Predictive value of malignancy of thyroid nodule ultrasound classification systems: a prospective study. J Clin Endocrinol Metab 2018;103(4):1359–68.

31. Singh Ospina N, Papaleontiou M. Thyroid nodule evaluation and management in older adults: a review of practical considerations for clinical endocrinologists. Endocr Pract 2021;27(3):261–8.

32. Cawood TJ, Mackay GR, Hunt PJ, et al. TIRADS management guidelines in the investigation of thyroid nodules; illustrating the concerns, costs, and performance. J Endocr Soc 2020;4(4):1–13.

33. Hoang JK, Middleton WD, Tessler FN. Update on ACR TI-RADS: successes, challenges, and future directions, from the AJR special series on radiology reporting and data systems. Am J Roentgenol 2021;1–9. https://doi.org/10.2214/ajr.20. 24608.

34. Middleton WD, Teefey SA, Reading CC, et al. Comparison of performance characteristics of American College of Radiology TI-RADS, Korean Society of Thyroid

Radiology TIRADS, and American Thyroid Association guidelines. Am J Roentgenol 2018;210(5):1148–54.

35. Han K, Kim EK, Kwak JY. 1.5-2 cm tumor size was not associated with distant metastasis and mortality in small thyroid cancer: a population-based study. Sci Rep 2017;7. https://doi.org/10.1038/srep46298.

36. Shin JJ, Caragacianu D, Randolph GW. Impact of thyroid nodule size on prevalence and post-test probability of malignancy: a systematic review. Laryngoscope 2014;125(1):263–72.

37. Park VY, Lee HS, Kim EK, et al. Frequencies and malignancy rates of 6-tiered Bethesda categories of thyroid nodules according to ultrasound assessment and nodule size. Head Neck 2018;40(9):1947–54.

38. Hong MJ, Na DG, Baek JH, et al. Impact of nodule size on malignancy risk differs according to the ultrasonography pattern of thyroid nodules. Korean J Radiol 2018;19(3):534–41.

39. Machens A, Holzhausen HJ, Dralle H. The prognostic value of primary tumor size in papillary and follicular thyroid carcinoma: a comparative analysis. Cancer 2005;103(11):2269–73.

40. Ha SM, Baek JH, Na DG, et al. Diagnostic performance of practice guidelines for thyroid nodules: thyroid nodule size versus biopsy rates. Radiology 2019; 291(1):92–9.

41. Yim Y, Baek JH, Chung SR, et al. Recurrence and additional treatment of cystic thyroid nodules after ethanol ablation: validation of three proposed criteria. Ultrasonography 2021;40(3):378–86.

42. Spencer-Bonilla G, Singh Ospina N, Rodriguez-Gutierrez R, et al. Systematic reviews of diagnostic tests in endocrinology: an audit of methods, reporting, and performance. Endocrine 2017;57(1):18–34.

43. Trimboli P, Castellana M, Piccardo A, et al. The ultrasound risk stratification systems for thyroid nodule have been evaluated against papillary carcinoma. A meta-analysis. Rev Endocr Metab Disord 2021;22(2):453–60.

44. Castellana M, Piccardo A, Virili C, et al. Can ultrasound systems for risk stratification of thyroid nodules identify follicular carcinoma? Cancer Cytopathol 2020; 128(4):250–9.

45. Itani M, Assaker R, Moshiri M, et al. Inter-observer variability in the American College of Radiology thyroid imaging reporting and data system: in-depth analysis and areas for improvement. Ultrasound Med Biol 2019;45(2):461–70.

46. Basha MAA, Alnaggar AA, Refaat R, et al. The validity and reproducibility of the thyroid imaging reporting and data system (TI-RADS) in categorization of thyroid nodules: Multicentre prospective study. Eur J Radiol 2019;117(February):184–92.

47. Persichetti A, DI Stasio E, Coccaro C, et al. Inter- and intraobserver agreement in the assessment of thyroid nodule ultrasound features and classification systems: a blinded multicenter study. Thyroid 2020;30(2):237–42.

48. Liu H, Ma AL, Zhou YS, et al. Variability in the interpretation of grey-scale ultrasound features in assessing thyroid nodules: a systematic review and meta-analysis. Eur J Radiol 2020;129:109050.

49. Kwong N, Medici M, Angell TE, et al. The influence of patient age on thyroid nodule formation, multinodularity, and thyroid cancer risk. J Clin Endocrinol Metab 2015;100(12):4434–40.

50. Cherella CE, Feldman HA, Hollowell M, et al. Natural history and outcomes of cytologically benign thyroid nodules in children. J Clin Endocrinol Metab 2018; 103(9):3557–65.

51. He LZ, Zeng TS, Pu L, et al. Thyroid hormones, autoantibodies, ultrasonography, and clinical parameters for predicting thyroid cancer. Int J Endocrinol 2016;2016. https://doi.org/10.1155/2016/8215834.

52. Al Dawish MA, Robert AA, Thabet MA, et al. Thyroid nodule management: thyroid-stimulating hormone, ultrasound, and cytological classification system for predicting malignancy. Cancer Inform 2018;17.

53. Frates MC, Benson CB, Doubilet PM, et al. Prevalence and distribution of carcinoma in patients with solitary and multiple thyroid nodules on sonography. J Clin Endocrinol Metab 2006;91(9):3411–7.

54. Angell TE, Maurer R, Wang Z, et al. A cohort analysis of clinical and ultrasound variables predicting cancer risk in 20,001 consecutive thyroid nodules. J Clin Endocrinol Metab 2019;104(11):5665–72.

55. Pazaitou-Panayiotou K, Capezzone M, Pacini F. Clinical features and therapeutic implication of papillary thyroid microcarcinoma. Thyroid 2007;17(11):1085–92.

56. Furuya-Kanamori L, Bell KJL, Clark J, et al. Prevalence of differentiated thyroid cancer in autopsy studies over six decades: a meta-analysis. J Clin Oncol 2016;34(30):3672–9.

57. Charkes ND. On the prevalence of familial nonmedullary thyroid cancer in multiply affected kindreds. Thyroid 2006;16(2):181–6.

58. Schneider AB. Dose-response relationships for radiation-induced thyroid cancer and thyroid nodules: evidence for the prolonged effects of radiation on the thyroid. J Clin Endocrinol Metab 1993;77(2):362–9.

59. Somerville HM, Steinbeck KS, Stevens G, et al. Thyroid neoplasia following irradiation in adolescent and young adult survivors of childhood cancer. Med J Aust 2002;176(12):584–7.

60. White MG, Cipriani NA, Abdulrasool L, et al. Radiation-induced differentiated thyroid cancer is associated with improved overall survival but not thyroid cancer-specific mortality or disease-free survival. Thyroid 2016;26(8):1053–60.

61. Pacini F, Vorontsova T, Demidchik EP, et al. Post-chernobyl thyroid carcinoma in Belarus children and adolescents: comparison with naturally occurring thyroid carcinoma in Italy and France. J Clin Endocrinol Metab 1997;82(11):3563–9.

62. Wang Z, Vyas CM, Van Benschoten O, et al. Quantitative analysis of the benefits and risk of thyroid nodule evaluation in patients $\geq$70 years old. Thyroid 2018; 28(4):465–71.

63. Stead WW. Clinical implications and challenges of artificial intelligence and deep learning. JAMA 2018;320(11):1107–8.

64. Matheny MS, Israni ST, Ahmed M, et al, Editors. Artificial Intelligence in Health Care: The Hope, the Hype, the Promise, the Peril. Washington, DC: National Academy of Medicine Special Publication; 2019.

65. Gubbi S, Hamet P, Tremblay J, et al. Artificial intelligence and machine learning in endocrinology and metabolism: the dawn of a new era. Front Endocrinol (Lausanne) 2019;10:185. Available at: http://www.embase.com/search/results?subaction=viewrecord&from=export&id=L627959380%0Ahttps://doi.org/10.3389/fendo.2019.00185.

66. Hinton G. Deep learning-a technology with the potential to transform health care. JAMA 2018;320(11):1101–2.

67. Liu Y, Chen P-HC, Krause J, et al. How to read articles that use machine learning. JAMA 2019;322(18):1806.

68. Nagendran M, Chen Y, Lovejoy CA, et al. Artificial intelligence versus clinicians: systematic review of design, reporting standards, and claims of deep learning studies in medical imaging. BMJ 2020;368. https://doi.org/10.1136/bmj.m689.

69. Li X, Zhang S, Zhang Q, et al. Diagnosis of thyroid cancer using deep convolutional neural network models applied to sonographic images: a retrospective, multicohort, diagnostic study. Lancet Oncol 2019;20(2):193–201.
70. Chambara N, Ying M. The diagnostic efficiency of ultrasound computer–aided diagnosis in differentiating thyroid nodules: a systematic review and narrative synthesis. Cancers (Basel) 2019;11(11). https://doi.org/10.3390/cancers 11111759.
71. Edwards MK, Singh Ospina N. Implementation of thyroid nodule risk stratification in a high volume clinic. Clin Thyroidol 2021;33(5):221–4.
72. Buda M, Wildman-Tobriner B, Hoang JK, et al. Management of thyroid nodules seen on us images: deep learning may match performance of radiologists. Radiology 2019;292(3):695–701.
73. Zhang B, Tian J, Pei S, et al. Machine learning-assisted system for thyroid nodule diagnosis. Thyroid 2019;29(6):858–67.
74. Hammad ARY, Noureldine SI, Hu T, et al. A meta-analysis examining the independent association between thyroid nodule size and malignancy. Gland Surg 2016; 5(3):312–7.
75. Wildman-Tobriner B, Buda M, Hoang JK, et al. Using artificial intelligence to revise ACR TI-RADS risk stratification of thyroid nodules: diagnostic accuracy and utility. Radiology 2019;292(1):112–9.
76. Xu L, Gao J, Wang Q, et al. Computer-aided diagnosis systems in diagnosing malignant thyroid nodules on ultrasonography: a systematic review and meta-analysis. Eur Thyroid J 2020;9(4):186–93.
77. Thomas J, Haertling T. AIBx, artificial intelligence model to risk stratify thyroid nodules. Thyroid 2020;30(6):878–84.
78. Doshi-Velez F, Perlis RH. Evaluating machine learning articles. JAMA 2019; 322(18):1777–9.
79. Amann J, Blasimme A, Vayena E, et al. Explainability for artificial intelligence in healthcare: a multidisciplinary perspective. BMC Med Inform Decis Mak 2020; 20(1). https://doi.org/10.1186/s12911-020-01332-6.

Minimally Invasive Techniques for the Management of Thyroid Nodules

Chelsey K. Baldwin, MD, ECNU[a,*], Michael B. Natter, MD[a],
Kepal N. Patel, MD[b], Steven P. Hodak, MD, ECNU[a]

KEYWORDS

- Thyroid nodule • Thyroid neoplasms • Minimally invasive therapy • Ethanol ablation
- Thermal ablation • Radiofrequency ablation • Laser ablation

KEY POINTS

- Data increasingly support the use of minimally invasive techniques (MITs) as nonsurgical options for the treatment of thyroid disease.
- MITs are typically performed in the ambulatory setting under local anesthesia. This facilitates rapid treatment and discharge postprocedure.
- Evidence supports the use of MIT for the treatment of select benign symptomatic and autonomously functional thyroid nodules. Recent literature demonstrates the potential for MIT in the treatment of primary papillary thyroid cancer as well as recurrent disease.
- These techniques require training, practice, and competent understanding of cervical anatomy to minimize risk and produce successful outcomes. When performed by an experienced operator, risks associated with RFA are typically lower than those associated with surgical management creating a favorable risk to benefit ratio.

Thyroid nodules are common and the majority are benign and do not require intervention.[1] A subset of benign thyroid nodules (BTN) may be symptomatic or autonomously functional requiring definitive treatment. Radioactive iodine (RAI) is effective in treating autonomously functional thyroid nodules (AFTN), but can render the patient permanently hypothyroid and presents risks of salivary and lacrimal gland injury as well as potential risks of secondary malignancy. Surgical management is appropriate for BTN and thyroid cancers requiring definitive management. Surgery requires hospital admission, general anesthesia, and even if the procedure is limited to lobectomy up to 23.6% of patients will remain permanently hypothyroid.[2] Surgery also conveys a

[a] Department of Medicine, Diabetes and Endocrinology Section, New York University School of Medicine, 222 East, 41st Street, Floor 23, NY 10016, USA; [b] Otolaryngology and Biochemistry, Division of Endocrine Surgery, Department of Surgery, Division of Endocrine Surgery, New York University School of Medicine, 530 1st Avenue, Floor 12, NY 10016, USA
* Corresponding author.
E-mail address: Chelsey.Baldwin@nyulangone.org

Endocrinol Metab Clin N Am 51 (2022) 323–349
https://doi.org/10.1016/j.ecl.2022.01.001
0889-8529/22/© 2022 Elsevier Inc. All rights reserved.

endo.theclinics.com

small risk of permanent hypoparathyroidism and voice changes. Alternatives to both surgery and RAI are appealing, and recent innovation in MIT for the management of thyroid nodules may provide such an alternative.

MIT uses a variety of ultrasound-guided percutaneous methods performed in the outpatient setting under local anesthesia with the optional addition of a mild sedative. MIT is associated with no or minimal scarring, rapid recovery, and almost never results in hypothyroidism in appropriately selected patients.

The composition, size, and functional status of thyroid nodules dictate both the selection and success of each modality of MIT. The goal of this article is to present the various MIT modalities, discussion of indications, techniques, risks, and outcomes.

MIT MODALITIES
Simple aspiration

Outcomes by indication
Cystic and predominantly cystic nodules. Predominantly cystic nodules are composed of greater than 50% fluid by volume and are overwhelmingly benign[3] but may still produce compressive and cosmetic symptoms. These symptoms can often be immediately relieved by simple aspiration and drainage. However without the use of sclerosing agent (typically 95%–98% dehydrated ethanol) cystic fluid reaccumulation occurs in 58%–81%[4,5] of cases. Despite the relatively high likelihood of fluid reaccumulation, the procedure is low risk and allows the acquisition of diagnostic cytology to confirm benignity before more definitive treatment such as ethanol ablation (EA), thermal ablation, or surgery. Simple aspiration (**Fig. 1**) is, therefore, often a reasonable first step in the management of predominantly cystic nodules.[6]

Technique
Please refer to the included Appendix 1 for the discussion of the technique for simple aspiration of predominantly cystic nodules.

Ethanol ablation

Outcomes by indication
Pure cyst and predominantly cystic nodules. In the case of reaccumulation of a predominantly cystic nodule, ethanol sclerotherapy commonly referred to as EA offers an effective means of therapeutic escalation after negative cytology has been verified[6] (**Fig. 2**). EA may be used as first-line therapy for the initial treatment of purely cystic nodules without confirming benign cytology given the risk of malignancy is less than 1%.[7] Injection of 95% to 99% ethanol into an evacuated cyst causes coagulative and ischemic necrosis of the cyst epithelium and small vessels in contact with ethanol including inducing reactive fibrosis that can prevent the reaccumulation of cystic contents. EA is 85% to 98% effective in pure cysts and 60% to 90% effective in predominantly cystic nodules (>50% cystic).[6] The ability to evacuate all cystic fluid contents before ethanol instillation has been shown to predict higher success rate (93.3%) versus nodules with a lesser degree of cystic fluid evacuation.[4] However it's noteworthy that even when EA sufficiently resolves the cystic component of a complex thyroid nodule, Jang and colleagues reported that patient satisfaction may decline when the initial solid component exceeds 20%.[8]

Autonomously functioning thyroid nodules. EA for AFTN was first proposed in 1990 by Livraghi and colleagues who reported that multiple and serial injections of 1 to 5 mL of 95% ethanol-induced coagulative necrosis leading to the normalization of thyroid function, nodule volume reduction, and normalization of nuclear scintigraphy.[9,10]

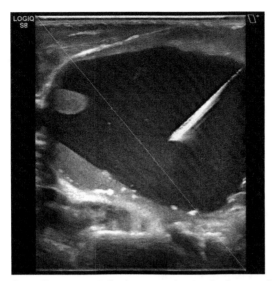

Fig. 1. Placement of Needle via transisthmic approach into the lumen of cyst.

Complete responses ranged from 64% to 85% and nodule volumes greater than 15 mL were associated with poor response.[11] Papini and colleagues subsequently suggested that EA might be particularly useful in young patients with nontoxic AFTN in which progression over lifetime is likely, nodules tend to be smaller, and as a way of avoiding hypothyroidism following surgical management or RAI.[12] Papini and colleagues reported EA success rates of greater than 90% in nontoxic AFTN.[11] A newer vascularity targeted ethanol injection technique has been described by Sharma and colleagues which requires fewer ethanol injections and smaller volumes of ethanol (median 0.46 mL/mL nodule volume), resulting in an increase in TSH in 83% of patients and TSH normalization in 61%, n = 18.[13] However, median nodule volume in this study was 5.7 mL and large nodule volume greater than 20 mL was cited as the cause for 2/5 reported procedure failures.

Despite the low rate of malignancy in AFTN we still recommend obtaining benign cytology on one occasion before EA since papillary thyroid carcinoma in these functional thyroid nodules may still rarely occur.[14]

Recurrent papillary thyroid cancer. A growing literature supports the use of EA as a 2nd line intervention for treated recurrent PTC in appropriately selected cases. Though there are no head-to-head comparisons of surgical management and EA, meta-analysis data including 27 studies with a total of 1617 patients that though the surgery was statistically superior to EA rates of posttreatment cervical recurrence as well as complications, both were low and statistically similar for both procedures. However, the authors note that cases in the surgery cohort represented more histologically aggressive PTC recurrence, and patients treated with EA were generally older with more clinically indolent disease underscoring the clinical superiority of surgical management. The authors conclude that though surgical management remains the most definitive management option for recurrent PTC, EA can be effective for treating selected lesions when a "berry picking" approach is reasonable.[15]

Long-term follow-up of patients following EA is relatively scant but Hay and colleagues report over 5 years of mean follow-up for 25 patients with recurrent PTC

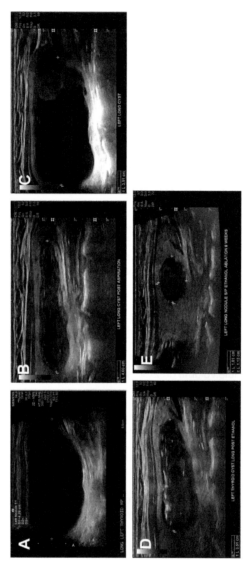

Fig. 2. Case of a 37-year-old female with cosmetic and compressive symptoms due to left-sided predominantly cystic nodule (*A*) Initial ultrasound evaluation (*B*) Status post simple aspiration (*C*) Reaccumulation of cystic fluid at 1-month follow-up (*D*) Immediately post ethanol aspiration (*E*) sustained benefit at 8-weeks post ethanol ablation.

with a total of 37 foci of cervical nodal recurrence.[16] Of 37 treated lesions 35 (95%) demonstrated a decrease in lesion size, 17 (46%) demonstrated complete ultrasonographic resolution, and all lesions seemed avascular by Doppler flow on follow-up. Subsequent disease recurrence at different sites was noted in 6 patients with a total of 18 new lesions of which 15 (83%) were successfully treated with additional EA. The authors further note that EA allowed avoidance of 40 neck reoperations at an aggregate cost savings of more than $61,000.

In patients with smaller foci of recurrent PTC, EA has been shown to have efficacy similar to the RFA with statistically similar outcomes both for VRR and complete disappearance of the targeted lesion. The rate of complications following RFA and EA were also statistically similar leading the authors to conclude that both RFA and EA are similarly effective interventions for patients with locally recurrent thyroid cancer who are not candidates for surgical management.

We agree that though surgery remains the most definitive method for control of locoregionally recurrent PTC EA may be effective for patients who are not ideal candidates for surgery, especially in the case of pauci-metastatic small volume locoregional recurrence, and may result in considerable cost savings when compared with surgery.

Technique
Please refer to the included Appendix 1 (**Figs. 3–6**) for the discussion of the technique for the EA of cystic lesions and recurrent PTC.

Thermal ablation

Thermal ablation includes a number of methods that generally employ the use of nonionizing electromagnetic energy to produce heat-induced coagulative necrosis of target tissue.

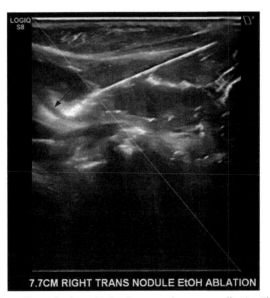

Fig. 3. Hyperechoic artifact of ethanol injection can obscure needle tip. Blue arrow demonstrates ethanol flow from the needle tip.

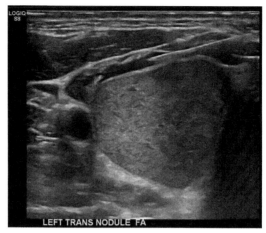

Fig. 4. Lidocaine 1% applied to anesthetize the thyroid capsule appears as an anechoic band separating the thyroid capsule and anterior lying sternothyroid muscle.

Radiofrequency ablation

Thyroid radiofrequency ablation (RFA) involved the percutaneous insertion of a 19 to 20 G internally water-cooled radiofrequency electrode to deliver electromagnetic energy in the range of 450 to 1200 kHz to cause friction between charged ions resulting in thermal injury and subsequent coagulative necrosis. Initially described for the treatment of hepatocellular disease, RFA was first used for the treatment of thyroid cancer lymph node metastasis in 1998. An early obstacle for thyroid RFA was unintended collateral tissue necrosis of nearby structures around the treatment target due to the distant propagation of heat generated during the procedure. Pivotal breakthroughs in thyroid RFA technique included the 1996 development of internally water-cooled electrodes that minimize thermal propagation,[17] and the transisthmic moving shot technique in 2008[18] which allows improved control of the treatment zone.. Though RFA has been successfully used in Asia and Europe for over a decade [19,20] whereby numerous guidelines have been developed (**Table 1**), FDA approval of RFA for the treatment of soft tissue disease including structural thyroid disease was only granted in 2018 making the procedure still relatively new in the US (RFA Approval

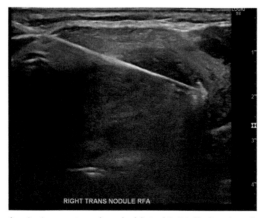

Fig. 5. The marginal vein is punctured and ablated initially by the electrode tip to avoid heat sink and promote peripheral treatment.

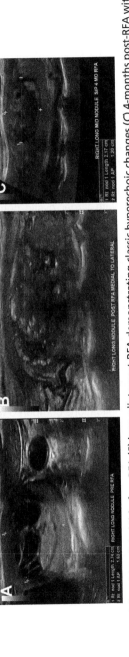

Fig. 6. Right-sided thyroid nodule (A) before RFA (B) immediate post-RFA demonstrating classic hyperechoic changes (C) 4-months post-RFA with classic dense hypoechoic appearance.

letter, March 14, 2018, Retrieved May 1, 2021 https://www.accessdata.fda.gov/cdrh_docs/pdf17/K172012.pdf). Additionally, RFA lacks a CPT billing code and is still considered an experimental procedure by most payers within the US limiting reimbursement and therefore access for many patients. Despite an extensive international literature demonstrating the efficacy and safety of RFA, the US experience has remained limited and further published studies using US populations will be needed to support the development of a CPT code that will allow reimbursement for what is now almost exclusively a cash-only procedure.

Outcomes by indication

Benign symptomatic predominantly solid thyroid nodules Benign nodules causing cosmetic or compressive symptoms can be effectively treated with RFA with an expected volume reduction rate (VRR) of 50%–88.2% over the course of 6 to 18 months.[21,22] Patients reported significant improvement in cosmetic scores[23,24] and compressive symptom scores.[25]

Factors impacting efficacy include the feasibility of complete nodule treatment impacted by proximity to high-risk structures, nodule size, and nodule composition. Smaller nodule size and those with larger cystic components are associated with the greatest VRR.[21,26] Though a single competently performed RFA is effective in most cases, multiple treatments may be necessary in nodules greater than 30 mL[25] or in the case of marginal regrowth of previously treated lesions.[27]

Compared with surgical management which is the traditional first-line treatment of symptomatic benign nodules, it is important to educate patients that the benefit of RFA is not immediate, and instead accrues over the course of months. The VRR within the first 3 to 6 months occurs at the most rapid rate with continued but more gradual volume reduction over the following 6 to 18 months, as shown in a prospective single-center Austrian study which demonstrated a VRR of 68% and 82% at 3 and 12 months, respectively.[26] Despite this delay in therapeutic benefit one retrospective study demonstrated the efficacy and safety of RFA (n = 200) compared with patients managed surgically (n = 200) for cytologic benign symptomatic or functional thyroid nodules. RFA treated nodules demonstrated a mean 84.8% volume reduction at 1 year and had a lower risk of complications compared with those managed surgically, 1% versus 6%, $P = .002$.[28] Notably, the risk of postprocedural hypothyroidism was significantly lower after RFA versus surgery, 0.13% versus 71.5%, respectively.[28] Cases of post-RFA hypothyroidism are rarely reported to occur in patients with high titer of TPO or Tg antibodies before RFA.[29,30] Costs of RFA and surgery were similar in this study but the cost of thyroid surgery in China was reported to be $2556.95 ± $171.88 compared with an average US Medicare cost of $5784 (https://www.medicare.gov/procedure-price-lookup/cost/60210 accessed 8/7/2021), suggesting that cost–benefit comparison is location dependent.

Bernardi and colleagues[24] compared RFA to hemithyroidectomy for the alleviation of nodule-related symptoms and found that though symptomatic and cosmetic outcomes were not statistically different following patients with RFA experienced significantly less procedure-related pain, hypothyroidism, and complications.

The sustainability of nodule volume reduction after RFA treatment was illustrated in a study of 111 patients with benign, nonfunctional thyroid nodules that demonstrated a mean volume reduction of 93.4% maintained over 3 years of follow-up with only a 5.6% rate of recurrence (increase of >50% of volume) attributed peripheral regrowth.[31]

Autonomous functioning thyroid nodules In 2008, Baek and colleagues[32] published the first case report of the successful use of RFA for AFTN. Subsequent studies

Table 1
Current RFA pre procedure requirements and indication by guidelines

Guidelines	Pre - Procedure Work up	First-Line Indications	Second-Line Indications
KSThR 2017	Two benign FNA/CNB Exception: One benign FNA/CNB in AFTN or K-TIRADS 2	Compressive or cosmetic symptomatic nonfunctional predominantly solid nodule Toxic or pretoxic AFTNs	Cystic/predominantly cystic nodule (after failed EA) Primary or recurrent thyroid neoplasms in patients refusing or unable to undergo surgery
AACE/ACE/AME 2016	Two benign FNA/CNB	Compressive or cosmetic symptomatic nonfunctional predominantly solid nodule	
NICE 2016	Two benign FNA/CNB	Compressive or cosmetic symptomatic benign thyroid nodules	
MITT group 2019	Two benign FNA/CNB Exception: One benign FNA/CNB in AFTN or EU-TIRADS 2, 3 Repeat FNA after initial RFA, before re-treatment in the setting of regrowth	Compressive or cosmetic symptomatic nonfunctional predominantly solid nodule	Cystic/predominantly cystic nodule (after failed EA) Dominant nodule in nontoxic MNG refusing surgery AFTN in patient refusing surgery or RAI Small AFTN in patients prioritizing sparing thyroid tissue and >80% of nodule ablation expected
Austrian professional associations 2019	Two benign FNA/CNB	Compressive or cosmetic symptomatic benign thyroid nodules Unifocal AFTN <15 mL	

(continued on next page)

Table 1
(continued)

Guidelines	Pre - Procedure Work up	First-Line Indications	Second-Line Indications
ETA 2020	Two benign FNA/CNB Exception: One benign FNA/CNB of spongiform or pure cystic lesions	Compressive or cosmetic symptomatic predominately solid benign thyroid nodules well defined dominant nodule of MNG Small AFTN and incomplete suppression of the perinodular thyroid issue	Cystic or predominantly cystic nodules that failed EA Large AFTN in patients who decline surgery or RAI Large AFTN with compressive symptoms may consider concurrent RAI and TA (RFA or LTA) for more rapid therapeutic response

Abbreviations: AACE/ACE/AME, American Association of Clinical Endocrinology/American College of Endocrinology/Associazione Medici Endocrinologi; AFTN, autonomous functioning thyroid nodule; CNB, Core needle biopsy; EA, ethanol ablation; ETA, European Thyroid Association; EU-TIRADS- European thyroid imaging reporting, and data system; FNA, fine needle aspiration; KSThR, Korean Society of Thyroid Radiology; K-TIRADS, Korean thyroid imaging reporting and data system; LTA, laser thermal ablation; MITT, minimally invasive treatment of thyroid; MNG, multinodular goiter; NICE, National Institute for Health and Care Excellence; RAI, radioactive iodine; TA, thermal ablation.

have reported variable efficacy of RFA for the treatment of AFTN with the improvement of thyroid function tests, discontinuation of antithyroidal medication, and scintigraphic evidence of response in66.7%–100%,[30,33,34] 22.7%–78.6%,[22,34–36] and44.4%–79.5%[30,34] of cases, respectively.

Cesareo and colleagues published a prospective study that demonstrated that RF outcomes for AFTN were dependent on nodule size: nodules less than 12 mL had larger VRR, greater increases in TSH, and significantly higher cure rate.[37] Additionally, they showed higher pretreatment AFTN volume was a negative predictor for the normalization of thyroid function.[38] This is consistent with the Austrian guidelines that support the use of RFA in AFTN less than 15 mL.[39]

Controversy still exists over whether initial nodule volume and the number of RFA treatments is accurate predictors of outcome as these findings have not been consistently significant.[40] Bernardi and colleagues reported that following RFA of patients with AFTN with complete normalization of thyroid function had an average of 81% volume reduction versus 68% volume reduction in those with only a partial response whereby thyroid function did not fully normalize,[36] suggesting that the ability to deliver complete treatment to the target nodule and not just initial nodule size is the critical factor impacting treatment outcome. This has been recognized by the Italian minimally invasive treatment of the thyroid group (MITT) group that recommends the consideration of RFA as a second-line intervention for AFTN when projected treated volume reduction will be at least 80%.[19]

Sung and colleagues demonstrate in a retrospective multi-institution study of 44 patients, that repeat sessions of RFA may be necessary for adequate response TSH normalization occurred in 81.7% of patients with AFTN with a mean initial nodule volume of 18.5 mL $\pm$ 30.1 mL. Treatment required a mean of 1.8 $\pm$ 0.9 sessions but up to 6 RFA sessions were necessary for the complete treatment of AFTN with attention to the adequate treatment of the marginal zones that could otherwise result in neoplastic regrowth of unabated tissue.[34]

Pretoxic nodules, defined as AFTN that do not suppress surrounding thyroid tissue on scintigraphy may respond to RFA better than more overtly functional thyroid nodules; Spiezia and colleagues reported 100% of patients with pretoxic nodules were able to discontinue antithyroid drugs following RFA versus 53% with toxic nodules.[35] Because of these findings, the European Thyroid Association 2020 guideline supports the first-line use of RFA for the treatment of pretoxic AFTN.[41]

Radioactive iodine (RAI) and surgery are the most commonly recommended first-line treatments for AFTN, though RFA is now recognized as a reasonable second-line option. There are a few studies in which RFA has been compared with these standards of care. To our knowledge, only a single retrospective study of 50 nodules compares RAI and RFA for the treatment of AFTN. Nodules were treated with fixed dose of 15 mCi of RAI (n = 25; mean pretreatment volume 11.0 mL) or 1 session of RFA (n = 25; mean pretreatment volume 14.3 mL).[33] The study demonstrated 100% efficacy restoring euthyroid function in both groups however RFA demonstrated a significantly larger VRR of 76.4% compared with RAI VRR of 68.4% ($P > .05$). Hypothyroidism occurred in 20% of patients treated with RAI and none of the patients treated with RFA leading the study authors to suggest that RFA may be a preferable option for the treatment of AFTN.

A 2014 retrospective study by Bernardi and colleagues comparing RFA to surgical management of thyroid nodules included a small subset of AFTN treated by RFA versus Surgery (n = 12; n = 20, respectively). Not surprisingly, the cure rate following thyroidectomy was 100% compared with only 33% of patients whose hyperthyroidism resolved following RFA.[24]

Predominantly cystic nodules (cystic component 50%–90%) Ethanol ablation of predominantly cystic nodules has demonstrated superior volume reduction compared with RFA, with a mean volume reduction of 81.1% versus 70.8%, respectively.[42] And Baek and colleagues did not demonstrate the superiority of RFA to EA in predominantly cystic nodules when superiority was defined as greater than 13% difference in VRR. Data suggest that EA is preferable first-line intervention for predominantly cystic nodules.[43] However, RFA may be considered as a second-line option after the failure of EA.[19,41,44] In 2011, Jang and colleagues showed that approximately a third of patients with predominantly cystic nodules, typically those with solid component greater than 20%, could be effectively treated with subsequent RFA leading to significant improvement in cosmetic and symptom scores as well as significant volume reduction of 92%, $P > .001$.[8]

Combined and simultaneous use of sclerotherapy and RFA has also been proposed. Shen and colleagues studied 119 patients with mixed solid cystic nodules treated with a combination of RFA for solid portions and polidocanol sclerotherapy in cystic portions resulting in VRR of 91.08%,[45] however the study is limited by lack of comparison to RFA or sclerotherapy only control groups.

Thyroid neoplasms Radiofrequency ablation (RFA) is also emerging as a useful tool for the management of small primary papillary thyroid cancers, follicular neoplasm, and locoregionally recurrent papillary thyroid cancer. Limited data do not support the use of RFA for the treatment of more aggressive thyroid carcinomas such as anaplastic carcinoma and medullary thyroid cancer.

Papillary thyroid cancer: The safety and efficacy of RFA for the treatment of papillary thyroid micro-carcinoma (PTMC) has been well demonstrated,[46,47] suggesting that in addition to observational management RFA may be another useful nonsurgical alternative for management. Complete or near-complete resolution of micro-PTC has been repeatedly demonstrated[47–49] including the treatment of bilateral PTMC foci.[50] Emerging data also show the efficacy of RFA treatment of larger primary tumors up to T1bN0.[51] These studies generally include cytologically confirmed solitary papillary thyroid carcinomas without aggressive clinical and ultrasonographic features in patients not otherwise suitable for surgical intervention.[46] Though literature is limited and additional studies are necessary, it still seems that RFA can be a useful alternative to surgery for small and otherwise low-risk papillary thyroid cancers.

Recurrent papillary thyroid cancer: A retrospective study by Choi and colleagues compared RFA and repeat surgical management for the treatment of patients with fewer than 3 foci of recurrent PTC. There was no statistically significant difference in recurrence-free survival between groups; however, there was a significantly higher risk of both hypocalcemia and overall complication rate among the patients managed with surgery.[52]

Chung and colleagues published a retrospective single institution study examining long-term outcomes among 29 patients with a total of 46 recurrent foci of PTC treated with RFA all of whom had a minimum of 5 years of posttreatment follow-up. Complete resolution was noted in 91% of cases. Though new locoregional recurrence and distant metastasis developed in 8 of 29 (28%), and 2 of 29 (7%) patients, respectively, 19 of 29 (66%) patients remained disease free with no long-term complications due to RFA at a mean of 80-months follow-up.[53]

Chung and colleagues also performed a meta-analysis including 24 studies, 2421 patients, and 2786 thyroid nodules to determine the safety of RFA for the treatment of benign nodules and recurrent thyroid cancers. Not surprisingly, complications occurred more frequently following the treatment of recurrent cancer compared with benign nodules. The authors suggest that the absence of normal thyroid tissue surrounding BTN and operator inexperience which could not be determined in the meta-analysis may explain the outcome differences. They nonetheless conclude that despite a slightly great risk of complication compared with the treatment of benign nodules, RFA is still a relatively safe and effective treatment of recurrent PTC.[54]

Follicular neoplasm: Surgery remains the standard of care for follicular neoplasms as only histologic examination can confirm the presence or absence of capsular and vascular invasion that distinguishes follicular thyroid carcinoma (FTC) from benign follicular neoplasm. However, as most of the follicular neoplasms are histologically benign great interest in less invasive methods such as RFA despite a generally sparse and controversial literature.[55] The use of RFA for follicular adenomas was discouraged by Dobrinja and colleagues who reported treatment of 6 ultrasonographically bland follicular neoplasms ranging in size from 2 to 40 mL. Of 6 treated nodules greater than 20 mL at the time of initial treatment regrew at 6 and 24 months of follow-up and were proven to be FTC following surgical excision. They conclude that RFA may delay surgical management for patients harboring follicular thyroid cancer and question whether RFA itself might induce neoplastic transformation.[56] Conversely, Ha and colleagues reported successful management of 1 to 2 cm nodules cytologic follicular neoplasms in 10 patients who refused surgery. Outcomes included 99.5% mean volume reduction, with 8/10 nodules completely disappearing, and no recurrence by final follow averaging more than 5 years.[57] Lesion size may be the critical factor differentiating the outcomes in these 2 small studies: Histologically follicular neoplasms greater than 4 cm have been shown to have a malignancy rate of 31% versus 13% for lesions less than 4 cm ($P = .05$)[58] and Machens and colleagues previously showed that the risk of all metastasis from FTC was nearly zero in tumors < 2 cm.[59] The noted differences in size may, therefore, explain the differences in outcomes noted by Dobrinja and Ha and colleagues and may suggest that for smaller follicular neoplasms that are very unlikely to have undergone malignant transformation RFA may be effective.

Though RFA is an alluring alternative for minimally invasive treatment of smaller follicular neoplasms, data remain extremely limited, and far more study is needed before an adequately supported recommendation can be made.

Device and techniques. Please refer to the included Appendix 1 for the discussion of the technique for RFA of thyroid nodules.

Laser ablation
Laser is a highly columnated, coherent, monochromatic energy source uniquely suited for thermal ablation because it can precisely deliver energy to an intended treatment target via an optical fiber. The feasibility of percutaneous laser ablation (LA) for the treatment of thyroid nodules was initially proposed by Pacella in 2000.[60]

Device and technique. Please refer to the included Appendix 1 for the discussion of the technique for LA of thyroid nodules.

Summary of clinical outcomes. A multicenter retrospective review by Pacella demonstrated that LA may be effectively and reproducibly provided in an ambulatory setting (n = 1531 patients) with a mean nodule volume reduction of 72% $\pm$ 11% (range 48%–96%), significant improvement in both compressive and cosmetic symptoms, and a low complication rate of 0.9%.[61]

Clinical outcomes following LA and RFA have also been compared with determine whether one method is conclusively superior. A large meta-analysis by Trimboli included 12 studies using RFA and an additional 12 studies using LA for the treatment of thyroid nodules.[62] Though a greater VRR was demonstrated with RFA the authors note that marked heterogeneity in the size and type of nodules limit the ability of the study to conclude RFA is a superior method. A more recent 6-month, single-center, randomized, open-label, parallel trial compared outcomes among 60 patients with nonfunctional benign thyroid nodules (NFBTN) randomly assigned to receive either a single session of RFA or LA. A successful procedure was defined as a >50% reduction in nodule volume at 6-month and both RFA and LA demonstrated statistically identical success rates of 86.7% and 66.7%, respectively ($P = .13$). Both methods also achieved similar reductions in compressive symptoms and cosmetic score; however, RFA demonstrated a statistically superior VRR of 64.3% compared with 53.2% for LA ($P = .02$).[63]

One group of authors has found that LA is more common in Europe but RFA is more widely used in Asia.[62] Our experience is that clinicians that routinely offer thermal ablation treatments for thyroid nodules are increasingly migrating away from LA in favor of RFA because of its superior VRR and relative ease of use. Nonetheless, LA remains a widely used and effective thermal ablation method.

High-intensity focused ultrasound

High-intensity focused ultrasound (HIFU) is a form of thermal ablation first introduced in the 1940s when it was observed that focusing high-power ultrasound beams at a distance from a source could cause complete necrosis of tissues lying within the focus.[64] It is a noninvasive modality that uses sound waves to cause intense vibrations which, in turn, generates frictional heat to cause necrosis within the target. For the thyroid gland, the first clinical report described the successful ablation of a 1 cm toxic adenoma that became cystic 2 weeks after the application.[65] Biochemical euthyroidism was attained within 3 months and maintained for up to 18 months. The target nodule also shrank and became a tiny hypoechoic scar with no demonstrable Doppler flow. The authors concluded that HIFU might be a safe and effective treatment of small-sized toxic thyroid adenomas.

Device and technique. Please refer to the included Appendix 1 for the discussion of the technique for HIFU of thyroid nodules.

Advantages and disadvantages of high-intensity focused ultrasound. One of the major advantages of HIFU ablation is that it is truly noninvasive. There is no skin or nodule puncture making infection and bleeding extremely rare. This benefit is particularly important for patients who are anticoagulated and HIFU ablation is reportedly safe to perform without withholding any of these agents before the procedure.[66] The major disadvantage of HIFU ablation is that the treatment efficacy is less predictable when compared with other forms of MITs. This is because the acoustic energy needs to propagate through multiple tissue layers before reaching the thyroid. As a result, the energy can become attenuated by the tissue layers on top of the target. HIFU ablation is less suited in patients with thick necks or deep-seated nodules because of energy attenuation. Unwanted prefocal heating to the skin, subcutaneous tissues, and muscles can also occur and both cause discomfort and reduce treatment efficacy. This is likely the main reason that treatment outcomes are variable in the literature. Fortunately, with currently available HIFU technology the frequency of skin burns has declined to 1%.[67–69]

Summary of clinical outcomes. HIFU lacks data from high-quality prospective studies. Two systematic reviews of HIFU for benign nonfunctional nodules reported pooled volume reductions of 45% to 70% ranging from 3 to 24 months of follow-up.[70] As with other thermal ablation techniques, there is an inverse correlation between initial nodule size and final volume reduction.[71,72] Thyroid function is rarely affected by HIFU treatment of an isolated nodule.[73]

Microwave ablation

Microwave ablation uses electromagnetic waves in the microwave energy spectrum (300 MHz to 300 GHz) to produce tissue-heating effects. The oscillation of polar molecules produces frictional heating, ultimately generating tissue necrosis within solid tumors.[74] Because an electromagnetic field is used instead of an electrical current, electrical conduction is not necessary. The effectiveness and safety of MWA has been demonstrated in many articles.[75–78]

Device and technique. Please refer to the included Appendix 1 for the discussion of the technique for MWA of thyroid nodules.

Advantages and disadvantages of Microwave ablation. Compared with RFA, MWA uses higher frequency waves and thus has higher speed of temperature rise and smaller ablation zones. The reduction in treatment time may be more valuable when treating larger tumors. The restricted ablation zone could help avoid injury to critical structures around the tumor. However, as a result of rapid temperature rise, the carbonization of tumor may be more severe than RFA and may block heat transmission. As a result, a moving-shot ablation technique should be used in large tumors.

Summary of clinical outcomes. A meta-analysis of 7 studies of MWA for BTN (1146 subjects and 1226 nodules) showed a pooled VRR of 63% (CI: 84.0%–100.6%, I2 = 24%) at 12 months postablation.[75] Symptom and cosmetic scores were significantly lower postablation with pooled mean differences of 1.50 (CI: −0.4, 3.42) and 1.20 (CI: 0.87, 1.52), respectively. In addition, the overall complication rate was low (0%–4.6%) with voice change and hematoma being the most common major complication. A more recent meta-analysis comparing MWA and RFA for BTN demonstrated a pooled VRR of 80.0% (CI: 76.6%–83.5%, I^2 = 74.1%) at 12 months postablation, and noted that VRR was not statistically different at 3 and 6 months, but was lower at 12 months when compared with RFA (80.0 vs 86.2%, P = .036).[76]

Complications and risks of minimally invasive techniques

The confines of neck anatomy and the numerous proximate critical structures such as the trachea, esophagus great vessels, nerve plexi, recurrent laryngeal nerves (**Fig. 7**), and parathyroid glands (**Fig. 8**) require the operator to have an understanding of the mechanism by which each MIT treatment is delivered as well as expertise with cervical ultrasound anatomy to avoid potentially serious complications.

A meta-analysis of randomized control trials of MIT modalities for the treatment of BTN found no significant difference in the rate of complications among the various modalities.[42] However, some complications, for example, rare reports of inebriated sensation after EA or transient hyperthyroidism after the treated of AFTN are unique to the modality and target lesion, respectively. **Table 2** summarizes the side effects of MIT by modality.

Anticoagulation and procedure-related bleeding complications

Retrospective studies have led to general agreement that conventional anticoagulation/antiplatelet therapy (AC/AP) including agents such as aspirin, clopidogrel, cilostazol, or warfarin both as monotherapy and in combination may be safely continued before FNA with no statistically significant difference in the rate of postprocedural hematoma, bleeding, nondiagnostic aspirates, or other complication.[79–83] A single report

Table 2
Reported risks of MIT by treatment modality (implied rates were not included)

Risks	Simple Aspiration	Ethanol Ablation • Cystic nodules • AFTN	RFA • Benign predominantly solid nodules • AFTN • Parathyroid • primary PTC • Recurrent PTC	Laser Ablation • Benign predominantly solid nodules • primary PTC • Recurrent PTC	HIFU • Benign predominantly solid nodules • Parathyroid	Microwave Ablation • Benign predominantly solid nodules • Cystic nodules • Parathyroid • primary PTC
Overall	1%[86]	8.2%-29%[87,88] 90%-100%[11,13]	3.3%[29] 2.4%-100%[34,38] 0%-10%[89-91] 3.0%-8.5%[47,50] 10.4%[52]	0%-15%[35,92-94] 91.9%[95] 8.3%[96]	0%-31.8%[69,97] 25%[98]	0%-36.3%[74,99] 10.3%[100] 28.6%[77] 5.2%[78]
Minor complications	1%[86]	19%-29%[10,88] 90%-100%[11,13]	1.9%[29] 100%[34] 2.3-4.1%[47,48]	0%-1.6%[92,93] 91.9%[95] 4.2%[96]	0%-31.8%[69,97]	0%-36.3%[74,99] 10.3%[100] 22.9%[77] 0.6%[78]
Pain[a]		19%-29%[10,88] 90%-100%[11,13]	2.6%[b,29] 100%[34] 8.5%[50]	91.9%[95]		
Extra-thyroidal hematoma		0.8%-3.9%[11,101]	0%-2.1%[18,28] 1.6%-2.7%[47,48]	0%[95]	0%[c,66]	36.3%[74]
Intra-nodular/thyroid hemorrhage/hematoma	1%[86]	6.5%[87]	5%[8]		0%[c,66]	10.3%[100]
Vomiting			0.09%-0.6%[29,31]		8%[68]	
Skin burns			0.3%[29] 0.8-1.4%[47,48]	0%[92] 4.2%[96]	0%-31.8%[67-69]	0%-10%[74,99]

Fever		6.0%[d,35] 0.02% - 8%[10,11]	0.3%[29]	2.7%[95]		27.3%[74]
Transient hyperthyroidism		0% -3.8%[88,102] 0% – 38%[10,11]	1.3% -2.7%[18,24]	1.6%[93]		
Vasovagal reaction			0.3%[29]			
Drunken sensation	1.6%[103]					
Development of thyroid autoantibody			2.3%[e,34]			
Major complications	0%[86]	0% - 3.4%[89,104] 3.2%[101]	1.4 %[29] 0% – 1.4%[8,30,34,35,38] 0% -10%[89-91] 0.8 - 1.4%[47,48] 3%[f,52]	0% - 15%[35,92-94] 0%[95] 4.2%[96]	0% - 3.9%[67,68,105] 25%[98]	0% - 9.1%[74,99,106] 5.7%[77] 4.6%[78]
Diffuse glandular hemorrhage or airway compromising hematoma	Case reports[107,108]					
Hypoparathyroidism			0%[28] 0%[52]			
Edema requiring steroid			9.1%[22]	15%[92]		
Nodule Rupture			0.2% - 0.5%[28,29] 0.07% requiring surgical intervention 9.[29]	Case series of 3[109]		
Hypothyroidism	0%[88]		0% – 0.3%[26,28,29,h] 0%[34] 0%[110]	1.6%[i,93]	0% - 1.4%[73,111]	

(continued on next page)

Table 2
(continued)

Transient voice change	0% -3.4%[9,87,112] 0% - 3.9%[11,13]	0.5% - 2.7%[18,24,28] 0% -10%[89-91] 0.8% - 1.4%[47,48] 8.3 %[52]	0% - 8.3%[92-94] 0%[95] 4.2%[96]	0% - 3.9%[67,68,105] 25%[98]	0% - 9.1%[74,99,106] 5.7%[77] 4.6%[78]
Permanent voice change	0%[87]	0% - 0.09%[28,31] 0%[52]	0%[92-94] 0%[95] 0%[96,113]	0%[67,105]	0%[74,99,106] 0%[77] 0%[78]
Brachial plexus injury		0% - 0.09%[28,31]			
Wound infection / abscess	0%[87] 0.8%[101]	0.3%[26]	0%[95]		
Arrhythmia	1.6%[87]	TC[i]	0.82%[93]		
Thrombus of Jugular Vein	0.23%[11]				
Carotid a. injury			TC	TC	TC
Tracheal injury	TC	AR	TC	TC	TC[114]
Esophageal injury	TC	TC	TC	TC	TC[114]
Spinal Accessory n. injury			TC	TC	TC[114]
sympathetic chain injury			TC	Case report[115]	

Abbreviations: AR, anecdotal risks are nonpublished risks but are known to have occurred; TC, theoretic complications have not yet been reported in literature nor known to have occurred but thought to be possible by expert opinion.

a The reporting of pain between studies is highly variable, ranging from reporting of all cases of intraprocedural pain regardless of severity to only pain requiring the discontinuation of procedure.
b Pain has been reported at ablation site or radiates to head, ear, teeth, shoulder, and chest.
c All patients in the study underwent HIFU while continuing anticoagulation or antiplatelet agent therapy.
d Study provided combined data for cold and pretoxic/toxic nodules.
e 1/44 patients treated with RFA for AFTN developed Tg Ab without hypothyroidism.
f Choi and colleagues only considered voice change a major complication if persistent greater than 1 mo, leading to a discrepancy between the reported frequency of voice change and major complications.
g Patient had an associated abscess formation.
h Patient was noted to have TPO or Tg positivity before thermal ablation.
i RF current passes through the heart use of monopolar electrode making cardiac electrical events a theoretic concern.

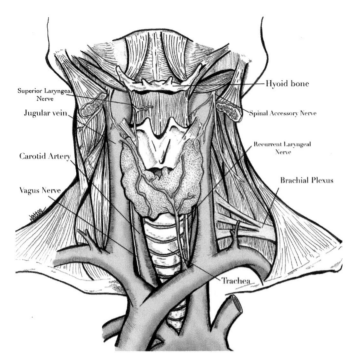

Fig. 7. At-risk structures of the neck during MIT. *(Courtesy of* Michael B. Natter, MD, New York, NY)

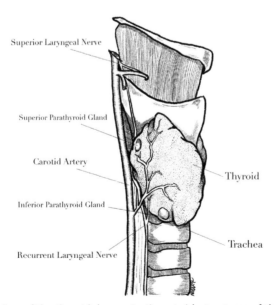

Fig. 8. Posterior view of the thyroid demonstrating at-risk structures of the neck. *(Courtesy of* Michael B. Natter, MD, New York, NY)

Table 3		
Timeline for the cessation of AC/AP/NOACs[44,85] for RFA, LA or other MIT in which increased risk of bleed is perceived		
Stop Before Procedure		Restart Medication Postprocedure
ASA, clopidogrel 7–10 d		24 h
warfarin 3–5 d		12 h
4–6 h for heparin		2–6 h
NOACs 3 d		24–48 h

that makes a notable exception to these generally positive findings is a retrospective study by Khan and colleagues that found that the rate of nondiagnostic aspirates among 47 patients receiving aspirin monotherapy was approximately double that of 500 patients receiving no AC/AP: 34% and 16%, respectively.[84]

We are not aware of studies that address procedure-related bleeding and nondiagnostic aspirate rates for patients treated with novel oral anticoagulants (NOACs) including dabigatran, rivaroxaban, and apixaban. However, Lyle and colleagues suggested that as the rate of bleeding complications associated with NOACs is similar to that of more conventional AC/AP for minor procedures such as dental and other minor surgeries which do not require the discontinuation of these agents, they are as safe as AC/AP and also do not require discontinuation before FNA.[85] We also agree that in routine cases, AC/AP/NOACs may be safely continued before FNA. For patients treated with warfarin, we prefer an INR of 2.5 or lower and will usually defer FNA in the case of supratherapeutic INRs.

For procedures using 19 to 21G CNB we consider the discontinuation of AC/AP/NOAC when feasible (**Table 3**) and when discontinuation is not considered high-risk based on the underlying indication for AC/AP/NOAC treatment. For procedures that involve repeated large bore needle insertion and movement through the target lesion such as LA and RFA AC/AP/NOACs must always be discontinued as small procedure-related hematoma in these cases is fairly common and in rare cases, clinically significant hematoma can occur. In this setting, we discontinue all AC/AP/NOACs for at least 3 days and in the select case of warfarin treatment ensure the INR is ~1. In all cases, when the discontinuation of AC/AP/NOAC is required, we request direction from the AC/AP/NOAC prescriber to advise the patient regarding specific instructions for medication discontinuation.

SUMMARY

The use of MITs for the treatment of thyroid disease is an exciting and rapidly developing field. These techniques offer attractive alternatives to surgical management and RAI and are changing the treatment paradigms for thyroid disease.

As with any novel technology, proper training, familiarity and experience are necessary to minimize serious complications. In appropriately selected patients, MITs offer advantages over the traditional surgical and medical management of patients with benign and malignant thyroid disease.

CLINICS CARE POINTS

- FNA documenting benign cytology x 2 before MIT
- The presence of antithyroid antibodies before RFA is a risk factor for postprocedure hypothyroidism

- 1% lidocaine infused along the pericapsular space provides adequate local anesthesia. General anesthesia and deep sedation are not necessary and may lead to inadvertent injury by preventing the patient from reporting pain associated with procedure-related thermal and mechanical injury.
- Postprocedural ultrasound at 1, 6, and 12 months should be performed to evaluate procedural outcomes.

DISCLOSURE

The authors have nothing to disclose.

SUPPLEMENTARY DATA

Supplementary data related to this article can be found online at https://doi.org/10.1016/j.pmr.2016.04.003.

REFERENCES

1. Mazzaferri EL. Management of a solitary thyroid nodule. N Engl J Med 1993; 328(8):553–9.
2. Lee DY, Seok J, Jeong WJ, et al. Prediction of thyroid hormone supplementation after thyroid lobectomy. J Surg Res 2015;193(1):273–8.
3. Frates MC, Benson CB, Doubilet PM, et al. Prevalence and distribution of carcinoma in patients with solitary and multiple thyroid nodules on sonography. J Clin Endocrinol Metab 2006;91(9):3411–7.
4. In HS, Kim DW, Choo HJ, et al. Ethanol ablation of benign thyroid cysts and predominantly cystic thyroid nodules: factors that predict outcome. Endocrine 2014;46(1):107–13.
5. Miller JM, Zafar SU, Karo JJ. The cystic thyroid nodule. Recognition and management. Radiology 1974;110(2):257–61.
6. Hahn SY, Shin JH, Na DG, et al. Ethanol ablation of the thyroid nodules: 2018 consensus statement by the Korean Society of Thyroid Radiology. Korean J Radiol 2019;20(4):609–20.
7. Kanematsu R, Hirokawa M, Higuchi M, et al. Risk of malignancy and clinical outcomes of cyst fluid only nodules in the thyroid based on ultrasound and aspiration cytology. Diagn Cytopathol 2020;48(1):30–4.
8. Jang SW, Baek JH, Kim JK, et al. How to manage the patients with unsatisfactory results after ethanol ablation for thyroid nodules: role of radiofrequency ablation. Eur J Radiol 2012;81(5):905–10.
9. Guglielmi R, Pacella CM, Bianchini A, et al. Percutaneous ethanol injection treatment in benign thyroid lesions: role and efficacy. Thyroid 2004;14(2):125–31.
10. Monzani F, Goletti O, Caraccio N, et al. Percutaneous ethanol injection treatment of autonomous thyroid adenoma: hormonal and clinical evaluation. Clin Endocrinol (Oxf) 1992;36(5):491–7.
11. Lippi F, Ferrari C, Manetti L, et al. Treatment of solitary autonomous thyroid nodules by percutaneous ethanol injection: results of an Italian multicenter study. The Multicenter Study Group. J Clin Endocrinol Metab 1996;81(9):3261–4.
12. Papini E, Pacella CM, Verde G. Percutaneous ethanol injection (PEI): what is its role in the treatment of benign thyroid nodules?. Thyroid 1995;5(2):147–50.

13. Sharma A, Abraham D. Vascularity-targeted percutaneous ethanol injection of toxic thyroid adenomas: outcomes of a feasibility study performed in the USA. Endocr Pract 2020;26(1):22–9.

14. Mon SY, Riedlinger G, Abbott CE, et al. Cancer risk and clinicopathological characteristics of thyroid nodules harboring thyroid-stimulating hormone receptor gene mutations. Diagn Cytopathol 2018;46(5):369–77.

15. Heilo A, Sigstad E, Fagerlid KH, et al. Efficacy of ultrasound-guided percutaneous ethanol injection treatment in patients with a limited number of metastatic cervical lymph nodes from papillary thyroid carcinoma. J Clin Endocrinol Metab 2011;96(9):2750–5.

16. Hay ID, Lee RA, Davidge-Pitts C, et al. Long-term outcome of ultrasound-guided percutaneous ethanol ablation of selected "recurrent" neck nodal metastases in 25 patients with TNM stages III or IVA papillary thyroid carcinoma previously treated by surgery and 131I therapy. Surgery 2013;154(6):1448–55 [discussion 1454-5].

17. Lorentzen T. A cooled needle electrode for radiofrequency tissue ablation: thermodynamic aspects of improved performance compared with conventional needle design. Acad Radiol 1996;3(7):556–63.

18. Jeong WK, Baek JH, Rhim H, et al. Radiofrequency ablation of benign thyroid nodules: safety and imaging follow-up in 236 patients. Eur Radiol 2008;18(6): 1244–50.

19. Papini E, Pacella CM, Solbiati LA, et al. Minimally-invasive treatments for benign thyroid nodules: a Delphi-based consensus statement from the Italian minimally-invasive treatments of the thyroid (MITT) group. Int J Hyperthermia 2019;36(1): 376–82.

20. Gharib H, Papini E, Garber JR, et al. American Association of Clinical Endocrinologists, American College of Endocrinology, and Associazione Medici Endocrinologi Medical Guidelines for Clinical Practice for the Diagnosis and Management of Thyroid Nodules - 2016 Update Appendix. Endocr Pract 2016;22:1–60.

21. Kim YS, Rhim H, Tae K, et al. Radiofrequency ablation of benign cold thyroid nodules: initial clinical experience. Thyroid 2006;16(4):361–7.

22. Deandrea M, Limone P, Basso E, et al. US-guided percutaneous radiofrequency thermal ablation for the treatment of solid benign hyperfunctioning or compressive thyroid nodules. Ultrasound Med Biol 2008;34(5):784–91.

23. Jawad S, Morley S, Otero S, et al. Ultrasound-guided radiofrequency ablation (RFA) of benign symptomatic thyroid nodules - initial UK experience. Br J Radiol 2019;92(1098):20190026.

24. Bernardi S, Dobrinja C, Fabris B, et al. Radiofrequency ablation compared to surgery for the treatment of benign thyroid nodules. Int J Endocrinol 2014; 2014:934595.

25. Guang Y, He W, Luo Y, et al. Patient satisfaction of radiofrequency ablation for symptomatic benign solid thyroid nodules: our experience for 2-year follow up. BMC Cancer 2019;19(1):147.

26. Dobnig H, Amrein K. Monopolar radiofrequency ablation of thyroid nodules: a prospective Austrian Single-Center Study. Thyroid 2018;28(4):472–80.

27. Sim JS, Baek JH. Long-term outcomes of thermal ablation for benign thyroid nodules: the issue of regrowth. Int J Endocrinol 2021;2021:9922509.

28. Che Y, Jin S, Shi C, et al. Treatment of benign thyroid nodules: comparison of surgery with radiofrequency ablation. AJNR Am J Neuroradiol 2015;36(7): 1321–5.

29. Baek JH, Lee JH, Sung JY, et al. Complications encountered in the treatment of benign thyroid nodules with US-guided radiofrequency ablation: a multicenter study. Radiology 2012;262(1):335–42.

30. Baek JH, Moon WJ, Kim YS, et al. Radiofrequency ablation for the treatment of autonomously functioning thyroid nodules. World J Surg 2009;33(9):1971–7.

31. Lim HK, Lee JH, Ha EJ, et al. Radiofrequency ablation of benign non-functioning thyroid nodules: 4-year follow-up results for 111 patients. Eur Radiol 2013;23(4): 1044–9.

32. Baek JH, Jeong HJ, Kim YS, et al. Radiofrequency ablation for an autonomously functioning thyroid nodule. Thyroid 2008;18(6):675–6.

33. Cervelli R, Mazzeo S, Boni G, et al. Comparison between radioiodine therapy and single-session radiofrequency ablation of autonomously functioning thyroid nodules: a retrospective study. Clin Endocrinol (Oxf) 2019;90(4):608–16.

34. Sung JY, Baek JH, Jung SL, et al. Radiofrequency ablation for autonomously functioning thyroid nodules: a multicenter study. Thyroid 2015;25(1):112–7.

35. Spiezia S, Garberoglio R, Milone F, et al. Thyroid nodules and related symptoms are stably controlled two years after radiofrequency thermal ablation. Thyroid 2009;19(3):219–25.

36. Bernardi S, Stacul F, Michelli A, et al. 12-month efficacy of a single radiofrequency ablation on autonomously functioning thyroid nodules. Endocrine 2017;57(3):402–8.

37. Cesareo R, Naciu AM, Iozzino M, et al. Nodule size as predictive factor of efficacy of radiofrequency ablation in treating autonomously functioning thyroid nodules. Int J Hyperthermia 2018;34(5):617–23.

38. Cesareo R, Palermo A, Benvenuto D, et al. Efficacy of radiofrequency ablation in autonomous functioning thyroid nodules. A systematic review and meta-analysis. Rev Endocr Metab Disord 2019;20(1):37–44.

39. Dobnig H, et al. Radiofrequency ablation of thyroid nodules: "Good Clinical Practice Recommendations" for Austria : An interdisciplinary statement from the following professional associations: Austrian Thyroid Association (ÖSDG), Austrian Society for Nuclear Medicine and Molecular Imaging (OGNMB), Austrian Society for Endocrinology and Metabolism (ÖGES), Surgical Endocrinology Working Group (ACE) of the Austrian Surgical Society (OEGCH). Wien Med Wochenschr 2020;170(1–2):6–14.

40. Kim HJ, Cho SJ, Baek JH, et al. Efficacy and safety of thermal ablation for autonomously functioning thyroid nodules: a systematic review and meta-analysis. Eur Radiol 2021;31(2):605–15.

41. Papini E, Monpeyssen H, Frasoldati A, et al. 2020 European Thyroid Association Clinical Practice Guideline for the Use of Image-Guided Ablation in Benign Thyroid Nodules. Eur Thyroid J 2020;9(4):172–85.

42. He L, Zhao W, Xia Z, et al. Comparative efficacy of different ultrasound-guided ablation for the treatment of benign thyroid nodules: Systematic review and network meta-analysis of randomized controlled trials. PLoS One 2021;16(1): e0243864.

43. Baek JH, Ha EJ, Choi YJ, et al. Radiofrequency versus Ethanol Ablation for Treating Predominantly Cystic Thyroid Nodules: A Randomized Clinical Trial. Korean J Radiol 2015;16(6):1332–40.

44. Kim JH, Baek JH, Lim HK, et al. 2017 Thyroid Radiofrequency Ablation Guideline: Korean Society of Thyroid Radiology. Korean J Radiol 2018;19(4):632–55.

45. Shen R, Cheng R, Zhou H, et al. Ultrasonography-guided radiofrequency ablation combined with lauromacrogol sclerotherapy for mixed thyroid nodules. Am J Transl Res 2021;13(5):5035–42.

46. Tufano RP, Pace-Asciak P, Russell JO, et al. Update of Radiofrequency Ablation for Treating Benign and Malignant Thyroid Nodules. The Future Is Now. Front Endocrinol (Lausanne) 2021;12:698689.

47. Lim HK, Cho SJ, Baek JH, et al. US-Guided Radiofrequency Ablation for Low-Risk Papillary Thyroid Microcarcinoma: Efficacy and Safety in a Large Population. Korean J Radiol 2019;20(12):1653–61.

48. Cho SJ, Baek SM, Lim HK, et al. Long-term follow-up results of ultrasound-guided radiofrequency ablation for low-risk papillary thyroid microcarcinoma: more than 5-year follow-up for 84 tumors. Thyroid 2020;30(12):1745–51.

49. Zhang C, Yin J, Hu C, et al. Comparison of ultrasound guided percutaneous radiofrequency ablation and open thyroidectomy in the treatment of low-risk papillary thyroid microcarcinoma: A propensity score matching study. Clin Hemorheol Microcirc 2021;80(2):73–81.

50. Yan L, Zhang M, Song Q, et al. The Efficacy and Safety of Radiofrequency Ablation for Bilateral Papillary Thyroid Microcarcinoma. Front Endocrinol (Lausanne) 2021;12:663636.

51. Xiao J, Lan Y, Yan L, et al. [Short-term Outcome of T1bN0M0 Papillary Thyroid Cancer after Ultrasonography-guided Radiofrequency Ablation]. Zhongguo Yi Xue Ke Xue Yuan Xue Bao 2020;42(6):771–5.

52. Choi Y, Jung SL, Bae JS, et al. Comparison of efficacy and complications between radiofrequency ablation and repeat surgery in the treatment of locally recurrent thyroid cancers: a single-center propensity score matching study. Int J Hyperthermia 2019;36(1):359–67.

53. Chung SR, Baek JH, Choi YJ, et al. Longer-term outcomes of radiofrequency ablation for locally recurrent papillary thyroid cancer. Eur Radiol 2019;29(9): 4897–903.

54. Chung SR, Suh CH, Baek JH, et al. Safety of radiofrequency ablation of benign thyroid nodules and recurrent thyroid cancers: a systematic review and meta-analysis. Int J Hyperthermia 2017;33(8):920–30.

55. Gulcelik NE, Gulcelik MA, Kuru B. Risk of malignancy in patients with follicular neoplasm: predictive value of clinical and ultrasonographic features. Arch Otolaryngol Head Neck Surg 2008;134(12):1312–5.

56. Dobrinja C, Bernardi S, Fabris B, et al. Surgical and Pathological Changes after Radiofrequency Ablation of Thyroid Nodules. Int J Endocrinol 2015;2015: 576576.

57. Ha SM, Sung JY, Baek JH, et al. Radiofrequency ablation of small follicular neoplasms: initial clinical outcomes. Int J Hyperthermia 2017;33(8):931–7.

58. Paramo JC, Mesko T. Age, tumor size, and in-office ultrasonography are predictive parameters of malignancy in follicular neoplasms of the thyroid. Endocr Pract 2008;14(4):447–51.

59. Machens A, Holzhausen HJ, Dralle H. The prognostic value of primary tumor size in papillary and follicular thyroid carcinoma. Cancer 2005;103(11):2269–73.

60. Pacella CM, Bizzarri G, Guglielmi R, et al. Thyroid tissue: US-guided percutaneous interstitial laser ablation-a feasibility study. Radiology 2000;217(3):673–7.

61. Pacella CM, Mauri G, Achille G, et al. Outcomes and Risk Factors for Complications of Laser Ablation for Thyroid Nodules: A Multicenter Study on 1531 Patients. J Clin Endocrinol Metab 2015;100(10):3903–10.

62. Trimboli P, Castellana M, Sconfienza LM, et al. Efficacy of thermal ablation in benign non-functioning solid thyroid nodule: a systematic review and meta-analysis. Endocrine 2020;67(1):35–43.

63. Cesareo R, Pacella CM, Pasqualini V, et al. Laser ablation versus radiofrequency ablation for benign non-functioning thyroid nodules: six-month results of a randomized, parallel, open-label, trial (LARA Trial). Thyroid 2020;30(6):847–56.

64. Lynn JG, Zwemer RL, Chick AJ. The biological application of focused ultrasonic waves. Science 1942;96(2483):119–20.

65. Esnault O, Rouxel A, Le Nestour E, et al. Minimally invasive ablation of a toxic thyroid nodule by high-intensity focused ultrasound. AJNR Am J Neuroradiol 2010;31(10):1967–8.

66. Lang BH, Woo YC, Chiu KW. High intensity focused ultrasound (HIFU) ablation of benign thyroid nodule is safe and efficacious in patients who continue taking an anti-coagulation or anti-platelet agent in the treatment period. Int J Hyperthermia 2019;36(1):186–90.

67. Lang BH, Woo YC, Wong CKH. High-intensity focused ultrasound for treatment of symptomatic benign thyroid nodules: a prospective study. Radiology 2017; 284(3):897–906.

68. Lang BHH, Woo YC, Chiu KW. Two sequential applications of high-intensity focused ultrasound (HIFU) ablation for large benign thyroid nodules. Eur Radiol 2019;29(7):3626–34.

69. Esnault O, Franc B, Ménégaux F, et al. High-intensity focused ultrasound ablation of thyroid nodules: first human feasibility study. Thyroid 2011;21(9):965–73.

70. Lang BH, Wu ALH. High intensity focused ultrasound (HIFU) ablation of benign thyroid nodules - a systematic review. J Ther Ultrasound 2017;5:11.

71. Sennert M, Happel C, Korkusuz Y, et al. Further Investigation on High-intensity Focused Ultrasound (HIFU) Treatment for Thyroid Nodules: Effectiveness Related to Baseline Volumes. Acad Radiol 2018;25(1):88–94.

72. Lang BH, Woo YC, Chiu KW. Single-Session High-Intensity Focused Ultrasound Treatment in Large-Sized Benign Thyroid Nodules. Thyroid 2017;27(5):714–21.

73. Lang BHH, Woo YC, Chiu KW. High-intensity focused ablation (HIFU) of single benign thyroid nodule rarely alters underlying thyroid function. Int J Hyperthermia 2017;33(8):875–81.

74. Feng B, Liang P, Cheng Z, et al. Ultrasound-guided percutaneous microwave ablation of benign thyroid nodules: experimental and clinical studies. Eur J Endocrinol 2012;166(6):1031–7.

75. Cui T, Jin C, Jiao D, et al. Safety and efficacy of microwave ablation for benign thyroid nodules and papillary thyroid microcarcinomas: a systematic review and meta-analysis. Eur J Radiol 2019;118:58–64.

76. Guo DM, Chen Z, Zhai YX, et al. Comparison of radiofrequency ablation and microwave ablation for benign thyroid nodules: A systematic review and meta-analysis. Clin Endocrinol (Oxf) 2021;95(1):187–96.

77. Zhuo L, Zhang L, Peng LL, et al. Microwave ablation of hyperplastic parathyroid glands is a treatment option for end-stage renal disease patients ineligible for surgical resection. Int J Hyperthermia 2019;36(1):29–35.

78. Cao XJ, Liu J, Zhu YL, et al. Efficacy and Safety of Thermal Ablation for Solitary T1bN0M0 Papillary Thyroid Carcinoma: A Multicenter Study. J Clin Endocrinol Metab 2021;106(2):e573–81.

79. Abu-Yousef MM, Larson JH, Kuehn DM, et al. Safety of ultrasound-guided fine needle aspiration biopsy of neck lesions in patients taking antithrombotic/anticoagulant medications. Ultrasound Q 2011;27(3):157–9.

80. Khadra H, Kholmatov R, Monlezun D, et al. Do anticoagulation medications increase the risk of haematoma in ultrasound-guided fine needle aspiration of thyroid lesions? Cytopathology 2018;29(6):565–8.

81. Denham SL, Ismail A, Bolus DN, et al. Effect of Anticoagulation Medication on the Thyroid Fine-Needle Aspiration Pathologic Diagnostic Sufficiency Rate. J Ultrasound Med 2016;35(1):43–8.

82. Kwon JH, Kim DB, Han YH, et al. Contributory Factors to Hemorrhage After Ultrasound-Guided Fine Needle Aspiration of Thyroid Nodules with an Emphasis on Patients Taking Antithrombotic or Anticoagulant Medications. Iran J Radiol 2018;15(2):e57231.

83. Cordes M, Schmidkonz C, Horstrup K, et al. Fine-needle aspiration biopsies of thyroid nodules. Nuklearmedizin 2018;57(6):211–5.

84. Khan TS, Sharma E, Singh B, et al. Aspirin Increases the Risk of Nondiagnostic Yield of Fine-Needle Aspiration and Biopsy of Thyroid Nodules. Eur Thyroid J 2018;7(3):129–32.

85. Lyle MA, Dean DS. Ultrasound-guided fine-needle aspiration biopsy of thyroid nodules in patients taking novel oral anticoagulants. Thyroid 2015;25(4):373–6.

86. Galvan G, Manzl M, Balcke C, et al. [Therapy of thyroid cysts with fine needle aspiration]. Schweiz Med Wochenschr 1982;112(26):926–30.

87. Cho W, Sim JS, Jung SL. Ultrasound-guided ethanol ablation for cystic thyroid nodules: effectiveness of small amounts of ethanol in a single session. Ultrasonography 2021;40(3):417–27.

88. Halenka M, Karasek D, Schovanek J, et al. Safe and effective percutaneous ethanol injection therapy of 200 thyroid cysts. Biomed Pap Med Fac Univ Palacky Olomouc Czech Repub 2020;164(2):161–7.

89. Hussain I, Ahmad S, Aljammal J. Radiofrequency Ablation of Parathyroid Adenoma: A Novel Treatment Option for Primary Hyperparathyroidism. AACE Clin Case Rep 2021;7(3):195–9.

90. Korkusuz H, Wolf T, Grünwald F. Feasibility of bipolar radiofrequency ablation in patients with parathyroid adenoma: a first evaluation. Int J Hyperthermia 2018; 34(5):639–43.

91. Khandelwal AH, Batra S, Jajodia S, et al. Radiofrequency Ablation of Parathyroid Adenomas: Safety and Efficacy in a Study of 10 Patients. Indian J Endocrinol Metab 2020;24(6):543–50.

92. Papini E, Guglielmi R, Bizzarri G, et al. Ultrasound-guided laser thermal ablation for treatment of benign thyroid nodules. Endocr Pract 2004;10(3):276–83.

93. Valcavi R, Riganti F, Bertani A, et al. Percutaneous laser ablation of cold benign thyroid nodules: a 3-year follow-up study in 122 patients. Thyroid 2010;20(11): 1253–61.

94. Spiezia S, Vitale G, Di Somma C, et al. Ultrasound-guided laser thermal ablation in the treatment of autonomous hyperfunctioning thyroid nodules and compressive nontoxic nodular goiter. Thyroid 2003;13(10):941–7.

95. Ji L, Wu Q, Gu J, et al. Ultrasound-guided percutaneous laser ablation for papillary thyroid microcarcinoma: a retrospective analysis of 37 patients. Cancer Imaging 2019;19(1):16.

96. Mauri G, Cova L, Ierace T, et al. Treatment of Metastatic Lymph Nodes in the Neck from Papillary Thyroid Carcinoma with Percutaneous Laser Ablation. Cardiovasc Intervent Radiol 2016;39(7):1023–30.

97. Kovatcheva RD, Vlahov JD, Stoinov JI, et al. Benign Solid Thyroid Nodules: US-guided High-Intensity Focused Ultrasound Ablation-Initial Clinical Outcomes. Radiology 2015;276(2):597–605.

98. Kovatcheva RD, Vlahov JD, Shinkov AD, et al. High-intensity focused ultrasound to treat primary hyperparathyroidism: a feasibility study in four patients. AJR Am J Roentgenol 2010;195(4):830–5.

99. Khanh HQ, Hung NQ, Vinh VH, et al. Efficacy of Microwave Ablation in the Treatment of Large (≥3 cm) Benign Thyroid Nodules. World J Surg 2020;44(7): 2272–9.

100. Dong S, Sun L, Xu J, et al. Intracystic Hemorrhage and Its Management During Ultrasound-Guided Percutaneous Microwave Ablation for Cystic Thyroid Nodules. Front Endocrinol (Lausanne) 2020;11:477.

101. Tarantino L, Francica G, Sordelli I, et al. Percutaneous ethanol injection of hyperfunctioning thyroid nodules: long-term follow-up in 125 patients. AJR Am J Roentgenol 2008;190(3):800–8.

102. Antonelli A, Campatelli A, Di Vito A, et al. Comparison between ethanol sclerotherapy and emptying with injection of saline in treatment of thyroid cysts. Clin Investig 1994;72(12):971–4.

103. Yasuda K, Ozaki O, Sugino K, et al. Treatment of cystic lesions of the thyroid by ethanol instillation. World J Surg 1992;16(5):958–61.

104. Kim YJ, Baek JH, Ha EJ, et al. Cystic versus predominantly cystic thyroid nodules: efficacy of ethanol ablation and analysis of related factors. Eur Radiol 2012;22(7):1573–8.

105. Lang BHH, Woo YC, Chiu KW. Vocal cord paresis following single-session high intensity focused ablation (HIFU) treatment of benign thyroid nodules: incidence and risk factors. Int J Hyperthermia 2017;33(8):888–94.

106. Yue W, Wang S, Wang B, et al. Ultrasound guided percutaneous microwave ablation of benign thyroid nodules: safety and imaging follow-up in 222 patients. Eur J Radiol 2013;82(1):e11–6.

107. Noordzij JP, Goto MM. Airway compromise caused by hematoma after thyroid fine-needle aspiration. Am J Otolaryngol 2005;26(6):398–9.

108. Roh JL. Intrathyroid hemorrhage and acute upper airway obstruction after fine needle aspiration of the thyroid gland. Laryngoscope 2006;116(1):154–6.

109. Tian P, Du W, Liu X, et al. Ultrasonographic characteristics of thyroid nodule rupture after microwave ablation: Three case reports. Medicine (Baltimore) 2021;100(9):e25070.

110. Ding M, Tang X, Cui D, et al. Clinical outcomes of ultrasound-guided radiofrequency ablation for the treatment of primary papillary thyroid microcarcinoma. Clin Radiol 2019;74(9):712–7.

111. Korkusuz H, Sennert M, Fehre N, et al. Localized Thyroid Tissue Ablation by High Intensity Focused Ultrasound: Volume Reduction, Effects on Thyroid Function and Immune Response. Rofo 2015;187(11):1011–5.

112. Negro R, Colosimo E, Greco G. Outcome, Pain Perception, and Health-Related Quality of Life in Patients Submitted to Percutaneous Ethanol Injection for Simple Thyroid Cysts. J Thyroid Res 2017;2017:9536479.

113. Spartalis E, Karagiannis SP, Plakopitis N, et al. Percutaneous laser ablation of cervical metastatic lymph nodes in papillary thyroid carcinoma: clinical efficacy and anatomical considerations. Expert Rev Med Devices 2021;18(1):75–82.

114. Yang YL, Chen CZ, Zhang XH. Microwave ablation of benign thyroid nodules. Future Oncol 2014;10(6):1007–14.

115. Ben Hamou A, Monpeyssen H. Horner's Syndrome During High-Intensity Focused Ultrasound Ablation for a Benign Thyroid Nodule. AACE Clin Case Rep 2021;7(3):164–8.

Less-Intensive Management Options for Low-Risk Thyroid Cancer

Joana Ochoa, MD[a], Susan C. Pitt, MD, MPHS[b],*

KEYWORDS

- Low-risk thyroid cancer • Lobectomy • Total thyroidectomy • Active surveillance

KEY POINTS

- The incidence of thyroid cancer continues to increase largely because of incidental findings, but given the excellent prognosis of these cancers, mortality has remained relatively stable.
- Surgical options for low-risk thyroid cancers include lobectomy and total thyroidectomy. Total thyroidectomy is associated with a higher complication rate with no significant added oncologic value over lobectomy.
- Active surveillance is an appropriate alternative to surgery for very-low-risk differentiated thyroid cancers. There remains reluctance to choosing active surveillance because of physician- and patient-driven factors.
- A patient's quality of life can be significantly affected by any given treatment. Patients must be counseled appropriately to choose the optimal treatment individualized to their tumor characteristics and personal needs.

INTRODUCTION

Over the last few decades, significant changes occurred in the incidence of thyroid cancer as well as in the paradigm of thyroid cancer management. In the 1990s, the incidence of thyroid cancer increased sharply, whereas the overall death rate remained stable. This pattern indicates overdiagnosis, which is largely attributed to incidental findings in the thyroid identified on imaging performed for other reasons.[1,2] Studies of autopsy results performed on people who died of other causes from the 1980s reported thyroid cancer in up to 36% of specimens.[3] More recent studies report this rate to be approximately 10% to 14%, which supports the presence of overdiagnosis and subsequent treatment of thyroid cancer.[4,5]

a Department of Surgery, University of Florida College of Medicine–Jacksonville, 653 West 8th Street, Faculty Clinic 3rd Floor, Jacksonville, FL 33209, USA; b Division of Endocrine Surgery, Department of Surgery, University of Michigan, 1500 East Medical Center Drive, Taubman 2920F, Ann Arbor, MI 48109, USA
* Corresponding author.
E-mail address: scpitt@med.umich.edu

Endocrinol Metab Clin N Am 51 (2022) 351–366
https://doi.org/10.1016/j.ecl.2021.11.018
0889-8529/21/© 2021 Elsevier Inc. All rights reserved.

Today, thyroid cancer represents 2.3% of all new cancer diagnoses in the United States and is the twelfth most commonly diagnosed cancer.[1] Although the overall rate of thyroid cancer diagnoses compared with all other new cancer diagnoses has decreased slightly in recent years, the absolute number of new cases of thyroid cancer continues to increase and was 15.5 per 100,000 people compared with 14.3 in 2019.[1,6] Approximately 30% to 40% of new thyroid cancer diagnoses are papillary thyroid microcarcinoma (PTMC), defined as papillary thyroid cancers (PTC) that measure 1 cm or smaller.[7,8] Given the excellent prognosis and indolent nature of most differentiated thyroid cancers (DTC), most of these microcarcinomas are unlikely to become clinically significant, and the possibility of associated complications from unnecessary treatment is not insignificant. In addition to devastating complications, such as permanent hypoparathyroidism or recurrent laryngeal nerve injuries, many studies indicate that quality of life (QOL) is significantly decreased because of the need for synthetic thyroid hormone replacement, scarring related to surgery, as well as health care costs.[8–12] Changes made in thyroid nodule biopsy guidelines by the American Thyroid Association (ATA) in 2015 will likely continue to decrease the rate of PTMC diagnosis, as many nodules do not meet biopsy criteria for further evaluation.[13] Although the "less is more" approach regarding treatment of low-risk thyroid cancers is not new, it is increasingly becoming more widely accepted as more data support its efficacy.

This review discusses treatment options for low-risk thyroid cancer focusing on options that are less intensive while exploring the benefits and limitations of each treatment. "Low-risk" according to the 2015 ATA guidelines refers to thyroid cancers that have a low risk of structural disease recurrence. Most low-risk cancers have less than 6% risk of recurrence, although this risk can be as high as 10%.[13] The ATA risk-stratification system has been proven to be a reliable predictor of outcomes in patients with DTC (**Fig. 1**).[14]

IDENTIFYING LOW-RISK THYROID CANCER

To determine the appropriate initial management option for thyroid cancer, clinicians must assess the clinical and histologic characteristics of the tumor. All thyroid nodules and cancers must be evaluated sonographically with a comprehensive neck ultrasound preoperatively to estimate their risk status, which is confirmed after surgical resection and pathologic evaluation. Specific nodule characteristics that can be detected on ultrasound include the size, location, extrathyroidal extension, and concern for invasion into adjacent structures (**Fig. 2**). Preoperative nodule characteristics indicative of low-risk thyroid cancer include size less than 4 cm, no evidence of lymph node metastasis, unifocal or multifocal PTMC, mutational status, completely intrathyroidal lesion (ie, no extrathyroidal extension or invasion into surrounding structures), and no aggressive cytologic findings. To be classified as low risk after reviewing final pathology, cancers must also have no aggressive histology, no vascular invasion (or <4 foci depending on the histologic type), and less than 5 lymph nodes with micrometastasis (<0.2 cm) (**Table 1**).[13] These features cannot be taken individually; the summation of these features must be taken under consideration.

A further subset of low-risk thyroid cancer is very low-risk cancer, which refers to PTMC with no clinical evidence of metastasis or local invasion as well as no cytologic evidence of aggressive disease.[13] Although microcarcinomas may be small, those that display extrathyroidal extension, nodal diseases, or distant metastases have high-risk features and may require more intensive or earlier treatment despite the small size of the primary tumor. Multifocal PTMC remain in the low-risk category despite the presence of multiple lesions.[13]

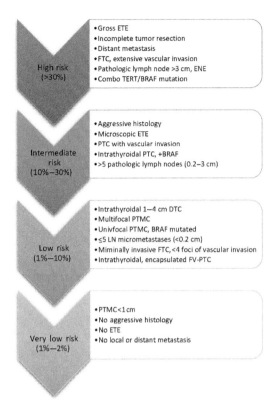

Fig. 1. Summary of risk of DTC recurrence. ENE, extranodal extension; ETE, extrathyroidal extension; FTC, follicular thyroid cancer; FV-PTC, follicular-variant papillary thyroid cancer. (*Data from* Haugen BR et al. 2015 American Thyroid Association Management Guidelines for Adult Patients with Thyroid Nodules and Differentiated Thyroid Cancer: The American Thyroid Association Guidelines Task Force on Thyroid Nodules and Differentiated Thyroid Cancer. Thyroid. 2016 Jan;26(1):1-133.)

LESS-INTENSIVE MANAGEMENT: THYROID LOBECTOMY

Although total thyroidectomy with or without a central neck dissection has long been the recommended treatment of choice for thyroid cancer, the 2015 ATA Guidelines established thyroid lobectomy (also referred to as hemithyroidectomy) as a legitimate, less-intensive management option for low-risk thyroid cancer. Many studies have evaluated the efficacy of lobectomy as an option for low-risk tumors compared with total thyroidectomy. These studies have established that there is no improvement in survival after total thyroidectomy compared with lobectomy alone,[15–17] as well as no differences in local or regional recurrence rates.[15] Benefits of thyroid lobectomy over total thyroidectomy make this treatment option preferable to some patients. These benefits include the potential to forgo the need for thyroid hormone replacement, no risk of hypoparathyroidism, decreased risk of recurrent laryngeal nerve injury and hematoma, as well as potentially improved QOL.[18] Studies show, however, that to achieve optimal thyroid-stimulating hormone (TSH) suppression, more than 70% of these patients may require levothyroxine replacement.[18] Limitations of this approach include challenges in following thyroglobulin levels and the potential for completion thyroidectomy if final pathology confirms intermediate or high risk for recurrence. As

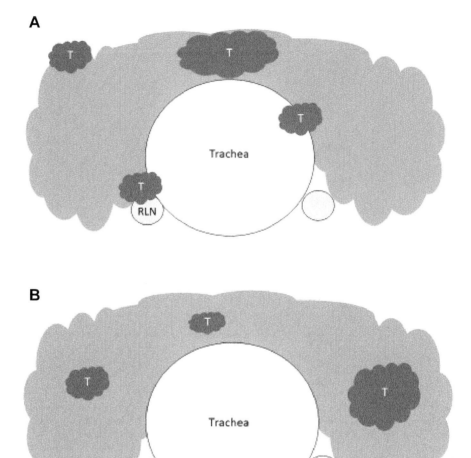

Fig. 2. Tumor locations where lobectomy or total thyroidectomy may be indicated (*A*) compared with locations where lobectomy versus active surveillance may be considered (*B*). RLN, recurrent laryngeal nerve; T, tumor.

many as 43% of patients who undergo initial lobectomy for what is thought to be a low-risk tumor have been shown to require completion thyroidectomy to facilitate radioactive iodine administration.[19] A thorough discussion of these pros and cons is important for informing patients and facilitating shared decision making to identify the optimal treatment and goals for each individual patient.

More recent studies further support the use of lobectomy for low-risk thyroid cancer and are establishing the efficacy of lobectomy for thyroid cancer with more aggressive features. Xu and colleagues[20] retrospectively evaluated 2059 patients who underwent lobectomy (n = 1224) and total thyroidectomy (n = 835) who had just 1 high-risk feature, which included tumor larger than 4 cm, known multifocal PTC, extrathyroidal extension, and confirmed nodal metastasis. No significant differences were found in

Table 1
Comparison of tumor, patient, and physician characteristics that contribute to choice of treatment for low-risk differentiated thyroid cancer

	Lobectomy Alone	Total or Completion Thyroidectomy	Active Surveillance	Radiofrequency or Ethanol Ablation
Preoperative findings (ultrasound or FNA)	Nodule ≤4 cm Intrathyroidal, may abut surrounding structures	Nodule ≥4 cm Extrathyroidal extension suspected	Nodule ≤1 cm[a] Intrathyroidal without invasion into surrounding structures	Nodule ≤1 cm[a] Intrathyroidal
	Contralateral lobe without nodules or with benign nodules	Large isthmus nodule or nodules with aggressive mutation	No concern for multifocality	Not adjacent to critical structures
	No evidence of nodal disease	Suspected/confirmed nodal disease	No evidence of nodal disease	No evidence of nodal disease
Postoperative findings (final pathology)	PTC-FV with <4 foci of vascular invasion	Extrathyroidal extension or vascular invasion present	N/A	N/A
	Micrometastasis of perithyroidal lymph node (<0.2 cm)	Aggressive variant with certain mutations (ie, TERT)		
		Extranodal extension or nodal metastases >0.2 cm in >5 nodes		
		Any feature that would indicate radioactive iodine		

(continued on next page)

Table 1
(continued)

	Lobectomy Alone	Total or Completion Thyroidectomy	Active Surveillance	Radiofrequency or Ethanol Ablation
Patient characteristics	Reliable	Unreliable	Reliable	Reliable
	Prefers to avoid thyroid hormone supplementation	Prefers to have the entire thyroid removed	Prefers to avoid thyroid hormone supplementation	Refuses surgery
	Not optimal surgical candidates—need to limit surgical dissection	Thyroid disease is present (hypothyroidism or hyperthyroidism)	Psychologically prepared to live with cancer	Previous neck surgery increasing risk for complications
	Older age (clinically significant recurrence unlikely during lifetime)	Significant family history of thyroid cancer	Accepts risk of cancer growth/metastasis	Poor surgical candidates
		Prior neck surgery or radiation exposure	No compressive symptoms	No compressive symptoms
Physician characteristics	Capable of performing surveillance of contralateral lobe	Unable to perform postoperative surveillance	Capable of performing surveillance of the cancer	Experience in providing these services and capable of performing surveillance

Abbreviation: N/A, not applicable.

[a] Larger cancers can be considered; however, long-term data on outcomes of this approach in larger cancers are pending.

disease-specific survival and recurrence-free survival within the 2 groups after a median follow-up of 93 months (range, 41–200 months). After stratifying by specific high-risk feature, still no significant differences existed between the lobectomy and total thyroidectomy groups, which supports the recent guidelines and use of lobectomy as an appropriate intervention in select patients.

Thyroid lobectomy is currently recommended by the ATA as the initial treatment for patients with very-low-risk thyroid cancer, such as PTMC. In 1 retrospective review of 255 patient in Korea who underwent a lobectomy or a total thyroidectomy for treatment of unilateral multifocal PTMC, there were no significant differences in recurrence after a median of almost 95 months (range, 24–209 months).[21] These findings were consistent regardless of patient age, tumor size, microscopic extrathyroidal extension, and lymphovascular invasion.[21] The only significant findings were the high incidence of complications, such as hypocalcemia and vocal cord paralysis, in the group total undergoing thyroidectomy.

MORE-INTENSIVE MANAGEMENT: TOTAL THYROIDECTOMY

Patients who do not meet the aforementioned criteria or who have a preference for more intensive management are candidates for a total thyroidectomy as their initial treatment. Specifically, tumor characteristics indicating total thyroidectomy as the initial intervention are size greater than 4 cm, large isthmus nodules, or a nodule that extends to the contralateral side, which may make it unsafe to transect without risking a contralateral nerve injury (see **Fig. 2**). Postoperative pathologic findings that may indicate need for a completion thyroidectomy include aggressive histology, lymph node involvement, positive margins, and significant vascular invasion.[13] Other factors that are important to consider are previous history of head/neck radiation, previous surgery, strong family history of thyroid cancer, and whether the patient would have a benefit from radioiodine ablation postoperatively. If there is a need to follow thyroglobulin levels closely as part of the surveillance plan, then total thyroidectomy would be beneficial, as thyroglobulin levels can be difficult to interpret after lobectomy alone (see **Table 1**).

An equally important but at times overlooked consideration in treatment decision making is considering the patient's own beliefs and thoughts regarding extent of surgery.[22] Some patients feel more comfortable having a total thyroidectomy, desire to avoid a future completion thyroidectomy, or prefer follow-up with accurate thyroglobulin monitoring. However, clinicians must keep in mind that fear of cancer and anxiety may be drivers of patient preference for total thyroidectomy and the desire for outcomes, such as peace of mind, that may not be achieved if they experience worry about recurrence. A detailed discussion that provides the necessary information and supports patients' emotional concerns is ideal to facilitate this decision. Studies have shown that emotions like fear and anxiety are associated with preference for more intensive treatment but may lead to decision regret.[23,24]

LESS-INTENSIVE, NONOPERATIVE MANAGEMENT: ACTIVE SURVEILLANCE

Active surveillance (AS) is the continued monitoring of a known cancer that delays or completely avoids thyroid surgery. Monitoring of these lesions is typically done with serial comprehensive ultrasounds. Although resistance to this approach hinders broad acceptance, the concept of AS is not new. The first study to propose AS as an efficacious alternative to surgery for treatment of PTMC began in 1993 in Japan at Kuma Hospital, a facility specializing in the treatment and management of thyroid disease. This initial study found more than 70% of PTMCs were stable or actually decreased in size.[25] Although the ATA does not routinely recommend fine needle aspiration (FNA) for 1-cm or smaller lesions, which may represent very low-risk cancers, multiple studies have supported AS, which led the ATA to include this option in the most recent guidelines for very-low-risk cancers with nonaggressive features.[26,27] These features include completely intrathyroidal lesions, no evidence of extrathyroidal extension or concern for positive cervical lymph nodes, and no evidence of distant disease.[28] Symptomatic lesions, such as voice changes indicating recurrent laryngeal nerve invasion, are a contraindication to AS. Other suspicious features not universally accepted as contraindications include calcifications. Macrocalcifications have been associated with a shorter tumor volume doubling time (TVDT, defined as time it takes for volume of the tumor to increase by 50%).[29] Nevertheless, other studies have not identified rim, macrocalcifications, abnd microcalcifications as aggressive features.[27,28]

Currently, no universally accepted protocol or standardized method exists for how and when to perform ultrasound monitoring for AS. The overall duration of ultrasound surveillance is also in question, particularly for young patients who will live a long time. In their original study, Miyauchi and colleagues[28] used ultrasound at 6 months after diagnosis and at least once a year afterward. Other options include ultrasound 3 months after initial diagnosis and then 6 months followed by yearly surveillance or ultrasound every 6 months for the first 2 years with yearly ultrasound surveillance thereafter. Consistency in the way the ultrasound is performed is crucial particularly with 3-dimensional measurements as well as nodal evaluation. This includes evaluation of the ultrasound by the same team with images readily available for comparison. Confidence in ultrasound quality is a potential barrier to AS. Any suspicious lymph nodes encountered during surveillance should be biopsied. This nonoperative approach would benefit from endorsement of an accepted algorithm, which may in turn increase a provider's comfort in their recommendations and management.

Active Surveillance: Patient Selection

Although the tumor characteristics described above drive patient eligibility for AS, other patient characteristics are also important in selection. Many studies have shown that younger age is associated with larger and early increases in size of PTMC as well as the development of lymph nodes metastasis.[26,29–31] One study found that age less than 50 years had TVDT of less than 5 years ($P<.001$), indicating that this age group has a faster tumor growth.[29] These findings are perhaps the opposite of what one would predict, as older age is generally considered a negative prognostic factor for PTC and highlights potential heterogeneity of thyroid cancer.[32] On the other hand, some studies indicate that older age is associated with reduced risk of tumor growth during AS.[33] Because this age group may have a shorter remaining lifespan during which a thyroid cancer would not be expected to grow substantially, those with advanced age or competing causes of death can be good candidates for AS.[34,35]

As the literature to investigate the effectiveness of AS increases, so too have the size criteria for inclusion, with cancers up to 2 cm being evaluated under research protocols.[36–39] In 1 meta-analysis, 9 studies evaluating the efficacy of AS, which included 4156 pooled patients, found that AS is a safe alternative to surgery without increased risk of recurrence or death with a 0.03% disease-specific mortality.[40] The meta-analysis found that 4.4% of these tumors increased in size ($\geq$3 mm) for both low-risk and very-low-risk cancers. Although not all included studies showed a decrease in tumor size, the pooled proportion of those that did reveal 6.7% of tumors decreased in size. Local metastasis to cervical lymph nodes was low at 1.2% for PTMCs. Although the growth increase of $\geq$3 mm is widely reported and used as an indication of progression and referral to surgery, TVDT has also gained traction as a more dynamic estimation of thyroid cancer size. In 1 study, the vast majority (71.8%) of patients had a TVDT of more than 5 years with only 10.3% of patients having a TVDT of less than 2 years. These findings may support the very slow growth of a large proportion of PTMCs and suggest that some patients who will fail AS will declare themselves early on.[29] Although there are some promising data in support of AS, more research is needed to fully evaluate its effectiveness and long-term outcomes.

Although AS is a less-intensive option for patients with low- and very-low-risk thyroid cancer, this approach can also be used in high-risk patients with multiple comorbidities, those with advanced age with a short expected life expectancy, or any patient wherein the risk of surgery outweighs the potential benefit.

Active Surveillance: Tumor Progression and Delayed Thyroid Surgery

Tumor progression and referral for surgery are typically indicated for growth ≥3 mm or when nodal metastasis is suspected or confirmed. In addition to these developments, lesions in close proximity to, but not invading, surrounding structures are recommended for surgical consideration. If the patient elects to proceed with AS despite progression, Miyauchi and colleagues recommend rescue surgery once the PTMC increases to 13 mm. As discussed previously, TVDT has become a useful indicator for tumor progression. One study containing 273 patients found that 29% had a significant volume increase (defined as ≥50%), but only 4.4% of patients had a significant maximal diameter increase of ≥3 mm.[29] In this cohort, the patients who had a tumor increase ≥3 mm all had TVDT of less than 3 years.[29] Studies are needed to determine the optimal measure of progression and maximal diameter alone versus TVDT.

In 1 meta-analysis containing 9 different studies, the pooled incidence of delayed thyroid surgery (DTS) for PTMCs was 11.2%.[40] This meta-analysis also evaluated if patient preference was the indication for DTS and found that at least half of DTS was performed because of patient preference (51.9%). The same meta-analysis found that only 29.1% of DTS was performed because of growth of the tumor.[40] Other studies have shown a higher rate of DTS (19.4%), with most of these owing to rapidly growing tumors (60.3%).[29]

Active Surveillance: Decision-Making Considerations

For a patient to undergo AS for management of PTMC, it is essential that a thorough discussion includes all options, risks of progression, and DTS. A multidisciplinary approach, including surgeons, endocrinologists, the patient, and their loved ones, that considers tumor factors is important and must be considered as the team comes to a *joint* conclusion regarding the patient's care. When evaluating data before the 2015 ATA Guidelines, Price and colleagues[22] found most patients with PTMC underwent a total thyroidectomy (70.8%). Those patients who were known to have a PTMC preoperatively had an even higher rate of total thyroidectomy (94.7%). Chart review revealed various reasons for the decision, but most were *surgeon*-driven decisions.[22] Interestingly, the only patient reasons given for choosing surgery was the "surgeon's recommendation." This finding highlights the considerable amount of weight that a physician has in swaying their patient's decision regarding treatment. In another survey of practice patterns, responses from 134 Japanese institutes that treat 72% of the thyroid cancer cases in Japan indicated that 38% of respondents provided the patient with all treatment options and did not provide their own recommendation so as not to influence a patient's decision.[41] Although other respondents also provided options, 31% recommended AS and 26% recommended surgery. AS was selected in 54% of the patients treated at these institutions.[41]

Active Surveillance: Patient Decision-Making Considerations

For a patient to be enrolled in AS management, he or she must ideally be committed to the process, be able to comply with routine visits and testing, and understand their disease. Inclusion of a nonbinding contract or consent form signed by the physician and patient may be considered a strategy to encourage patient dedication to AS. Despite patients having an excellent prognosis because their cancer is small and slow growing, noncompliance with AS has the potential to cause unnecessary morbidity. A full discussion of the potential psychological effects of living with cancer is important, as the sequelae can substantially influence a patient's QOL.

Even with considerable evidence supporting AS and some studies indicating a 3% risk of tumor progression, the decision to proceed to thyroid surgery is most often patient-driven.[42] In 1 QOL assessment comparing patients who selected AS versus immediate surgery, the surgery group experienced more fatigue, changes in voice and appearance, and more severe health deterioration. Patients who selected AS for management had higher baseline psychological health scores and had better physical and psychological health scores 8 months after intervention.[43] The type of procedure completed in the surgery group varied from lobectomy to a total thyroidectomy with modified radical neck dissection, which may have affected the QOL scores if patients experienced higher levels of morbidity. Another QOL survey of patients with PTMC undergoing AS versus lobectomy showed that the lobectomy group had more neuromuscular problems, complaints involving the throat/mouth, and scar complaints than the AS group with no difference in fear of progression of their disease.[44] Additional long-term data from a large cohort are needed, as these studies were all limited by their size.

Active Surveillance: Provider Decision-Making Considerations

Although patient factors are important to consider in the decision to pursue AS, provider-related factors also affect the decision-making process. A survey of 448 physicians who treat thyroid cancer revealed that 76% thought AS was appropriate management for some patients.[45] Despite this result, only 44% recommended AS in their practice with increasing age of the patient and smaller tumor size associated with increased AS recommendations. When asked about barriers to AS, the most common responses were related to *patient factors* with subsequent *physician factors* being related to malpractice, diagnosis concerns, and unknown length of time for follow-up.[45] These results likely relate to physicians' discomfort with AS and lack of knowledge of the literature that often occurs when a new approach to a well-established disease process is being adopted. The lack of randomized controlled trials evaluating the efficacy of AS may be another barrier to the acceptance by some physicians.

Interestingly, despite resistance to AS, many providers are likely performing surveillance of nodules that have not yet been identified as malignant. The 2015 ATA Guidelines indicate that many of the PTMCs that would qualify for AS do not meet biopsy criteria based on size or degree of suspicion. The provider may then elect for the patient to return in a 3-, 6-, or 12-month timeframe to monitor for stability. For example, a 6-mm hypoechoic completely intrathyroidal lesion with normal borders does not meet biopsy criteria and would be followed with repeat ultrasound.[13]

Active Surveillance: Costs

When choosing treatment, patients and physicians must also consider the costs of treatment. For AS, costs include continued clinic visits, ultrasounds, and laboratory tests. The adequate duration of this monitoring is unknown, particularly for younger patients with long life expectancy. Although the costs for patients who undergo surgery appear to be isolated to the event itself, these patients still require postoperative clinic visits, surveillance ultrasounds, and thyroglobulin monitoring, although the duration may not be as long as that for AS. Other cost considerations not often discussed in the literature are that of surgical complications, postoperative medications (thyroid suppression/replacement, calcitriol, and persistent calcium use), and the associated laboratory tests to monitoring these. As a result, the literature is mixed, with some studies indicating that AS increases cost of care,[46–48] whereas others indicate surgery is drastically more expensive that AS.[8] These results change based on country of origin and may not be generalized to other nations with varying forms of reimbursement/health care. Ultimately, cost should not be the primary driver of care. The best management option for each individual patient should be in line with his or her goals of care. The influence of treatment on QOL should also be considered.

LESS-INTENSIVE, NONOPERATIVE MANAGEMENT: ABLATION

Although AS is a key nonoperative option and alternative to surgery, other management options exist for patients with very-low- or low-risk DTC who may not be comfortable with as passive an option as AS. In patients who are not surgical candidates or seek a less-invasive option (ie, refuse surgery), ethanol ablation (EA) and radiofrequency ablation (RFA) have been found to be effective in treatment of FNA-confirmed metastatic disease to cervical lymph nodes or locally recurrent cancer that is not near critical structures in the neck.[13] These options have been heavily studied for benign thyroid disease, such as EA for thyroid cysts or RFA of thyroid nodules, but have limited evidence in the treatment of primary DTC.[49] EA is performed by percutaneously directly injecting the index mass with the goal of causing atrophy and often requires several treatment sessions (1–6 injections), but does not require general anesthesia. EA, also called ethanol injection or sclerotherapy, has a pooled success rate of 87.5% for the treatment of recurrence with a 1.2% pooled risk of complications.[50] RFA is also a percutaneous treatment performed under local anesthesia but results in thermal tissue necrosis and fibrosis. In a study of 152 primary intrathyroidal PTMCs treated with ultrasound-guided RFA, 91.4% of tumors completely disappeared and had no evidence of recurrence or need for surgery with a mean follow-up of 39 months. The overall complication rate was 3%, including a voice change.[51] Other types of ablation, such as laser and microwave, have also been used for first-line treatment of PTMC. Much research is still needed to determine the efficacy of these ablative techniques in treatment of primary thyroid cancer. Their role is likely to be highest for very-low-risk disease like PTMC, or smaller low-risk cancers. Much like the multidisciplinary approach needed when pursuing AS, consultation with a surgeon before selecting these nonoperative managements may aid in patient selection and appropriately inform the patient of their surgical options so the patient may decide on an individualized treatment plan.

AREAS FOR FURTHER INVESTIGATION

In addition to expanding research on ablation of low-risk cancer, data are needed to determine if molecular testing is beneficial in deciding whether it is more appropriate to perform AS, primary surgery, or another less-invasive technique. Although molecular testing may increase costs, the findings could help minimize unnecessary surgery in some and inform extent of treatment in others. Consider a young patient with a 3.5-cm PTC. If this patient was found to have a dual TERT/BRAF mutation, which is associated with more aggressive disease, this result could factor into the decision to undergo a more invasive index surgery like a total thyroidectomy. The lack of a high-risk mutation could also potentially save a patient from a larger surgery and decrease associated perioperative costs and postoperative complications. Research on the role of molecular testing on guiding postoperative surveillance of patients with low-risk cancer is also needed. The role of TSH suppression also needs to be further evaluated as an adjunct to AS, as does the effectiveness of AS for tumors greater than 1 cm. Decreasing the duration and intensity of surveillance may be possible for some patients. In addition, high-quality randomized data are needed to determine the efficacy and long-term outcomes of the various treatments for low-risk thyroid cancer.

SUMMARY

Less-intensive management options, including AS and thyroid lobectomy, can be safely performed in patients with low-risk thyroid cancer and with excellent results. The decision to proceed with either of these options, as opposed to total thyroidectomy or ablation, relies on the characteristics of the tumor, the patient's desires, and a physician's ability to manage the patient. To increase utilization of AS, a consensus statement outlining specific indications and an algorithm would help ensure patients receive appropriate care and standardize the process. Ultimately, high-quality, head-to-head comparative effectiveness research is needed to support the uptake and adoption of less-intensive treatment strategies for low-risk thyroid cancer.

CLINICS CARE POINTS

- Low-risk papillary thyroid cancers have a recurrence rate of less than 10%. Less-intensive management may be warranted to decrease risks of morbidity. Total thyroidectomy, thyroid lobectomy, active surveillance, ethanol ablation, and radiofrequency ablation are all potentially effective treatments for thyroid cancer depending on the setting.

- In low-risk papillary thyroid cancers, lobectomy has been shown to have equal survival outcomes with decreased risks of complications, such as hypoparathyroidism and recurrent laryngeal nerve injury.

- Papillary thyroid microcarcinomas are a subset of papillary thyroid cancer that measures 1 cm or smaller and whose risk of recurrence in many cases is less than 2%.

- In papillary thyroid microcarcinomas without high-risk features, active surveillance should be discussed as an option with patients who are able to commit to the necessary follow-up and who can cope with living with cancer.

- Physicians have a substantial influence on patients and their treatment decisions. All viable treatment options should be discussed with patients, and physicians should make an effort to ensure patients have an active role in decision making that honors the patient's goals and preferences.

- Thyroid cancers that have many high-risk features, such as greater than 4 cm, extrathyroidal extension, invasion of adjacent structures, known disease to cervical lymph nodes or distant metastasis, are not ideal candidates for less-intensive management.

DISCLOSURE

The authors have nothing to disclose.

REFERENCES

1. SEER. Cancer stat facts: thyroid cancer. National Cancer Institute. Available at: https://seer.cancer.gov/statfacts/html/thyro.html. Accessed April 19, 2021.

2. Walgama E, Sacks WL, Ho AS. Papillary thyroid microcarcinoma: optimal management versus overtreatment. Curr Opin Oncol 2020;32(1):1–6. https://doi.org/10.1097/CCO.0000000000000595.

3. Harach HR, Franssila KO, Wasenius VM. Occult papillary carcinoma of the thyroid. A "normal" finding in Finland. A systematic autopsy study. Cancer 1985;56(3):531–8. https://doi.org/10.1002/1097-0142(19850801)56:3<531::aid-cncr2820560321>3.0.co;2-3.

4. Mohorea IS, Socea B, Şerban D, et al. Incidence of thyroid carcinomas in an extended retrospective study of 526 autopsies. Exp Ther Med 2021;21(6):607. https://doi.org/10.3892/etm.2021.10039.

5. LeClair K, Bell KJL, Furuya-Kanamori L, et al. Evaluation of gender inequity in thyroid cancer diagnosis: differences by sex in US thyroid cancer incidence compared with a meta-analysis of subclinical thyroid cancer rates at autopsy. JAMA Intern Med 2021;181(10):1351–8. https://doi.org/10.1001/jamainternmed.2021.4804.

6. McDow AD, Pitt SC. Extent of surgery for low-risk differentiated thyroid cancer. Surg Clin North Am 2019;99(4):599–610. https://doi.org/10.1016/j.suc.2019.04.003.

7. Molinaro E, Campopiano MC, Elisei R. Management of endocrine disease: papillary thyroid microcarcinoma: towards an active surveillance strategy. Eur J Endocrinol 2021. https://doi.org/10.1530/EJE-21-0256.

8. Oda H, Miyauchi A, Ito Y, et al. Comparison of the costs of active surveillance and immediate surgery in the management of low-risk papillary microcarcinoma of the thyroid. Endocr J 2017;64(1):59–64. https://doi.org/10.1507/endocrj.EJ16-0381.

9. White C, Weinstein MC, Fingeret AL, et al. Is less more? A microsimulation model comparing cost-effectiveness of the revised American Thyroid Association's 2015 to 2009 guidelines for the management of patients with thyroid nodules and differentiated thyroid cancer. Ann Surg 2020;271(4):765–73. https://doi.org/10.1097/SLA.0000000000003074.

10. Miyauchi A, Ito Y. Conservative surveillance management of low-risk papillary thyroid microcarcinoma. Endocrinol Metab Clin North Am 2019;48(1):215–26. https://doi.org/10.1016/j.ecl.2018.10.007.

11. Goldfarb M, Casillas J. Thyroid cancer-specific quality of life and health-related quality of life in young adult thyroid cancer survivors. Thyroid 2016;26(7):923–32. https://doi.org/10.1089/thy.2015.0589.

12. Hughes DT, Reyes-Gastelum D, Kovatch KJ, et al. Energy level and fatigue after surgery for thyroid cancer: a population-based study of patient-reported outcomes. Surgery 2020;167(1):102–9. https://doi.org/10.1016/j.surg.2019.04.068.

13. Haugen BR, Alexander EK, Bible KC, et al. 2015 American Thyroid Association management guidelines for adult patients with thyroid nodules and differentiated thyroid cancer: the American Thyroid Association Guidelines Task Force on thyroid nodules and differentiated thyroid cancer. Thyroid 2016;26(1):1–133. https://doi.org/10.1089/thy.2015.0020.

14. Grani G, Zatelli MC, Alfò M, et al. Real-world performance of the American Thyroid Association risk estimates in predicting 1-year differentiated thyroid cancer outcomes: a prospective multicenter study of 2000 patients. Thyroid 2021;31(2):264–71. https://doi.org/10.1089/thy.2020.0272.

15. Nixon IJ, Ganly I, Patel SG, et al. Thyroid lobectomy for treatment of well differentiated intrathyroid malignancy. Surgery 2012;151(4):571–9. https://doi.org/10.1016/j.surg.2011.08.016.

16. Adam MA, Pura J, Goffredo P, et al. Impact of extent of surgery on survival for papillary thyroid cancer patients younger than 45 years. J Clin Endocrinol Metab 2015;100(1):115–21. https://doi.org/10.1210/jc.2014-3039.

17. Haigh PI, Urbach DR, Rotstein LE. Extent of thyroidectomy is not a major determinant of survival in low- or high-risk papillary thyroid cancer. Ann Surg Oncol 2005;12(1):81–9. https://doi.org/10.1007/s10434-004-1165-1.

18. Cox C, Bosley M, Southerland LB, et al. Lobectomy for treatment of differentiated thyroid cancer: can patients avoid postoperative thyroid hormone supplementation and be compliant with the American Thyroid Association guidelines? Surgery 2018;163(1):75–80. https://doi.org/10.1016/j.surg.2017.04.039.

19. Kluijfhout WP, Pasternak JD, Lim J, et al. Frequency of high-risk characteristics requiring total thyroidectomy for 1-4 cm well-differentiated thyroid cancer. Thyroid 2016;26(6):820–4. https://doi.org/10.1089/thy.2015.0495.

20. Xu S, Huang H, Wang X, et al. Long-term outcomes of lobectomy for papillary thyroid carcinoma with high-risk features. Br J Surg 2021;108(4):395–402. https://doi.org/10.1093/bjs/znaa129.

21. Jeon YW, Gwak HG, Lim ST, et al. Long-term prognosis of unilateral and multifocal papillary thyroid microcarcinoma after unilateral lobectomy versus total thyroidectomy. Ann Surg Oncol 2019;26(9):2952–8. https://doi.org/10.1245/s10434-019-07482-w.

22. Price AK, Randle RW, Schneider DF, et al. Papillary thyroid microcarcinoma: decision-making, extent of surgery, and outcomes. J Surg Res 2017;218: 237–45. https://doi.org/10.1016/j.jss.2017.05.054.

23. Pitt SC, Saucke MC, Wendt EM, et al. Patients' reaction to diagnosis with thyroid cancer or an indeterminate thyroid nodule. Thyroid 2021;31(4):580–8. https://doi.org/10.1089/thy.2020.0233.

24. Bongers PJ, Greenberg CA, Hsiao R, et al. Differences in long-term quality of life between hemithyroidectomy and total thyroidectomy in patients treated for low-risk differentiated thyroid carcinoma. Surgery 2020;167(1):94–101. https://doi.org/10.1016/j.surg.2019.04.060.

25. Ito Y, Uruno T, Nakano K, et al. An observation trial without surgical treatment in patients with papillary microcarcinoma of the thyroid. Thyroid 2003;13(4):381–7. https://doi.org/10.1089/105072503321669875.

26. Ito Y, Miyauchi A, Kihara M, et al. Patient age is significantly related to the progression of papillary microcarcinoma of the thyroid under observation. Thyroid 2014;24(1):27–34. https://doi.org/10.1089/thy.2013.0367.

27. Sugitani I, Toda K, Yamada K, et al. Three distinctly different kinds of papillary thyroid microcarcinoma should be recognized: our treatment strategies and outcomes. World J Surg 2010;34(6):1222–31. https://doi.org/10.1007/s00268-009-0359-x.

28. Miyauchi A, Ito Y, Oda H. Insights into the management of papillary microcarcinoma of the thyroid. Thyroid 2018;28(1):23–31. https://doi.org/10.1089/thy.2017.0227.

29. Oh H-S, Kwon H, Song E, et al. Tumor volume doubling time in active surveillance of papillary thyroid carcinoma. Thyroid 2019;29(5):642–9. https://doi.org/10.1089/thy.2018.0609.

30. Fukuoka O, Sugitani I, Ebina A, et al. Natural history of asymptomatic papillary thyroid microcarcinoma: time-dependent changes in calcification and vascularity during active surveillance. World J Surg 2016;40(3):529–37. https://doi.org/10.1007/s00268-015-3349-1.

31. Miyauchi A, Kudo T, Ito Y, et al. Estimation of the lifetime probability of disease progression of papillary microcarcinoma of the thyroid during active surveillance. Surgery 2018;163(1):48–52. https://doi.org/10.1016/j.surg.2017.03.028.
32. Haser GC, Tuttle RM, Su HK, et al. Active surveillance for papillary thyroid microcarcinoma: new challenges and opportunities for the health care system. Endocr Pract 2016;22(5):602–11. https://doi.org/10.4158/EP151065.RA.
33. Koshkina A, Fazelzad R, Sugitani I, et al. Association of patient age with progression of low-risk papillary thyroid carcinoma under active surveillance. JAMA Otolaryngol Neck Surg 2020;146(6):552. https://doi.org/10.1001/jamaoto.2020.0368.
34. Papaleontiou M, Norton EC, Reyes-Gastelum D, et al. Competing causes of death in older adults with thyroid cancer. Thyroid 2021;31(9):1359–65. https://doi.org/10.1089/thy.2020.0929.
35. Lohia S, Gupta P, Curry M, et al. Life expectancy and treatment patterns in elderly patients with low-risk papillary thyroid cancer: a population-based analysis. Endocr Pract 2021;27(3):228–35. https://doi.org/10.1016/j.eprac.2020.12.004.
36. Tuttle RM, Fagin JA, Minkowitz G, et al. Natural history and tumor volume kinetics of papillary thyroid cancers during active surveillance. JAMA Otolaryngol Neck Surg 2017;143(10):1015. https://doi.org/10.1001/jamaoto.2017.1442.
37. Sanabria A. Active surveillance in thyroid microcarcinoma in a Latin-American cohort. JAMA Otolaryngol Neck Surg 2018;144(10):947. https://doi.org/10.1001/jamaoto.2018.1663.
38. Sakai T, Sugitani I, Ebina A, et al. Active surveillance for T1bN0M0 papillary thyroid carcinoma. Thyroid 2019;29(1):59–63. https://doi.org/10.1089/thy.2018.0462.
39. Griffin A, Brito JP, Bahl M, et al. Applying criteria of active surveillance to low-risk papillary thyroid cancer over a decade: how many surgeries and complications can be avoided? Thyroid 2017;27(4):518–23. https://doi.org/10.1089/thy.2016.0568.
40. Saravana-Bawan B, Bajwa A, Paterson J, et al. Active surveillance of low-risk papillary thyroid cancer: a meta-analysis. Surgery 2020;167(1):46–55. https://doi.org/10.1016/j.surg.2019.03.040.
41. Sugitani I, Ito Y, Miyauchi A, et al. Active surveillance versus immediate surgery: questionnaire survey on the current treatment strategy for adult patients with low-risk papillary thyroid microcarcinoma in Japan. Thyroid 2019;29(11):1563–71. https://doi.org/10.1089/thy.2019.0211.
42. Molinaro E, Campopiano MC, Pieruzzi L, et al. Active surveillance in papillary thyroid microcarcinomas is feasible and safe: experience at a single Italian center. J Clin Endocrinol Metab 2020;105(3):e172–80. https://doi.org/10.1210/clinem/dgz113.
43. Lan Y, Cao L, Song Q, et al. The quality of life in papillary thyroid microcarcinoma patients undergoing lobectomy or total thyroidectomy: a cross-sectional study. Cancer Med 2021;10(6):1989–2002. https://doi.org/10.1002/cam4.3747.
44. Jeon MJ, Lee Y-M, Sung T-Y, et al. Quality of life in patients with papillary thyroid microcarcinoma managed by active surveillance or lobectomy: a cross-sectional study. Thyroid 2019;29(7):956–62. https://doi.org/10.1089/thy.2018.0711.
45. Hughes DT, Reyes-Gastelum D, Ward KC, et al. Barriers to the use of active surveillance for thyroid cancer: results of a physician survey. Ann Surg 2020. https://doi.org/10.1097/SLA.0000000000004417.
46. Venkatesh S, Pasternak JD, Beninato T, et al. Cost-effectiveness of active surveillance versus hemithyroidectomy for micropapillary thyroid cancer. Surgery 2017;161(1):116–26. https://doi.org/10.1016/j.surg.2016.06.076.

47. Lin JF, Jonker PKC, Cunich M, et al. Surgery alone for papillary thyroid microcarcinoma is less costly and more effective than long term active surveillance. Surgery 2020;167(1):110–6. https://doi.org/10.1016/j.surg.2019.05.078.

48. Kandil E, Noureldine SI, Tufano RP. Thyroidectomy vs active surveillance for sub-centimeter papillary thyroid cancers—the cost conundrum. JAMA Otolaryngol Neck Surg 2016;142(1):9. https://doi.org/10.1001/jamaoto.2015.2852.

49. Ntelis S, Linos D. Efficacy and safety of radiofrequency ablation in the treatment of low-risk papillary thyroid carcinoma: a review. Hormones (Athens) 2021;20(2): 269–77. https://doi.org/10.1007/s42000-021-00283-5.

50. Fontenot TE, Deniwar A, Bhatia P, et al. Percutaneous ethanol injection vs reoperation for locally recurrent papillary thyroid cancer. JAMA Otolaryngol Neck Surg 2015;141(6):512. https://doi.org/10.1001/jamaoto.2015.0596.

51. Lim HK, Cho SJ, Baek JH, et al. US-guided radiofrequency ablation for low-risk papillary thyroid microcarcinoma: efficacy and safety in a large population. Korean J Radiol 2019;20(12):1653–61. https://doi.org/10.3348/kjr.2019.0192.

Novel Therapeutics for Advanced Differentiated Thyroid Cancer

Leedor Lieberman, MD[a], Francis Worden, MD[b],*

KEYWORDS

- Thyroid • Cancer • Radioactive iodine • Refractory • Sorafenib • Lenvatinib
- Immunotherapy • Next-generation sequencing

KEY POINTS

- Treatment of radioactive iodine (RAI) -refractory differentiated thyroid cancer is evolving.
- Current Food and Drug Administration–approved therapies include the tyrosine kinase inhibitors sorafenib and lenvatinib.
- Next-generation sequencing is used to guide individualized targeted therapies.
- Selective kinase therapies have promising outcomes as targeted therapy.
- Treatment invoking RAI sensitivity and immunotherapy is under investigation.

INTRODUCTION

Differentiated thyroid cancer (DTC) refers to papillary thyroid cancer, follicular thyroid cancer, and Hurthle cell thyroid cancer. DTC may be cured with thyroidectomy, radioactive iodine (RAI) therapy, and thyroid-stimulating hormone (TSH) suppression in most cases.[1] Recurrence can be treated with RAI therapy using iodine-131 (^{131}I) in both locoregional and metastatic disease.[1] Disease not responsive to ^{131}I is considered RAI-refractory and carries a poor prognosis.[1] Treatment for RAI-refractory DTC is evolving, and therapeutic choice should be individualized with consideration of adverse effects and tumor genomics (**Fig. 1**).

DEFINITION

The definition of RAI-refractory disease is controversial. In the 2015 American Thyroid Association Guidelines, RAI-refractory DTC was classified into the following categories[2,3]:

---

[a] Department of Metabolism, Endocrinology and Diabetes, University of Michigan, Lobby C #1300, 4029 Avenue Maria Drive, Ann Arbor, MI 48105, USA; [b] Department of Hematology and Oncology, University of Michigan, 1500 East Medical Center Drive Med Inn Building, Room C369, Ann Arbor, MI 48109, USA
* Corresponding author.
E-mail address: fworden@med.umich.edu

Endocrinol Metab Clin N Am 51 (2022) 367–378
https://doi.org/10.1016/j.ecl.2021.11.019
0889-8529/21/© 2021 Elsevier Inc. All rights reserved.

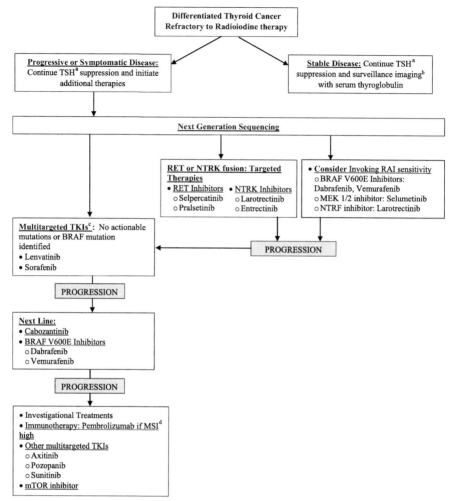

Fig. 1. Treatment algorithm for RAI-refractory DTC. Treatment of progressive or symptomatic disease includes the currently FDA-approved therapies: lenvatinib and sorafenib. Consideration of adverse effects is necessary in deciding an agent of choice. Selective kinases should be considered as the literature is evolving. Tumor-specific genomic alterations should be used to determine selective kinase therapy. Investigational treatments may be considered in progressive disease, including immunotherapy, targeted kinase inhibitors to invoke RAI avidity, and other targeted pathways. [a] TSH. [b] FDG-PET-CT, MRI, or CT scan of the neck, chest, abdomen, pelvis. [c] TKI. [d] Microsatellite instability.

1. Disease that does not concentrate ^{131}I at the time of initial diagnostic whole-body scan
2. Disease that previously concentrated [131]I
3. Disease that concentrates ^{131}I at some lesions, but not at others
4. Disease that has metastasized despite significant ^{131}I uptake

Some also consider patients to be RAI refractory if they have received greater than 600 mCi of RAI.[2]

Once disease is determined to be RAI refractory, surveillance for disease progression should be pursued with fluorodeoxyglucose-18 (^{18}FDG)-PET-computed tomography (CT), MRI, or CT of the neck, chest, abdomen, and pelvis with contrast, as ^{131}I whole-body scans may be futile.[2,3] Once the tumor burden is large and progressive or causes symptoms, systemic therapies should be considered.[2,3] However, if disease burden is minimal, treatment may not be warranted, owing to an indolent clinical course.[2–4]

CURRENT THERAPEUTICS

Targeted therapeutic agents for progressive or symptomatic RAI-refractory metastatic DTC emerged from genetic research in the field of thyroid cancer biology.[4] Following clinical investigations, multitargeted tyrosine kinase inhibitors (mTKIs) are now the first-line therapy for RAI-refractory metastatic DTC.[4] Currently, there are 2 tyrosine kinase inhibitors (TKIs) approved by the Food and Drug Administration (FDA) for RAI-refractory metastatic DTC: sorafenib and lenvatinib. Although sorafenib and lenvatinib share some targets, they differ in others, including tyrosine kinase inhibition of RAF, including BRAF-V6000E in sorafenib and FGFRs in lenvatinib.[5,6] Both treatments target multiple kinases and have been shown to improve progression-free survival, although with significant treatment-related adverse effects.[5,6]

Sorafenib

Sorafenib is a TKI with multiple targets, including VEGF-1 to 3, RET, PDGFR-B, and RAF, including BRAF-V600E.[5] In a phase 2 clinical study, Schneider and colleagues[7] found that in patients with RAI-refractory DTC treatment with sorafenib resulted in a median progression-free survival of 18 months. A phase 3 randomized, double-blinded, placebo-controlled, multicenter trial performed by the DECISION investigators was subsequently pursued.[5] In this study, patients with RAI-refractory DTC were randomized to sorafenib 400 mg twice daily (n = 207) versus placebo (n = 210).[5] The median progression-free survival was significantly improved in the sorafenib versus placebo group, with 10.8 months versus 5.8 months, respectively ($P<.0001$).[5] No statistically significant difference in overall survival between the treatment groups was found ($P = .14$).[5] The overall response rate in the sorafenib group was 12.2%, all partial response, versus 0.5% in the placebo group ($P<.0001$).[5] Patients had an improvement in progression-free survival regardless of BRAF and RAS tumor mutation status, although tumor mutation data were only available in a portion of the patients (61.4%).[5] With regards to safety, 98.6% of patients treated with sorafenib experienced treatment-related adverse effects, compared with the 87.6% of patients treated with placebo.[5] Most of the sorafenib adverse effects were grade 1 or grade 2, including hand-foot-skin reaction, diarrhea, and alopecia; the most common adverse effects in the placebo group were fatigue, diarrhea, and cough.[5] Serious adverse effects were reported in 37.2% in the sorafenib group versus 26.3% in the placebo group.[5]

Lenvatinib

Lenvatinib is a TKI with multiple targets, including VEGF-1 to 3, FGFR-1 to 4, PDGFR-a, RET, and KIT pathways.[8] The phase 2 study of lenvatinib showed positive response, after which the phase 3 Study of Lenvatinib in Differentiated Cancer of the Thyroid (SELECT) was developed.[8,9] In the phase 3 randomized, double-blinded, placebo-controlled, international multicenter trial, patients with RAI-refractory DTC were randomized to lenvatinib 24 mg daily (n = 261) versus placebo (n = 131).[8] The median progression-free survival was 18.3 months in the lenvatinib group versus 3.6 months in the placebo group (P<.001).[8] Furthermore, patients had an improved progression-free survival despite tumor BRAF or RAS mutation status.[8] Tumor response by RECIST criteria was significantly improved in the lenvatinib group: complete response was achieved in 1.5% (n = 4) and partial response in 63.2% (n = 165) in lenvatinib-treated patients versus 0% and 1.5%, respectively, in the placebo group.[8] Despite these promising outcomes, 97.3% of patients treated with lenvatinib experienced treatment-related adverse effects, including grade 3 or higher (75.9%) adverse effects, such as hypertension, proteinuria, and arterial and venous thromboembolic effects.[8] Furthermore, treatment with lenvatinib was terminated because of adverse effects in 14.2% of patients compared with 2.3% of placebo.[8]

Although both sorafenib and lenvatinib led to an improvement in progression-free survival in patients with RAI-refractory DTC, the investigators of SELECT think that the longer progression-free survival seen in lenvatinib may be due to the specific FGFR inhibition.[8]

Cabozantinib is an additional multikinase inhibitor that is on the horizon for potential future FDA approval for RAI-refractory DTC. In a recently published phase 3, multi-center, randomized, double-blind, placebo-control trial (COSMIC-311), patients with RAI-refractory DTC and prior treatment with lenvatinib or sorafenib were randomized to cabozantinib 60 mg (n = 125) or placebo (n = 62).[10] In the intention-to-treat population, the median progression-free survival at the interim analysis was not met in patients treated with cabozantinib versus 1.9 months in the placebo treatment group (P<.001).[10] Grade 3 or 4 adverse effects, including plantar-palmar erythrodysesthesia, hypertension and fatigue occurred in 57% of patients treated with cabozantinib versus 26% of those treated with placebo.[10] The investigators concluded that the limited progression-free survival in the placebo group is suggestive of an aggressive disease, for which cabozantinib is a promising treatment with a reasonable adverse effect profile.[10]

INVOKING RADIOACTIVE IODINE SENSITIVITY

Although the current treatments above represent an improvement in progression-free survival, the overall survival benefit is limited. Therefore, there is interest in developing therapies to invoke RAI sensitivity, which may impart survival benefit.

Specifically, BRAF inhibition via direct BRAF inhibitors or downstream MAPK kinase (MEK) inhibitors reestablishes iodine concentration in thyroid tumor cells.[6,11,12] Investigations of MEK1/2 inhibitors (selumetinib) and BRAF inhibitors (dabrafenib) have promising outcomes in invoking RAI sensitivity over a relatively short treatment course, allowing for additional treatment with ^{131}I with minimal drug exposure and associated adverse effects.[11,12]

MAPK kinase 1 and 2 Inhibitor

Selumetinib is a selective, allosteric MEK1 and 2 inhibitor.[11] Ho and colleagues[11] treated patients (n = 20) with RAI-refractory DTC with selumetinib 75 mg twice daily for 4 weeks. Pretreatment and posttreatment [124]I PET-CT were obtained and compared by blinded reviewers. If the posttreatment [124]I PET-CT suggested that an ^{131}I of 2000 cGy could be given, then a therapeutic dose was administered. Of the patients enrolled, 9 had BRAF-V600E and 5 had NRAS tumor genetic mutations.[11] Twelve (60%) patients treated with selumetinib had new and/or increased [124]I uptake on posttreatment PET-CT, 8 of whom underwent additional therapy with 300 mCi of radioiodine and had a decrease in the size of target lesions at 6 months.[11]

Furthermore, all 5 of the patients with NRAS tumor genetic mutation had an increase in ^{124}I uptake following treatment with selumetinib; only 1 patient with BRAF tumor mutation received additional radioiodine therapy.[11] This treatment may be of specific interest in patients with NRAS mutations and offers a short treatment course with potential clinical benefit.[11] However, ASTRA, a phase 3 trial randomizing patients to treatment with selumetinib or placebo for adjuvant RAI therapy, found no significant difference in complete remission rates.[13] The trial was terminated early because of futility.[14]

BRAF Inhibitor

Dabrafenib is a selective BRAF-V600E inhibitor.[12] Rothenberg and colleagues[12] treated patients (n = 10) with BRAF-V600E mutated RAI-refractory papillary thyroid cancer with dabrafenib 150 mg twice daily for 25 days. Posttreatment ^{131}I whole-body scans were performed, and if imaging showed new target lesions, then patients were continued on dabrafenib and received treatment with ^{131}I 150 mCi.[12] Six patients were found to have increased RAI uptake following treatment with dabrafenib and subsequently received additional ^{131}I treatment.[12] Of those treated with ^{131}I, 5 had a reduction in the size of target lesions on 6-month follow-up CT-scan imaging,[12] which by RECIST criteria was consistent with stable disease (n = 4) and partial response (n = 2).[12] The investigators concluded that dabrafenib can be used to induce RAI uptake in patients with BRAF-V600E mutated RAI-refractory papillary thyroid cancer.[12] More recently, Dunn and colleagues[15] found that treatment with vemurafenib, an alternative BRAF inhibitor, reestablishes RAI avidity in BRAF-mutated RAI-refractory thyroid cancer. Of note, treatment with BRAF inhibition remains experimental and has not universally been accepted as standard of care.

UTILITY OF NEXT-GENERATION SEQUENCING

The emergence of next-generation sequencing (NGS) has led to a broader understanding of cancer genomics and the development of target-specific therapeutics for various malignancies. NGS allows for identification of common and less-common genomic alterations that are potential targets of individualized therapeutics based on biopsy results.[16] Furthermore, in a recent retrospective study, Moore and colleagues[17] showed the potential for thyroid tumor control with NGS-guided therapy.

In DTC, specific genomic alterations have been identified in high frequency, including BRAF-V600E, RET, NTRK, and ALK.[17] The signal pathways involved in these genes have been exploited by the first-line therapy mTKI. However, the considerable side-effect profiles of mTKIs may be related to the nonspecific target affinity of these drugs.[18] As a result, there is interest in developing more specific signal-pathway targeted therapeutics that would focus treatment and limit side effects. Phase 1 and 2 trials have been completed, with additional studies in the future.

BRAF Inhibitors

The most common genetic alteration in thyroid cancer is the BRAF mutation, found in nearly 45% of sporadic papillary thyroid cancer.[19] Naturally, BRAF has evolved as a target of therapeutic interest. Vemurafenib and dabrafenib are both ATP-competitive BRAF inhibitors studied in the treatment of BRAF-mutated RAI-refractory DTC.[14,20–22]

Vemurafenib
In a phase 2 multicenter trial, Brose and colleagues[20] investigated the safety and efficacy of vemurafenib in patients with BRAF-V600E–positive RAI-refractory metastatic

or unresectable papillary thyroid cancer. Patients were enrolled into 2 cohorts based on prior treatment with a VEGFR multikinase inhibitor. In the VEGFR multikinase inhibitor treatment-naive group (n = 26), 38.5% of patients achieved a partial response and 35% of patients achieved stable disease for at least 6 months, with a median progression-free survival of 18.2 months.[20] In patients previously treated with a VEGFR multikinase inhibitor (n = 25), 27.3% of patients achieved a partial response and an additional 27.3% of patients achieved stable disease for at least 6 months, with a median progression-free survival of 8.9 months.[20]

Dabrafenib

In a phase 1 clinical trial by Falchook and colleagues,[21] 14 patients with BRAF-V600E–positive metastatic thyroid cancer were treated with dabrafenib. Partial response was achieved in 29% of patients, with a median progression-free survival of 11.3 months at the time of study completion. Most of treatment-related adverse effects were grade 2 or lower.[21] In an additional study by Shah and colleagues,[23] patients with BRAF-mutated, RAI-refractory papillary thyroid cancer were randomized to dabrafenib or dabrafenib with trametinib, a MEK inhibitor. The responses, based on modified RECIST criteria, showed a similar objective response rate of 50% versus 54% (P = .78), respectively, whereas the true overall response rates (complete, partial, and minor response) were 15% versus 35%, respectively.[23]

These findings suggest that vemurafenib and dabrafenib may have a therapeutic role in BRAF-mutated RAI-refractory thyroid cancer, as both first- or second-line therapy, especially as precision medicine evolves.[14,20–22]

RET inhibitors

Alterations in the RET protooncogene play a key role in tumorigenesis. More commonly associated with medullary thyroid cancer, RET alterations can also be found in less than 10% of DTC.[18] Studies investigating various RET-targeted therapeutics, including selpercatinib[18] and pralsetinib,[24] show promising results, which have led to their FDA approval in 2020.[25,26] In LIBRETTO-001, a phase 1/2 trial investigating selpercatinib (LOXO-292), 19 patients with previously treated, RET-fusion–positive, nonmedullary thyroid cancer were treated with selpercatinib 160 mg twice daily.[18] The results showed a 79% objective response.[18] The most common grade 3 or 4 adverse effects attributed to selpercatinib included edema, elevated liver function tests, and hyponatremia.[18] Treatment-related adverse effects with selpercatinib prompted dose reduction in 30% of patients and treatment discontinuation in 2% of patients.[18] In ARROW, a phase 1/2 clinical trial investigating the safety and efficacy of pralsetinib (BLU-667), 9 patients with previously treated, RET-fusion–positive, nonmedullary thyroid cancer were treated with pralsetinib 400 mg once daily and were included in the study.[24] The overall response rate was 89%, all partial responses by RECISTv1.1 criteria. The median progression-free survival was not reached, with an estimated 1-year progression-free survival rate of 81% after median follow-up of 12.9 months.[24] Concerning adverse effects attributed to pralsetinib included anemia, musculoskeletal pain, elevated liver function tests, hypertension, and pneumonitis; treatment-related adverse effects resulted in pralsetinib discontinuation in 4% of patients.[24]

The investigators concluded that for patients with thyroid cancer with RET-related genomic alterations, selpercatinib and pralsetinib are promising therapeutic options.[18,24]

NTRK inhibitors

NTRK genes encode tropomyosin receptor kinase (TRK) proteins, and rearrangements of the NTRK genes have been seen in papillary cancer among other solid malignancies.[17,27] Drilon and colleagues[27] investigated the efficacy and safety of larotrectinib, a TRK inhibitor, in patients with TRK-fusion-positive cancers. Of the 55 patients enrolled, 5 had thyroid cancers.[27] The overall response rate in all tumors was 75%.[27] Similar findings were seen in a pooled analysis of 3 clinical trials, where patients (n = 159) with TRK-fusion–positive cancers were enrolled and treated with larotrectinib.[28] Twenty-four patients with thyroid cancer were evaluated and found to have an objective response rate of 79%.[28] Recently, in an abstract by Cabanillas and colleagues,[29] treatment with larotrectinib in NTRK-fusion–positive DTC had an overall response rate of 90%. This emerging data suggest a potential role for TRK-target-specific treatment in RAI-refractory DTC with larotrectinib.[27–29]

FUTURE DIRECTIONS
Tyrosine Kinase Inhibitors Tolerability: Lenvatinib Dose Adjustment

The current mTKIs have encouraging outcomes in progression-free survival in RAI-refractory DTC at the cost of significant treatment-related adverse effects.[5,8] This has led to investigation into the consequences of treatment interruption and determination of the optimal lenvatinib dose. In a post hoc analysis of the phase 3 clinical trial investigating lenvatinib in RAI-refractory DTC (SELECT), longer duration of treatment dose interruptions owing to grade 3 or intolerable grade 2 adverse effects were associated with reduced treatment efficacy.[30] Lower doses have been suggested to improved drug tolerability. Alternative dosing of lenvatinib 14 mg with dose-uptitration or 18 mg without uptitration was found to have similar efficacy at 24 weeks with potential advantageous adverse effect profiles.[31] Clinically, this has been modeled in a recent trial comparing starting dose of lenvatinib 18 mg versus 24 mg (NCT02702388). An abstract with the findings did not show noninferiority in objective response rate of lenvatinib 18 mg versus 24 mg at 24 weeks with similar rates of grade 3 or higher treatment-related adverse effects.[32]

Invoke Radioactive Iodine Sensitivity with NTRK Inhibition

Future studies investigating the use of additional target-specific therapies to regain RAI avidity are necessary. In a case report, Groussin and colleagues[33] found that treatment with larotrectinib, a selective NTRK inhibitor, reestablished RAI uptake on diagnostic imaging that was previously inapparent. However, additional treatment with RAI was not pursued because of previous high levels of RAI exposure.

Enhancer of BRAF Inhibitor with Erb-3 Inhibition

It is hypothesized that the limited effect of BRAF inhibitors on restoration of iodine avidity in thyroid cancers is due to drug resistance from activation of the HER2/HER3 signaling pathway.[34] Cheng and colleagues[34] found that lapatinib, an HER inhibitor, added to BRAF/MEK inhibitors dabrafenib/selumetinib resulted in increased radioiodine uptake in BRAF-V600E–mutated cells in vitro when compared with treatment with BRAK/MEK inhibitors alone. A clinical trial (NCT01947023) assessing the safety and efficacy of treatment of dabrafenib with lapatinib in BRAF-V600E–mutated thyroid cancer is underway.[35] In their abstract, Sherman and colleagues[36] report 21 patients with BRAF-mutated DTC treated with various doses of lapatinib in combination with dabrafenib with overall response rate of 58% with a median progression-free survival of 18 months.

Immunotherapy

The development of immunotherapy targeting immune checkpoints, such as CTLA-4 and PD-L1, has led to encouraging outcomes in cancer therapy. In papillary thyroid cancer, PD-L1 overexpression is associated with increased risk of recurrence and shortened disease-free survival.[37] In a clinical trial (KEYNOTE-028), patients with 20 types of advanced solid malignancies were treated with pembrolizumab, a PD-L1 antibody, including 22 patients with papillary and follicular thyroid cancer.[38] In their abstract, Mehnert and colleagues[38] report that the 6-month overall survival was 100% with a 6-month median progression-free survival of 58.7%. More recently, Leboulleux and colleagues[39] published an abstract from a phase 2 clinical trial (NCT03012620) investigating pembrolizumab in RAI-refractory DTC. They found a median overall survival of 12.7 months and median progression-free survival of 2.6 months. At 6 months, the overall survival was 73.3% and progression-free survival was 16.9%.[39] In a study conducted by the International Thyroid Oncology Group (ITOG), 2 cohorts of immunotherapy and lenvatinib were studied in patients with RAI-refractory DTC. In cohort A, lenvatinib in combination with pembrolizumab as front-line therapy was shown to have a 74% median progression-free survival at 12 months.[40] In cohort B, pembrolizumab was added to lenvatinib on disease progression at whatever dose the patient progressed on. The median progression-free survival in this group was 12.6 months, and the overall response rate was 15%.[41]

Other Targets: mTOR

Additional tumorigenesis signal pathway inhibitors may play a role in augmenting outcomes of currently available therapies. For example, inhibition of the mTOR signaling pathway was found to reduce follicular cell thyroid tumor proliferation in a mouse model.[42] Subsequently, Sherman and colleagues[43] investigated the safety and efficacy of combining temsirolimus, an mTOR inhibitor, with sorafenib in patients with thyroid cancer. Of the 36 patients enrolled, 22% had a partial response and 58% had stable disease, with the median progression-free survival of 30.5% at 1 year.[43] The results of the Alliance A091302/ITOG 1706 randomized phase 2 study (NCT02143726) of sorafenib with or without everolimus in patients with RAI-refractory Hurthle cell thyroid cancer were reported at the ASCO 2021 annual meeting. The progression-free survival was significantly improved in the sorafenib and everolimus treatment group (24.7 months) as compared with the sorafenib-treatment-alone (10.9 months) group ($P = .1662$).[44]

SUMMARY

Treatment of RAI-refractory DTC has rapidly evolved with advancements in tumor genomics. Individualized treatment should consider specific tumor characteristics and balance the adverse effects of treatment. Additional studies are necessary to define treatment benefits and outcomes.

CLINICS CARE POINTS

- Sorafenib and lenvatinib are the only current Food and Drug Administration–approved therapies for radioactive iodine-refractory progressive differentiated thyroid cancer and are shown to improve progression-free survival.
- Lenvatinib may improve overall survival in older adults.
- Multitargeted tyrosine kinase inhibitors have significant adverse effects, which limit their use: skin reactions, diarrhea, hypertension, proteinuria, and thromboembolic events.
- Cabozantinib has promising outcomes for patients with disease progression on multitargeted tyrosine kinase inhibitors and may be a first-line therapy in the near future.

- Next-generation sequencing guides treatment via personalized tumor mutation genomics.
- Selective kinase inhibitors, including BRAF, RET, and NTRK, may improve progression-free survival in those with specific targeted alterations.
- Treatments invoking radioactive iodine sensitivity remain under investigation.
- The role of immunotherapy in radioactive iodine-refractory differentiated thyroid cancer may benefit patients who have disease progression on multitargeted tyrosine kinase inhibitors therapy.

DISCLOSURE

Dr L. Lieberman receives support from grant T32DK007245-45 from the National Institute of Diabetes and Digestive and Kidney Diseases. Dr F. Worden: Exilexis, Eisai, Pfizer, Merck, BMS, CUE Biopharmaceuticals.

REFERENCES

1. Busaidy NL, Cabanillas ME. Differentiated thyroid cancer: management of patients with radioiodine nonresponsive disease. J Thyroid Res 2012;2012:1–12. https://doi.org/10.1155/2012/618985.
2. Schlumberger M, Brose M, Elisei R, et al. Definition and management of radioactive iodine-refractory differentiated thyroid cancer. Lancet Diabetes Endocrinol 2014;2(5):356–8. https://doi.org/10.1016/S2213-8587(13)70215-8.
3. Haugen BR, Alexander EK, Bible KC, et al. 2015 American Thyroid Association Management Guidelines for adult patients with thyroid nodules and differentiated thyroid cancer: the American Thyroid Association Guidelines Task Force on thyroid nodules and differentiated thyroid cancer. Thyroid 2016;26(1):1–133. https://doi.org/10.1089/thy.2015.0020.
4. Gruber JJ, Colevas AD. Differentiated thyroid cancer: focus on emerging treatments for radioactive iodine-refractory patients. Oncologist 2015;20(2):113–26. https://doi.org/10.1634/theoncologist.2014-0313.
5. Brose MS, Nutting CM, Jarzab B, et al. Sorafenib in locally advanced or metastatic, radioactive iodine-refractory, differentiated thyroid cancer: a randomized, double-blind, phase 3 trial. Lancet 2014;384(9940):319–28. https://doi.org/10.1016/S0140-6736(14)60421-9.
6. Aashiq M, Silverman DA, Na'ara S, et al. Radioiodine-refractory thyroid cancer: molecular basis of redifferentiation therapies, management, and novel therapies. Cancers 2019;11(9):1382. https://doi.org/10.3390/cancers11091382.
7. Schneider TC, Abdulrahman RM, Corssmit EP, et al. Long-term analysis of the efficacy and tolerability of sorafenib in advanced radio-iodine refractory differentiated thyroid carcinoma: final results of a phase II trial. Eur J Endocrinol 2012; 167(5):643–50. https://doi.org/10.1530/EJE-12-0405.
8. Schlumberger M, Tahara M, Wirth LJ, et al. Lenvatinib versus placebo in radioiodine-refractory thyroid cancer. N Engl J Med 2015;372(7):621–30. https://doi.org/10.1056/NEJMoa1406470.
9. Sherman SI, Jarzab B, Cabanillas ME, et al. A phase II trial of the multitargeted kinase inhibitor E7080 in advanced radioiodine (RAI)-refractory differentiated thyroid cancer (DTC). J Clin Orthod 2011;29(15_suppl):5503. https://doi.org/10.1200/jco.2011.29.15_suppl.5503.
10. Brose MS, Robinson B, Sherman SI, et al. Cabozantinib for radioiodine-refractory differentiated thyroid cancer (COSMIC-311): a randomised, double-blind,

placebo-controlled, phase 3 trial. Lancet Oncol 2021. https://doi.org/10.1016/S1470-2045(21)00332-6.

11. Ho AL, Grewal RK, Leboeuf R, et al. Selumetinib-enhanced radioiodine uptake in advanced thyroid cancer. N Engl J Med 2013;368(7):623–32. https://doi.org/10.1056/NEJMoa1209288.

12. Rothenberg SM, McFadden DG, Palmer EL, et al. Redifferentiation of iodine-refractory *BRAF* V600E-mutant metastatic papillary thyroid cancer with dabrafenib. Clin Cancer Res 2015;21(5):1028–35. https://doi.org/10.1158/1078-0432.CCR-14-2915.

13. Ho A, Dedecjus M, Wirth L, et al. ASTRA: a phase III, randomized, placebo-controlled study evaluating complete remission rate (CRR) with short-course selumetinib plus adjuvant radioactive iodine (RAI) in patients (pts) with differentiated thyroid cancer (DTC). In: Proceedings of the 88th annual meeting of the American thyroid association. 2018. p. 3–7.

14. Kirtane K, Roth MY. Emerging therapies for radioactive iodine refractory thyroid cancer. Curr Treat Options Oncol 2020;21(3):18. https://doi.org/10.1007/s11864-020-0714-6.

15. Dunn LA, Sherman EJ, Baxi SS, et al. Vemurafenib redifferentiation of *BRAF* mutant, RAI-refractory thyroid cancers. J Clin Endocrinol Metab 2019;104(5):1417–28. https://doi.org/10.1210/jc.2018-01478.

16. Friedman AA, Letai A, Fisher DE, et al. Precision medicine for cancer with next-generation functional diagnostics. Nat Rev Cancer 2015;15(12):747–56. https://doi.org/10.1038/nrc4015.

17. Moore A, Bar Y, Maurice-Dror C, et al. Next-generation sequencing in thyroid cancers: do targetable alterations lead to a therapeutic advantage? Medicine (Baltimore) 2021;100(25):e26388. https://doi.org/10.1097/MD.0000000000026388.

18. Wirth LJ, Sherman E, Robinson B, et al. Efficacy of selpercatinib in RET-altered thyroid cancers. N Engl J Med 2020;383(9):825–35. https://doi.org/10.1056/NEJMoa2005651.

19. Xing M. BRAF mutation in thyroid cancer. Endocr Relat Cancer 2005;12(2):245–62. https://doi.org/10.1677/erc.1.0978.

20. Brose MS, Cabanillas ME, Cohen EEW, et al. Vemurafenib in patients with BRAFV600E-positive metastatic or unresectable papillary thyroid cancer refractory to radioactive iodine: a non-randomised, multicentre, open-label, phase 2 trial. Lancet Oncol 2016;17(9):1272–82. https://doi.org/10.1016/S1470-2045(16)30166-8.

21. Falchook GS, Millward M, Hong D, et al. BRAF inhibitor dabrafenib in patients with metastatic BRAF-mutant thyroid cancer. Thyroid 2015;25(1):71–7. https://doi.org/10.1089/thy.2014.0123.

22. Cabanillas ME, Patel A, Danysh BP, et al. BRAF inhibitors: experience in thyroid cancer and general review of toxicity. Horm Cancer 2015;6(1):21–36. https://doi.org/10.1007/s12672-014-0207-9.

23. Shah MH, Wei L, Wirth LJ, et al. Results of randomized phase II trial of dabrafenib versus dabrafenib plus trametinib in BRAF-mutated papillary thyroid carcinoma. J Clin Orthod 2017;35(15_suppl):6022. https://doi.org/10.1200/JCO.2017.35.15_suppl.6022.

24. Subbiah V, Hu MI, Wirth LJ, et al. Pralsetinib for patients with advanced or metastatic RET-altered thyroid cancer (ARROW): a multi-cohort, open-label, registrational, phase 1/2 study. Lancet Diabetes Endocrinol 2021;9(8):491–501. https://doi.org/10.1016/S2213-8587(21)00120-0.

25. Bradford D, Larkins E, Mushti SL, et al. FDA approval summary: selpercatinib for the treatment of lung and thyroid cancers with RET gene mutations or fusions. Clin Cancer Res 2021;27(8):2130–5. https://doi.org/10.1158/1078-0432.CCR-20-3558.

26. Kim J, Bradford D, Larkins E, et al. FDA approval summary: pralsetinib for the treatment of lung and thyroid cancers with *RET* gene mutations or fusions. Clin Cancer Res 2021;27(20):5452–6. https://doi.org/10.1158/1078-0432.CCR-21-0967.

27. Drilon A, Laetsch TW, Kummar S, et al. Efficacy of larotrectinib in TRK fusion–positive cancers in adults and children. N Engl J Med 2018;378(8):731–9. https://doi.org/10.1056/NEJMoa1714448.

28. Hong DS, DuBois SG, Kummar S, et al. Larotrectinib in patients with TRK fusion-positive solid tumours: a pooled analysis of three phase 1/2 clinical trials. Lancet Oncol 2020;21(4):531–40. https://doi.org/10.1016/S1470-2045(19)30856-3.

29. Cabanillas ME, Drilon A, Farago AF, et al. 1916P Larotrectinib treatment of advanced TRK fusion thyroid cancer. Ann Oncol 2020;31:S1086. https://doi.org/10.1016/j.annonc.2020.08.1404.

30. Tahara M, Brose MS, Wirth LJ, et al. Impact of dose interruption on the efficacy of lenvatinib in a phase 3 study in patients with radioiodine-refractory differentiated thyroid cancer. Eur J Cancer 2019;106:61–8. https://doi.org/10.1016/j.ejca.2018.10.002.

31. Hayato S, Shumaker R, Ferry J, et al. Exposure–response analysis and simulation of lenvatinib safety and efficacy in patients with radioiodine-refractory differentiated thyroid cancer. Cancer Chemother Pharmacol 2018;82(6):971–8. https://doi.org/10.1007/s00280-018-3687-4.

32. Brose MS, Panaseykin Y, Konda B, et al. 426P A multicenter, randomized, double-blind, phase II study of lenvatinib (LEN) in patients (pts) with radioiodine-refractory differentiated thyroid cancer (RR-DTC) to evaluate the safety and efficacy of a daily oral starting dose of 18 mg vs 24 mg. Ann Oncol 2020;31:S1409. https://doi.org/10.1016/j.annonc.2020.10.418.

33. Groussin L, Clerc J, Huillard O. Larotrectinib-enhanced radioactive iodine uptake in advanced thyroid cancer. N Engl J Med 2020;383(17):1686–7. https://doi.org/10.1056/NEJMc2023094.

34. Cheng L, Jin Y, Liu M, et al. HER inhibitor promotes BRAF/MEK inhibitor-induced redifferentiation in papillary thyroid cancer harboring BRAFV600E. Oncotarget 2017;8(12):19843–54. https://doi.org/10.18632/oncotarget.15773.

35. National Cancer Institute (NCI). A phase 1 study of dabrafenib in combination with lapatinib in BRAF mutant thyroid cancer. clinicaltrials.gov. 2021. Available at: https://clinicaltrials.gov/ct2/show/study/NCT01947023. Accessed July 22, 2021.

36. Sherman EJ, Ho AL, Fagin JA, et al. Combination of dabrafenib (DAB) and lapatinib (LAP) for the treatment of BRAF-mutant thyroid cancer. J Clin Orthod 2018;36(15_suppl):6087. https://doi.org/10.1200/JCO.2018.36.15_suppl.6087.

37. Chowdhury S, Veyhl J, Jessa F, et al. Programmed death-ligand 1 overexpression is a prognostic marker for aggressive papillary thyroid cancer and its variants. Oncotarget 2016;7(22):32318–28. https://doi.org/10.18632/oncotarget.8698.

38. Mehnert JM, Varga A, Brose M, et al. Pembrolizumab for advanced papillary or follicular thyroid cancer: preliminary results from the phase 1b KEYNOTE-028 study. J Clin Orthod 2016;34(15_suppl):6091. https://doi.org/10.1200/JCO.2016.34.15_suppl.6091.

39. Leboulleux S, Godbert Y, Penel N, et al. Benefits of pembrolizumab in progressive radioactive iodine refractory thyroid cancer: results of the AcSé Pembrolizumab Study from Unicancer. J Clin Orthod 2021;39(15_suppl):6082. https://doi.org/10.1200/JCO.2021.39.15_suppl.6082.

40. Haugen B, French J, Worden FP, et al. Lenvatinib plus pembrolizumab combination therapy in patients with radioiodine-refractory (RAIR), progressive differentiated thyroid cancer (DTC): results of a multicenter phase II International Thyroid Oncology Group trial. J Clin Orthod 2020;38(15_suppl):6512. https://doi.org/10.1200/JCO.2020.38.15_suppl.6512.

41. Haugen B, French JD, Worden F, et al. 1917P Pembrolizumab salvage add-on therapy in patients with radioiodine-refractory (RAIR), progressive differentiated thyroid cancer (DTC) progressing on lenvatinib: results of a multicenter phase II International Thyroid Oncology Group Trial. Ann Oncol 2020;31:S1086–7. https://doi.org/10.1016/j.annonc.2020.08.1405.

42. Guigon CJ, Fozzatti L, Lu C, et al. Inhibition of mTORC1 signaling reduces tumor growth but does not prevent cancer progression in a mouse model of thyroid cancer. Carcinogenesis 2010;31(7):1284–91. https://doi.org/10.1093/carcin/bgq059.

43. Sherman EJ, Dunn LA, Ho AL, et al. Phase 2 study evaluating the combination of sorafenib and temsirolimus in the treatment of radioactive iodine-refractory thyroid cancer. Cancer 2017;123(21):4114–21. https://doi.org/10.1002/cncr.30861.

44. Sherman EJ, Foster NR, Su YB, et al. Randomized phase II study of sorafenib with or without everolimus in patients with radioactive iodine refractory Hürthle cell thyroid cancer (HCC) (Alliance A091302/ITOG 1706). J Clin Orthod 2021;39(15_suppl):6076. https://doi.org/10.1200/JCO.2021.39.15_suppl.6076.

Novel Therapeutics and Treatment Strategies for Medullary Thyroid Cancer

Evan Walgama, MD[a], Naifa Busaidy, MD[b], Mark Zafereo, MD[c],*

KEYWORDS

- Medullary thyroid carcinoma • Surgery • Neoadjuvant therapy • RET mutation
- Immunotherapy

KEY POINTS

- Medullary Thyroid Carcinoma is an aggressive thyroid cancer that requires a distinct approach to workup and management.
- Testing for germline mutations in the RET proto-oncogene is used to identify hereditary forms of disease. Testing for somatic RET mutations should be performed in cases of locally advanced or metastatic sporadic disease.
- Selpercatinib and Pralsetinib are super-selective RET inhibitors with decreased toxicity and increased efficacy compared to multitarget kinase inhibitors.

INTRODUCTION

Medullary thyroid cancer (MTC) is a rare thyroid malignancy with unique management considerations. In general, small intrathyroidal tumors are cured by total thyroidectomy with central compartment dissection, while large tumors and those with disease spread to regional lymph nodes and distant organs (most commonly lung, liver, and bone) are more difficult to cure. The last decade has seen significant progress in the treatment of advanced MTC, largely due to the discovery and availability of novel targeted therapies, including new drugs specifically targeting the RET protooncogone.

Epidemiology

Medullary thyroid cancer (MTC) makes up approximately 2% of thyroid cancers,[1] but despite its relative rarity, MTC accounts for about 14% of deaths from thyroid cancer.[2,3] MTC occurs sporadically 80% of the time, while hereditary MTC accounts for 20%, as part of the multiple endocrine neoplasia (MEN) type 2 syndromes. In

[a] Saint John's Cancer Institute & Pacific Neuroscience Institute, Providence Health System, 2125 Arizona Avenue, Santa Monica, CA 90404, USA; [b] Department of Endocrine Neoplasia, MD Anderson Cancer Center, 1515 Holcombe Boulevard #853, Houston, TX 77030, USA; [c] Department of Head and Neck Surgery, MD Anderson Cancer Center, 1515 Holcombe Boulevard Unit 1445, Houston, TX 77030, USA
* Corresponding author.
E-mail address: mzafereo@mdanderson.org

Endocrinol Metab Clin N Am 51 (2022) 379–389
https://doi.org/10.1016/j.ecl.2022.02.001
0889-8529/22/Published by Elsevier Inc.

hereditary MTC cases, a germline mutation of the RET protooncogene is almost always present (>98%).[4–6] Sporadic MTC is associated with a somatic mutation of the RET protooncogene in 50% to 60% of cases.[6,7]

The RET protooncogene encodes a transmembrane receptor of the tyrosine kinase family. It represents an unusual circumstance in which gain of function, rather than loss of function, results in neoplastic disease.[6] RET translocations (fusions) are not seen in MTC, but are associated with papillary thyroid cancer (<10%, and more common among pediatric PTC) and anaplastic thyroid cancers (<1%).[8] RET alterations (mutations and fusions) are associated with, and sometimes a therapeutic target, in other human diseases, including lung cancer, certain leukemias, and Hirschsprung's disease.[9,10]

Sporadic Medullary Thyroid Cancer

Sporadic MTC is defined by the absence of a germline RET mutation, but is frequently associated with somatic RET mutations. Somatic RET mutations can be ascertained by molecular testing of tumor (via needle biopsy or surgery) for the RET protooncogene. The most common somatic mutation of the RET protooncogene is M918 T, a codon substitution-type mutation associated with a more aggressive disease course.[3] The M918 T mutation is generally absent in small MTC tumors.[11] RAS mutations are associated with RET wild-type sporadic MTC in approximately 25% of cases.[6,12]

Hereditary Medullary Thyroid Cancer

Almost all hereditary MTC is associated with a germline RET mutation and autosomal dominant pattern of inheritance with high penetrance in all known types. Hereditary MTC occurs as part of the MEN type 2 syndromes. MEN 2 A is 20 times as common as MEN 2B.[13] The germline RETc634 mutation is the most common overall hereditary RET mutation, and the most common mutation seen in MEN2A. Classical MEN 2A is characterized by MTC plus pheochromocytoma, hyperparathyroidism, or both. Other subtypes of MEN 2A are MTC plus cutaneous lichen amyloidosis, an itchy rash in the scapular region characterized by amyloid deposition, and MTC plus Hirschsprung's disease, whereby patients present with a toxic megacolon.[13] MEN 2A is associated with a variety of RET mutations which are classified by the ATA according to risk.[1]

Familial MTC (FMTC) is defined as an individual or family with a germline MTC mutation, when neither pheochromocytoma nor primary hyperparathyroidism is present. Previously considered a separate heritable type of MTC, it is now considered a subtype of MEN 2A It is characterized by a later age at the presentation of MTC and, usually, less aggressive tumor behavior.[14]

MEN 2B is almost always associated with an M918 T mutation.[15] Patients are at risk for MTC starting at a few years of age. Patients have neuromas to the lips, eyes, tongue, and GI tract, and the majority have a marfanoid body habitus. There is a high penetrance of MTC. A large number, approximately 75%, of cases result from de novo mutations, and diagnosis is often made from extra-endocrine features (predominantly constipation from intestinal neurogangliomatosis or tearless crying) by astute pediatricians.[15,16]

Biomarkers

Most MTC tumors secrete calcitonin and CEA, the 2 most important biomarkers in MTC, relevant in diagnosis, surgical planning, prognosis, and surveillance.[17] On diagnosis, the calcitonin level correlates with the overall prognosis and risk of metastatic disease.[18] Calcitonin levels more than 200 pg/mL are generally correlated with lymph node metastasis and may influence the decision for an elective lateral neck dissection at some centers. Patients presenting with preoperative calcitonin levels more than 1000 pg/mL are often associated with distant disease, and these patients have less than a 50% chance of biochemical cure after surgery.[18]

CLINICAL PRESENTATION

Sporadic MTC tends to occur in adults in the fourth and fifth decades of life, with older patients having worse outcomes.[19] A thyroid nodule or neck mass is usually the presenting sign. Less commonly, high levels of calcitonin can cause flushing or diarrhea. The discovery of an MTC neoplasm should prompt a genetic evaluation for a germline RET mutation in all cases, as up to 7% of apparently sporadic MTC cases will in fact harbor germline mutations.[1,20] If a hereditary condition is confirmed, first-degree relatives should be offered genetic molecular testing for the RET mutation.

When a pheochromocytoma is present, this must be managed before any thyroid surgery.[15] When hyperparathyroidism is present, enlarged parathyroid glands are removed at the time of the thyroid operation. Compared with MEN type 1, the hyperparathyroidism for MEN 2A is usually mild.[1]

In MEN 2B, Thyroidectomy should be performed at or before 1 year of age to improve disease-free survival. In a recent international series, thyroidectomy at or before 1 year resulted in 83% disease control, compared with 15% for those who had surgery after 1 year of age.[15]

Management

Evaluation and staging

As most sporadic MTC tumors present as a thyroid nodule, the initial evaluation proceeds according to established guidelines.[21] Fine needle aspiration biopsy is sufficient to establish the diagnosis in most of the cases.[22] When the result is equivocal, serum calcitonin levels may be checked.[23] Before FNA, serum calcitonin levels, while strongly suggestive of MTC when elevated in the setting of a suspicious nodule, are infrequently obtained on a routine basis in the United States. However, serum calcitonin screening in association with thyroid nodules is more common in Europe. In patients with suspicious nodules, a basal serum calcitonin greater than 100 pg/mL carries a positive predictive value for MTC of about 75%.[24]

In all cases of sporadic MTC, baseline serum calcitonin and CEA should be obtained, and genetic screening for a germline RET mutation should be performed. If a mutation is found, pheochromocytoma and hyperparathyroidism should be excluded. Workup for distant metastatic MTC should be considered when calcitonin is greater than 500 pg/mL, in the presence of cervical nodal disease, or when symptoms of possible metastatic disease (eg, bone pain) are present.[1]

In general, patients with a new diagnosis of MTC should receive a high-definition ultrasound of the neck, with a low threshold to obtain a contrast-enhanced CT of the neck, especially if the primary tumor is > 2 cm or if the serum calcitonin is > 20 pg/mL. If distant metastases are suspected, additional imaging may include: a contrast-enhanced CT of the chest, abdomen (3 phase or liver protocol), and pelvis; an MRI of the spine; and/or a bone scan. FDG PET/CT is not preferred in the workup for patients with MTC, although 68Ga-Dotatate may be considered for patients with advanced/recurrent disease.[25,26]

MTC should be staged according to the AJCC 8th edition for thyroid cancer, which is shared in common with differentiated thyroid cancer. A weakness of this staging system for MTC is its failure to account for number of nodes and calcitonin levels, which have been indicated as strong prognostic factors in MTC.[27,28] Otherwise, the main prognostic features are age, tumor size and TNM stage, presence of the M918 T mutation (germline or somatic), and calcitonin and CEA doubling times.[29–31]

Early stage disease

The best chance for cure lies in total surgical removal of intrathyroidal disease. At minimum, patients with early stage MTC should undergo a total thyroidectomy and bilateral central compartment dissection. A lateral compartment neck dissection is generally not performed in the absence of structural disease,[32] but can be considered in the setting of high calcitonin levels.[33,34]

When a prophylactic thyroidectomy is performed in a child with MEN 2 syndrome and normal calcitonin, a lymph node dissection is not usually performed.[15] The specific mutation is the strongest factor in determining the timing of thyroidectomy. Patients with ATA-highest risk mutation (M918 T or clinical MEN 2B) should undergo thyroidectomy usually before 1 year of age. Patients with ATA-high-risk mutations (patients with RET codon C634 mutations and the RET codon A883 F mutation) should undergo thyroidectomy at or before 5 years of age. Pediatric patients with ATA-MOD risk mutations (RET codon mutations other than M918 T, C634, and A883 F) should begin cervical ultrasound and calcitonin screenings by age 5.[35]

In hereditary MTC, the recommendation for the timing of thyroidectomy is based on the specific RET mutation present.[1] Those patients determined to have a germline M918 T mutation (in addition to those with clinical MEN 2B) are defined as "highest risk" and require thyroidectomy within the first year of life. Those patients with RET codon A883 F or with mutations at C634 are defined as "high risk" and are recommended for thyroidectomy within the first 5 years of life. To date, there are over 100 other mutations or translocations associated with hereditary MTC, of which the remainder are considered "moderate risk" and generally do not require prophylactic thyroidectomy until after puberty, unless there is radiographic or biochemical disease progression before puberty.[16]

Advanced Disease

Approximately 80% of patients with MTC present with greater than stage 1 disease.[2] Patients with nodal metastases detected on imaging should be treated with surgery, when feasible. Even when nodal metastases are present, a biochemical cure is often attainable, though this likelihood is inversely proportional to the number of affected nodes.[27] In most cases, surgery to control central compartment disease and lateral neck disease is required, and is generally performed in cases of distant metastasis, as the likelihood of morbidity from central and/or lateral neck disease is likely to precede morbidity from most metastatic disease.

Some patients with a limited volume of recurrent disease in the neck are candidates for revision surgery. However, in cases with extensive disease, and/or evidence of widespread metastasis, systemic therapy should be considered.[36] Symptom burden, extent of disease, calcitonin doubling time, presence of targetable mutations, feasibility of local therapies, and patient preference must all be taken into consideration, and the treatment plan must be individualized. Many of these patients are best served in tertiary centers. Enrollment in clinical trials is preferred, when available. Radiotherapy or zoledronic acid therapy should be considered for symptomatic and/or threatening (eg, spine) bone disease.[37] Bone modifying agents such as zoledronic acid or denosumab can be given for painful bony lesions or those at risk for fracture and may reduce skeletal-related events. Although there is no consensus data regarding frequency of administration, most providers treat every 3 to 6 months and monitor bone turnover markers (eg, CTX). Radiotherapy has very limited role in the management of locoregional disease, given its lack of durability, side effects, and the availability of better alternative options including surgery and targeted therapy.[38,39] Rarely, patients with extensive locoregional disease invasive of visceral structures (eg, trachea, esophagus, prevertebral or floor of neck musculature) may be considered for postoperative radiation therapy. Radioactive iodine treatment has no role in the treatment of MTC,[40] and traditional cytotoxic chemotherapy does not have a role in the modern treatment of MTC, given the availability of multiple targeted agents with good efficacy. Fortunately, successful experience with targeted therapies has significantly expanded in the last decade.

Targeted Therapy

Multitargeted kinase inhibitors

Vandetanib was the first multitargeted kinase inhibitor (MKI) approved by the United States Food and Drug Administration (FDA) (2011) for advanced MTC. The drug is administered orally and selectively targets RET, VEGF, and EGF receptors. A 2012 study randomized 331 patients with metastatic MTC to either vandetinib 300 mg daily or placebo.[41] Over the mean follow-up period of 24 months, the vandetanib cohort showed improved progression-free survival (30.2 vs 19.2 months in placebo group). The drug showed efficacy for both hereditary and sporadic disease. There was a higher objective response rate when a somatic M918 T mutation was present (55 vs 32%).[3,41]

Cabozantinib is a c-MET, VEGF2R, and RET inhibitor, the second MKI US FDA-approved for use in MTC (2012). A phase 3 trial compared cabozantinib to placebo in 330 patients with radiographically progressive MTC and showed greater PFS in the cabozantinib group.[42] Patients were enrolled regardless of mutational status; however, those with RET mutations fared better than those without (PFS of 60 vs 20 weeks); the subset of patients with somatic M918 T mutations experienced the greatest benefit.[42] Overall, the objective response rate (RECIST) was low, at 28%. A follow-up analysis of the cohort at a mean of 42 months did not demonstrate a significant difference in overall survival.[42]

Use of MKI is poorly tolerated by some patients due to off-target inhibition, often limiting effective dosing.[41,42] Diarrhea, rash, nausea, vomiting, fatigue, and hypertension are frequent complaints/side effects, with need for the reduction of dose in some cases. Of particular concern are those patients with disease adjacent to vascular structures or those with recent surgery, as MKIs carry risk of poor wound healing and fistula formation, which can be life-threatening in some cases.[43] Overall, few patients experience a complete response with MKIs, and acquired drug resistance is common.[3]

RET-specific inhibitors

There are currently 2 RET-specific inhibitors with FDA approval for patients with advanced, RET-mutant MTC. The first, selpercatinib, is an orally administered medication with greater specificity for the RET protooncogene compared with MKI. The reduction in off-target inhibition results in an improvement in tolerance compared with the MKI.[44,45] It has a half-life of 8 hours. The most common adverse events related to treatment, though seldom severe, and rare in comparison to MKIs, are hypertension, elevated liver enzymes, hyponatremia, and diarrhea.[44]

In 2020, Wirth and colleagues[44] published a phase 1 to 2 trial treated 143 patients with advanced MTC with selpercatinib. All patients harbored RET mutations. 88 patients were previously treated with systemic therapy, including multitarget kinase inhibitors. In those not previously treated with systemic therapy, 73% had an objective response, with 10% of the cohort demonstrating a complete response. Remarkably, in those previously treated with systemic therapy including MKI, 69% had an objective response, with 5% having a complete response. At 1 year, 86% of responses were durable. The results of this trial resulted in FDA approval of selpercatinib in 2020 for the treatment of advanced or metastatic MTC and other advanced thyroid malignancies with RET mutations (MTC) or fusions (PTC and ATC).

Pralsetinib, another super-selective RET inhibitor, gained FDA approval for use in RET-mutant MTC in December 2020. This orally administered drug was trialed in an open label phase 1 to 2 trial including 79 patients with advanced RET-mutant MTC, the overall response rate was 66%, with 5% having a complete response.[46,47] 79% of patients who responded had durable effect for greater than 6 months. Similar to selpercatinib, patients with prior MKI therapy had comparable rates of objective

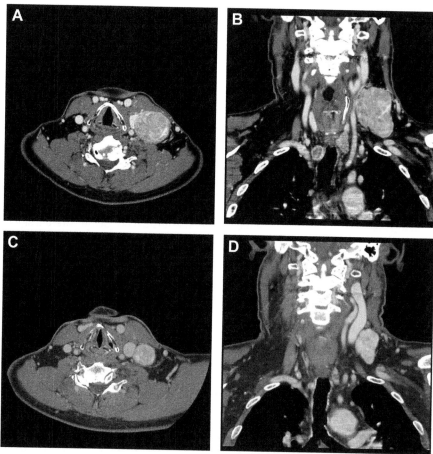

Fig. 1. Neoadjuvant response of recurrent lateral neck MTC to RET-specific inhibitor. Axial (*A*) and coronal (*B*) computed tomography images of patient presenting with localized recurrent disease to the left lateral compartment of the neck, extending to threaten the left internal jugular vein and involve the left sternocleidomastoid muscle. Axial (*C*) and coronal (*D*) images demonstrating partial RECIST response after 6 months of selpercatinib monotherapy. The neoadjuvant RET-specific inhibitor facilitated safe surgical removal of this lateral neck disease with extranodal extension.

response (60% vs 74%). In general, pralsetinib seems to be well tolerated, efficacious regardless of RET genotype and despite prior treatment with MKI therapy.

Patients with MTC with locally advanced disease, with or without metastatic disease, may benefit from upfront systemic treatment to facilitate surgical resection, especially those with a somatic RET mutation. Selpercatinib has been given in the neoadjuvant setting in select patients with advanced RET-mutated MTC[48] (**Fig. 1**). This strategy may reduce tumor size to allow for less morbid surgical treatment. There is currently an ongoing clinical trial (NCT04759911) for the evaluation of neodjuvant therapy for patients with locoregionally advanced RET-mutated MTC with or without distant metastases.[49]

Surveillance and Prognosis

Postoperative TSH should be monitored and maintained in the euthyroid range. There is no role for thyroid hormone suppression therapy.[1] For patients who undergo surgery, calcitonin and CEA should be checked approximately 3 months postoperatively, and an undetectable calcitonin following surgery is considered a biochemical cureand supports a favorable chance of disease-free survival.[50,51] Regardless of biochemical cure, serum calcitonin and CEA should be checked at least every 6 months (may be more often with patients with more biologically aggressive disease), and doubling time should be calculated.[1] Those patients with an incomplete biochemical response (calcitonin >10 pg/mL) are at higher risk for structural recurrence.[27] In patients with a postthyroidectomy calcitonin of less than 10 pg/mL, only 4% will eventually demonstrate recurrence.[52] For patients with postoperative serum calcitonin less than 150 pg/mL, disease sites outside of the neck are uncommon,[27] and ultrasound is the most sensitive study to detect structural disease in the neck.[53] Postoperative calcitonin level greater than 150 pg/mL should prompt workup for distant metastatic disease (including the cross-sectional imaging of the chest/abdomen/pelvis, MRI spine and/or bone scan; see section Management: Evaluation and Staging).[1]

In routine surveillance, the calcitonin doubling time is an important measure of disease aggression. Metastatic MTC may follow either an aggressive or indolent course. In addition to radiographic or symptomatic progression, calcitonin doubling time is a useful differentiating test. As an example, in a retrospective study of 65 patients with MTC, a doubling time of less than 6 months carried a poor prognosis (8% 10-year cause-specific survival), whereas a doubling time greater than 24 months was a positive prognostic sign (100% 10-year cause-specific survival).[29]

The 10-year mean overall survival for sporadic MTC is about 73%, substantially worse compared with differentiated thyroid cancers.[2,54]

SUMMARY

The treatment of MTC has seen remarkable advances in recent years, particularly with the addition of multi-target kinase inhibitors and selective RET inhibitors. Upfront germline testing for the RET mutation remains a key component of initial evaluation and staging, while somatic RET testing for germline RET-negative patients with advanced disease is increasingly common. Surgery remains a mainstay of therapy for the vast majority of patients with MTC, although some patients with significantly locoregionally advanced or large burden distant disease may move directly to upfront targeted therapy. External beam radiation therapy to the neck is very rarely used for MTC, while focal radiation to threatening bone lesions is common. Many patients with RET mutations (somatic or germline) who require systemic therapy are now being treated first-line with FDA-approved RET-specific inhibitors, while RET-negative patients are still treated with MKI (eg, cabozantinib, vanetanib). Ongoing clinical trials are continuing to compare RET-specific inhibitors versus MKI regimens for the treatment of advanced/metastatic RET-mutated disease.

CLINICS CARE POINTS

- All patients with medullary thyroid carcinoma should undergo immediate germline (blood) testing for the RET protooncogene, as 20% of medullary thyroid carcinomas are hereditary and associated with MEN types 2A and 2B.
- Approximately 50% of patients with sporadic (nonhereditary) MTC will have a RET somatic tumor mutation.
- The management for the vast majority of patients with MTC without structural distant disease is surgery, consisting of total thyroidectomy and central compartment lymph node dissection.
- Prophylactic (elective) lateral neck dissection for patients undergoing surgery for MTC is controversial, with many surgeons basing decision for lateral neck surgery only on the presence or absence of radiographically apparent structural disease in the lateral neck, while others suggest using calcitonin cutoffs as an indication for elective unilateral or bilateral lateral neck dissection.
- Two new RET-specific inhibitors have shown decreased toxicity and increased efficacy (as historically compared with other multikinase inhibitors) in recent clinical trials for patients with medullary thyroid carcinoma, leading to FDA approval for patients with advanced or metastatic MTC.
- Patients presenting with locoregionally advanced and/or metastatic sporadic (nonhereditary) MTC should be considered for somatic RET testing of their tumor as part of their initial work-up, as the presence of a RET mutation may alter treatment considerations including initial choice of systemic therapy and/or a neoadjuvant approach to therapy.

DISCLOSURE

E. Walgama: none. N. Busaidy: none. Dr. Zafereo receives industry support for clinical trials from Eli Lilly

REFERENCES

1. Wells SA, Asa SL, Dralle H, et al. Revised american thyroid association guidelines for the management of medullary thyroid carcinoma. Thyroid 2015;25(6): 567–610.
2. Modigliani E, Cohen R, Campos J-M, et al. Prognostic factors for survival and for biochemical cure in medullary thyroid carcinoma: results in 899 patients. Clin Endocrinol 1998;48(3):265–73.
3. Ceolin L, Duval MADS, Benini AF, et al. Medullary thyroid carcinoma beyond surgery: advances, challenges, and perspectives. Endocrine-Related Cancer 2019; 26(9):R499–518.
4. Raue F, Bruckner T, Frank-Raue K. Long-term outcomes and aggressiveness of hereditary medullary thyroid carcinoma: 40 years of experience at one center. J Clin Endocrinol Metab 2019;104(10):4264–72.
5. Elisei R, Tacito A, Ramone T, et al. Twenty-five years experience on ret genetic screening on hereditary MTC: an update on the prevalence of germline RET mutations. Genes 2019;10(9):698.

6. Larouche V, Akirov A, Thomas CM, et al. A primer on the genetics of medullary thyroid cancer. Curr Oncol 2019;26(6):389–94.

7. Romei C, Ciampi R, Elisei R. A comprehensive overview of the role of the RET proto-oncogene in thyroid carcinoma. Nat Rev Endocrinol 2016;12(4):192–202.

8. Prescott JD, Zeiger MA. TheREToncogene in papillary thyroid carcinoma. Cancer 2015;121(13):2137–46.

9. Drilon A, Oxnard GR, Tan DSW, et al. Efficacy of selpercatinib in RET fusion–positive non–small-cell lung cancer. N Engl J Med 2020;383(9):813–24.

10. Li AY, McCusker MG, Russo A, et al. RET fusions in solid tumors. Cancer Treat Rev 2019;81:101911.

11. Romei C, Ugolini C, Cosci B, et al. Low prevalence of the somatic M918T RET mutation in micro-medullary thyroid cancer. Thyroid 2012;22(5):476–81.

12. Agrawal N, Jiao Y, Sausen M, et al. Exomic sequencing of medullary thyroid cancer reveals dominant and mutually exclusive oncogenic mutations in RET and RAS. J Clin Endocrinol Metab 2013;98(2):E364–9.

13. Moline J, Eng C. Multiple endocrine neoplasia type 2: an overview. Genet Med 2011;13(9):755–64.

14. Wells SA, Pacini F, Robinson BG, et al. Multiple endocrine Neoplasia Type 2 and familial medullary thyroid carcinoma: an update. J Clin Endocrinol Metab 2013; 98(8):3149–64.

15. Castinetti F, Waguespack SG, Machens A, et al. Natural history, treatment, and long-term follow up of patients with multiple endocrine neoplasia type 2B: an international, multicentre, retrospective study. Lancet Diabetes Endocrinol 2019; 7(3):213–20.

16. Hedayati M, Zarif Yeganeh M, Sheikholeslami S, et al. Diversity of mutations in the RET proto-oncogene and its oncogenic mechanism in medullary thyroid cancer. Crit Rev Clin Lab Sci 2016;53(4):217–27.

17. Zheng-Pywell R, Cherian AJ, Enman M, et al. Carcinoembryonic antigen should be concurrently checked with calcitonin to identify distant metastases in medullary thyroid cancer. Int J Endocr Oncol 2020;7(1):IJE27.

18. Machens A, Dralle H. Biomarker-based risk stratification for previously untreated medullary thyroid cancer. J Clin Endocrinol Metab 2010;95(6):2655–63.

19. Sahli ZT, Canner JK, Zeiger MA, et al. Association between age and disease specific mortality in medullary thyroid cancer. Am J Surg 2021;221(2):478–84.

20. Elisei R, Romei C, Cosci B, et al. RET genetic screening in patients with medullary thyroid cancer and their relatives: experience with 807 individuals at one center. J Clin Endocrinol Metab 2007;92(12):4725–9.

21. Haugen BR, Alexander EK, Bible KC, et al. 2015 American thyroid association management guidelines for adult patients with thyroid nodules and differentiated thyroid cancer: the american thyroid association guidelines task force on thyroid nodules and differentiated thyroid cancer. Thyroid 2016;26(1):1–133.

22. Choi N, Moon W-J, Lee JH, et al. Ultrasonographic findings of medullary thyroid cancer: differences according to tumor size and correlation with fine needle aspiration results. Acta Radiol 2011;52(3):312–6.

23. Bugalho MJM, Santos JR, Sobrinho L. Preoperative diagnosis of medullary thyroid carcinoma: Fine needle aspiration cytology as compared with serum calcitonin measurement. J Surg Oncol 2005;91(1):56–60.

24. Turk Y, Makay O, Ozdemir M, et al. Routine calcitonin measurement in nodular thyroid disease management: is it worthwhile? Ann Surg Treat Res 2017; 92(4):173.

25. Werner RA, Schmid J-S, Higuchi T, et al. Predictive value of 18F-FDG PET in patients with advanced medullary thyroid carcinoma treated with vandetanib. J Nucl Med 2018;59(5):756–61.

26. Tuncel M, Kılıçkap S, Süslü N. Clinical impact of 68Ga-DOTATATE PET-CT imaging in patients with medullary thyroid cancer. Ann Nucl Med 2020;34(9):663–74.

27. Machens A, Lorenz K, Dralle H. Prediction of biochemical cure in patients with medullary thyroid cancer. Br J Surg 2020;107(6):695–704.

28. Esfandiari NH, Hughes DT, Yin H, et al. The effect of extent of surgery and number of lymph node metastases on overall survival in patients with medullary thyroid cancer. J Clin Endocrinol Metab 2014;99(2):448–54.

29. Barbet J, Campion L, Kraeber-Bodéré F, et al. Prognostic impact of serum calcitonin and carcinoembryonic antigen doubling-times in patients with medullary thyroid carcinoma. J Clin Endocrinol Metab 2005;90(11):6077–84.

30. Chen L, Wang Y, Zhao K, et al. Postoperative nomogram for predicting cancer-specific and overall survival among patients with medullary thyroid cancer. Int J Endocrinol 2020;2020:1–13.

31. Ho AS, Wang L, Palmer FL, et al. Postoperative nomogram for predicting cancer-specific mortality in medullary thyroid cancer. Ann Surg Oncol 2015;22(8):2700–6.

32. Pena I, Clayman GL, Grubbs EG, et al. Management of the lateral neck compartment in patients with sporadic medullary thyroid cancer. Head & Neck 2018;40(1):79–85.

33. Spanheimer PM, Ganly I, Chou JF, et al. Prophylactic lateral neck dissection for medullary thyroid carcinoma is not associated with improved survival. Ann Surg Oncol 2021;28(11):6572–9.

34. Szabo Yamashita T, Rogers RT, Foster TR, et al. Medullary thyroid cancer: What is the optimal management of the lateral neck in a node negative patient at index operation? Surgery 2021. https://doi.org/10.1016/j.surg.2021.04.052.

35. Machens A, Lorenz K, Weber F, et al. Genotype-specific progression of hereditary medullary thyroid cancer. Hum Mutat 2018;39(6):860–9.

36. Geller G, Laskin J, Cheung WY, et al. A retrospective review of the multidisciplinary management of medullary thyroid cancer: eligibility for systemic therapy. Thyroid Res 2017;10(1):6.

37. Andrade F, Probstner D, Decnop M, et al. The impact of Zoledronic acid and radioactive iodine therapy on morbi-mortality of patients with bone metastases of thyroid cancer derived from follicular cells. Eur Thyroid J 2019;8(1):46–55.

38. Nocera M, Baudin E, Pellegriti G, et al. Treatment of advanced medullary thyroid cancer with an alternating combination of doxorubicin-streptozocin and 5 FU-dacarbazine. Br J Cancer 2000;83(6):715–8.

39. Groen AH, Beckham TH, Links TP, et al. Outcomes of surgery and postoperative radiation therapy in managing medullary thyroid carcinoma. J Surg Oncol 2020;121(2):234–43.

40. Meijer JAA, Bakker LEH, Valk GD, et al. Radioactive iodine in the treatment of medullary thyroid carcinoma: a controlled multicenter study. Eur J Endocrinol 2013;168(5):779–86.

41. Wells SA, Robinson BG, Gagel RF, et al. Vandetanib in patients with locally advanced or metastatic medullary thyroid cancer: a randomized, double-blind phase III trial. J Clin Oncol 2012;30(2):134–41.

42. Schlumberger M, Elisei R, Müller S, et al. Overall survival analysis of EXAM, a phase III trial of cabozantinib in patients with radiographically progressive medullary thyroid carcinoma. Ann Oncol 2017;28(11):2813–9.

43. Blevins DP, Dadu R, Hu M, et al. Aerodigestive fistula formation as a rare side effect of antiangiogenic tyrosine kinase inhibitor therapy for thyroid cancer. Thyroid 2014;24(5):918–22.
44. Wirth LJ, Sherman E, Robinson B, et al. Efficacy of Selpercatinib in RET-altered thyroid cancers. New Engl J Med 2020;383(9):825–35.
45. Markham A. Selpercatinib: first approval. Drugs 2020;80(11):1119–24.
46. Hu M, Subbiah V, Wirth LJ, et al. 1913O Results from the registrational phase I/II ARROW trial of pralsetinib (BLU-667) in patients (pts) with advanced RET mutation-positive medullary thyroid cancer (RET+ MTC). Ann Oncol 2020;31: S1084.
47. Subbiah V, Hu MI, Wirth LJ, et al. Pralsetinib for patients with advanced or metastatic RET-altered thyroid cancer (ARROW): a multi-cohort, open-label, registrational, phase 1/2 study. Lancet Diabetes Endocrinol 2021;9(8):491–501.
48. Jozaghi Y, Zafereo M, Williams MD, et al. Neoadjuvant selpercatinib for advanced medullary thyroid cancer. Head & Neck 2021;43(1). https://doi.org/10.1002/hed.26527.
49. Available at: https://clinicaltrials.gov/ct2/show/NCT04759911. Accessed 08,2022.
50. Kwon H, Kim WG, Jeon MJ, et al. Dynamic risk stratification for medullary thyroid cancer according to the response to initial therapy. Endocrine 2016;53(1):174–81.
51. Engelbach M, Görges R, Forst T, et al. Improved diagnostic methods in the follow-up of medullary thyroid carcinoma by highly specific calcitonin measurements. J Clin Endocrinol Metab 2000;85(5):1890–4.
52. Franc S, Niccoli-Sire P, Cohen R, et al. Complete surgical lymph node resection does not prevent authentic recurrences of medullary thyroid carcinoma. Clin Endocrinol (Oxf) 2001;55(3):403–9.
53. Giraudet AL, Vanel D, Leboulleux S, et al. Imaging medullary thyroid carcinoma with persistent elevated calcitonin levels. J Clin Endocrinol Metab 2007;92(11):4185–90.
54. Bhattacharyya N. A population-based analysis of survival factors in differentiated and medullary thyroid carcinoma. Otolaryngol Head Neck Surg 2003;128(1):115–23.

Anaplastic Thyroid Cancer

New Horizons and Challenges

Anastasios Maniakas, MD, MSc[a,b], Mark Zafereo, MD[b],
Maria E. Cabanillas, MD[c,*]

KEYWORDS

- Anaplastic thyroid cancer • Targeted therapy • BRAF/MEK inhibitor • Surgery
- Multidisciplinary • Immunotherapy • Clinical trial

KEY POINTS

- Anaplastic thyroid cancer (ATC) remains a highly aggressive and deadly disease, requiring rapid referral to a highly specialized center
- *BRAF* mutation status must be obtained rapidly to determine BRAF/MEK inhibitor eligibility
- Enrollment in clinical trials may offer the best chance for survival and overall quality of life to a patient with ATC
- With the advent of novel therapeutics and rapid/favorable response to systemic therapy, patients with initial locoregional and/or metastatic disease may become eligible for surgery

BACKGROUND

Historically, anaplastic thyroid cancer (ATC) has been considered one of the most aggressive and lethal malignancies, which presents itself at a median age of 65 to 70 years,[1,2] with median overall survival (OS) of 4 months and a 6-month OS of 35%,[1] whereas disease-specific mortality approaches 100%.[3,4] Therefore, although ATC comprises 1% to 1.5% of all thyroid cancers, it represents more than half of the annual thyroid cancer-related mortality[5] because of its deadly and rapidly progressing nature. It is primarily due to this aggressiveness that the American Joint Committee on Cancer has classified all ATC as stage IV.[6]

Funding source: There was no funding source associated with this article.
[a] Division of Otolaryngology–Head and Neck Surgery, Hôpital Maisonneuve-Rosemont, Université de Montréal, 5415 Boul, Assomption, Montreal, QC H1T 2M4, Canada; [b] Department of Head and Neck Surgery, The University of Texas MD Anderson Cancer Center, 1400 Pressler Road, Unit 1465, Houston, TX 77030, USA; [c] Department of Endocrine Neoplasia and Hormonal Disorders, Division of Internal Medicine, The University of Texas MD Anderson Cancer Center, 1400 Pressler Road, Unit 1461, Houston, TX 77030, USA
* Corresponding author.
E-mail address: mcabani@mdanderson.org

Endocrinol Metab Clin N Am 51 (2022) 391–401
https://doi.org/10.1016/j.ecl.2021.11.020
0889-8529/21/© 2021 Elsevier Inc. All rights reserved.

Part of the challenge of understanding and treating ATC is that its tumorigenesis remains unclear. At present, the 2 main theories are that ATC arises either following the dedifferentiation of differentiated thyroid cancer (DTC) and poorly differentiated thyroid cancer (PDTC) or de novo[7] and the following are associated risk factors: a long-standing goiter, history of prior radiation, and history of prior treated DTC or PDTC with a rapidly evolving recurrence. Recent evidence on the coexistence of BRAF-mutated ATC with PTC suggests a potential likely common PTC origin for most of these tumors.[8–10] Although thyroid cancer, in general, is not considered a malignancy with a high tumor mutational burden (TMB), it has been shown that ATC has a higher relative mutational burden,[7] although TMB is low when compared when other solid tumors. Accumulation of genetic variations for ATC tend to occur in tumor suppressor genes (*p53*, *PTEN*), oncogenes (*TERT* promoter, *RAS*, *BRAF*, *PIK3CA*), oncofusions (*NTRK*, *RET*, *ALK*), or through mismatch repairs (**Fig. 1**).

Traditionally, ATC treatment provided minimal survival benefit, often being disease palliation oriented and seldom curative. Surgery alone is rarely beneficial, because patients' locoregional and metastatic tumor burden is often a significant factor at presentation, rendering them inoperable. Conventional cytotoxic chemotherapy has been shown to provide little to no benefit, even when combined with external beam radiation therapy, while causing significant side effects. Fortunately, recent advances in ATC treatment have shown remarkable shifts in outcomes and OS rates in the last decade,[2] which have also prompted the scientific community to update the American Thyroid Association Guidelines for ATC[11] for the first time in a decade to better transmit these changes and options for patients.

EXPERT MULTIDISCIPLINARY MANAGEMENT AND ACCESS TO CLINICAL TRIALS

Considering the rapidly evolving nature of ATC and its slight increased incidence in the United States in the past few decades,[12] it is important that physicians identify these cases in a timely fashion to ensure prompt clinical, radiologic, and molecular workup. With current median survival rates estimated at 9 months,[2] any delays in diagnosis and disease extent evaluation can be detrimental for patients and their OS. Having access to highly specialized multidisciplinary teams in cancer centers allows patients to receive thorough tumor workups, including rapid immunohistochemistry and cell-free DNA analyses,[13] while giving them access to select clinical trials specific to ATC, seldom found in most community and even tertiary centers. One such highly specialized program was developed in 2014 at the University of Texas MD Anderson Cancer Center, where patients are fast-tracked for multidisciplinary evaluation along with imaging and tumor molecular testing within 7 days. This Facilitating Anaplastic Thyroid Cancer Specialized Treatment (FAST) team[14] has increased clinical trial participation for patients with ATC 4-fold in less than 5 years,[2] allowing for ATC-specific trials to rapidly reach accrual and timely completions. Such trials[15] led to the US Food and Drug Administration (FDA) approval of dabrafenib with trametinib in May 2018 for patients with *BRAF*V600E-variant ATC, representing the first drug therapy approved by the FDA for ATC. Since then, several clinical trials are underway or have been completed, and are further discussed in this review.

Overall, what remains evident is that when dealing with such an advanced and deadly disease, physicians should always strive to treat patients on protocol, as much as possible, because this will not only ensure patients receive the most promising therapeutics but also allow us to learn as much as we can on disease evolution and its response to treatment. Through patient biopsies and/or surgical specimens, we are able to collect the highest level of clinical data possible, allowing us to further

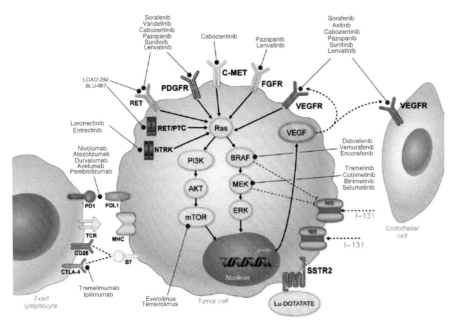

Fig. 1. Anaplastic thyroid cancer therapy according to pathway targeted. (*From* Cabanillas ME, Ryder M, Jimenez C. Targeted Therapy for Advanced Thyroid Cancer: Kinase Inhibitors and Beyond. Endocr Rev. 2019 Dec 1;40(6):1573–1604; with permission.)

study the disease and develop preclinical models for translational research and novel therapeutics development.[16,17]

MODERN THERAPIES FOR ANAPLASTIC THYROID CANCER

Initial treatment decisions for ATC start with determining resectability of the primary tumor. Although rare (10%[2]), patients with stage IVA (confined to the thyroid gland) disease should undergo upfront surgery followed by chemoradiation. Owing to the recognition that patients with *BRAF*V600E-mutated ATC respond favorably to BRAF-directed therapy, identification of those with a *BRAF*V600E mutation is now the pivotal decision point when determining initial treatment in patients with stage IVB (extends outside the thyroid gland and/or metastatic to regional lymph nodes) and IVC (distant metastatic disease) disease. Patients with stage IVB disease who are resectable can either undergo upfront surgery or, in select cases, neoadjuvant targeted therapy treatment before surgery. These patients should then undergo chemoradiation. Patients with stage IVC disease (>50%[2]) are the most difficult to treat. *BRAF*V600E-mutated patients should be initiated on BRAF-directed therapy. Non-*BRAF*V600E-mutated patients should, preferably, be offered a clinical trial when available, immunotherapy-based treatment if programmed death-ligand 1 (PD-L1) score is high, or supportive care/hospice.

Testing for BRAFV600E Mutation

Rapid identification of a *BRAF*V600E mutation must be a priority. Immunohistochemistry (IHC) staining for *BRAF*V600E, which tests for protein expression, may yield results in 24 to 72 hours, depending on the availability of the antibody. Of note, multiple biopsies, preferably core biopsies, should be performed because ATC tumors often present with large, nonviable, highly necrotic tissue, which may be difficult to adequately sample. Tissue-based next-generation sequencing (NGS) is, however, the gold standard for determination of BRAF status, although NGS through circulating cell-free DNA (cfDNA) liquid biopsy is also useful for results in approximately 1 week.[18] The latter has gained significant grounds in cancer genotyping because it offers a minimally invasive and reliable method to gain real-time tumor molecular profiling.[19] The use of cfDNA in ATC was first described in 2017 by Sandulache and colleagues[20] where the Guardant360 platform was used and had a 100% concordance rate for the *BRAF*V600E mutation between blood-drawn liquid biopsy and tumor molecular testing in untreated patients. A follow-up study showed 93% concordance between these.[18] This tool has since been used to not only evaluate the molecular profiling of patients with ATC at presentation and help guide treatment selection but has also recently been shown to aid in evaluating patient prognosis.[18]

BRAFV600E-Mutated Anaplastic Thyroid Cancer

The most significant targeted therapy to truly shift the pendulum for ATC management was the combinatorial use of BRAF/MEK inhibitors in patients harboring a *BRAF*V600E mutation.[15] Once a *BRAF*-mutated ATC has been identified, BRAF-directed therapy or chemoradiation therapy should be started in patients presenting with tumor burdens that are not amenable to upfront complete surgical resection. When successful, BRAF-directed therapy has been shown to induce rapid and significant tumor regression, potentially rendering patients, who were previously inoperable as, candidates for surgery. In the first such report, Wang and colleagues[8] demonstrated the remarkable tumor response to dabrafenib + trametinib in 6 patients who then underwent standard surgical resection of their thyroids and neck disease, even though they were either inoperable at presentation or would have required morbid surgeries involving the laryngopharyngoesophageal complex. The ability to offer complete locoregional surgical resections has been associated with some of the highest survival rates ever reported for advanced ATC to date, with a 94% 1-year survival and an unmet median OS in a cohort of 20 patients (8 of 20 having stage IVC disease) having received BRAF-directed therapy followed by surgery.[2] These findings have prompted the conception of a multicenter phase 2 clinical trial (NCT04675710) that will study the effect of dabrafenib + trametinib in combination with pembrolizumab before surgery, with the primary aim to attain complete gross surgical resection (R0: clear, or R1: microscopically positive surgical margins).[21]

Resistance to BRAF-Directed Therapy

Unfortunately, as reported with melanoma[22] and non–small cell lung cancer,[23] patients on BRAF/MEK inhibitors will invariably develop resistance that is frequently caused by the upregulation of growth factor receptors, the use of alternative pathways, or the reactivation of the mitogen-activated protein kinase and/or the PI3K/AKT pathways, which were initially inhibited.[24–26] More recently, de novo *RAS* mutations in *BRAF*-mutated thyroid cancer have been reported in an in vitro setting[27] following long-term vemurafenib exposure, whereas case reports have also been published in which patients with *BRAF*V600E-mutated thyroid cancers previously on BRAF/MEK inhibitors developed de novo *RAS* mutations in conjunction with disease progression.[28,29] Thus, what was previously believed to be a mutually exclusive path to tumorigenesis,[30] there is clear evidence that *RAS* mutations can occur in this population, and accurately identifying them may allow physicians to offer further therapeutic options with the advent of 2 new molecules being actively studied for *RAS*-mutated cancers.[31,32] Immunotherapy, in conjunction with the BRAF/MEK inhibitor therapy has also gained significant interest in the quest for inhibiting resistance, with reported results showing favorable outcomes.[33,34]

Immunotherapy for Anaplastic Thyroid Cancer

Despite the initial favorable antitumoral effect of combination therapy, patients will often develop resistance to therapy, whether it be through upregulation of growth factor receptors, development and/or use of alternative pathways, or mutation of proteins in signaling cascades. Therefore, combination therapy not only helps combat the disease but also helps combat treatment resistance development. Furthermore, because the *BRAF*V600E mutation is only found in approximately 30% to 40% of ATC tumors,[2,35] a significant proportion of patients will be ineligible to receive dabrafenib + trametinib, and other effective systemic agents are needed for the locoregional advanced and/or metastatic disease.

Human ATC tissue analyses have shown that there is a high PD-L1 expression and high frequency of tumor-infiltrating lymphocytes, suggesting an active immunogenic environment that may be targetable with immunotherapy.[36,37] To date, the use of immunotherapy in a monotherapy setting for ATC has shown modest results, with spartalizumab offering a 19% overall response rate[38] in a mixed *BRAF*-mutated and nonmutated cohort. Patients with tumors having higher PD-L1 scores had more favorable response rates and OS. Lower-than-expected responses in this trial may have been associated with the low PD-L1 expression scores seen on IHC in several of the patients enrolled in the trial (as low as <1%).

In contrast to monotherapy, combining targeted therapy with immunotherapy has shown great promise, both in in vivo preclinical trials in which anti PD-L1 therapy was shown to potentiate the effect of BRAF-directed therapy[39] and in the clinical setting with multiple retrospective reports.[2,33,40–42] Another checkpoint receptor, cytotoxic T lymphocyte antigen 4, is also being targeted in patients with ATC with a checkpoint inhibitor, ipilimumab, in a trial involving the combination of nivolumab (PD-L1 inhibitor) and ipilimumab. Ten patients with ATC received the combination, of which 30% had profound partial responses and 2 remain without any evidence of disease after 13 and 26 months of follow-up.[43]

Upfront use of lenvatinib in combination with checkpoint inhibitors can offer an adequate tumor response, as seen in the in vivo preclinical murine model by Gunda and colleagues.[44] Retrospective data on this combination showed extremely favorable responses, although the cohorts remained small (4 of 6 complete remission, 1 of 6 stable disease, and 1 of 6 disease progression).[45] This prompted the same investigators to commence a prospective phase 2 trial (ATLEP trial), evaluating the efficacy and safety of this combination treatment, with the primary end point being reached thanks to a best overall response of 37.5% for patients with ATC.[46] Recently, the investigators presented their interim results from this trial with an ATC-specific overall response rate of 68% and a clinical benefit rate of 100%. However, the elevated rate (53%) of severe (grade III/IV) adverse events, such as fistula development (11%), arterial hemorrhage (11%), and aspergillus pneumonia (11%), among others, should be noted and followed closely as the trial nears completion.[47]

At present, several prospective clinical trials are underway to evaluate the individual and synergistic effect of targeted therapies and checkpoint inhibitors, including one of the largest that is enrolling BRAF-mutated, RAS-mutated, and non-BRAF/non-RAS-mutated patients to try and capture as large an ATC population as possible.[34]

Other Therapies

Apart from immunotherapy and BRAF-directed therapies, other targetable genetic variations have been identified in ATC, for which the FDA has recently granted drug approvals. Although seldom found in ATC, these include the NTRK[48,49] (2%–4% of ATCs), ALK[50] (4% of ATCs), and RET fusions[51] (1% of ATCs). Specifically for the NTRK-directed therapy using larotrectinib, 7 patients with ATC have received it, of which 2 had a partial response (29%), whereas 1 had stable disease, 1 could not be determined, and 3 progressed.[52] Although the response was notable in 2 of 7, the effect was short lived because disease progressed within a few months.[53] Recent findings demonstrated that short-lived RET fusion-positive thyroid cancers have been treated with selpercatinib[54] or pralsetinib,[55] showing encouraging tumor response rates, although the number of ATC cases treated have been limited to allow for robust conclusions for the time being. In general, these drugs should be used in the setting of a clinical trial when possible.

Pazopanib, a tyrosine kinase inhibitor, was evaluated in a multicenter randomized placebo-controlled phase 2 trial of concurrent intensity-modulated radiation therapy (IMRT) and paclitaxel, as prior preclinical in vivo data had shown a potential synergistic mechanism.[56] Although the randomized trial reported no increase in adverse events, there was also no difference in OS (1, 2, and 3-year) when adding pazopanib to IMRT + paclitaxel.[57] Of note, both the placebo and pazopanib cohorts had significantly lower OS rates than those reported in studies using BRAF/MEK inhibitors with or without checkpoint inhibitors, further strengthening the argument that classic cytotoxic chemotherapy with IMRT should not be the initial treatment of patients with ATC, with or without a tyrosine kinase inhibitor.

Following a favorable response in a small-scale phase 2 trial conducted in Japan evaluating the efficacy of the multikinase inhibitor lenvatinib in patients with ATC (24% partial response rate),[58] a larger-scale, single-arm multicenter phase 2 trial[59] was conducted to further evaluate the role of this drug for ATC. Although the safety profile of lenvatinib was acceptable, the interim analysis overall response rate was 0%, halting the study altogether, with one patient ultimately achieving partial response (overall response rate of 2.9%).[59] Similar findings have been reported with other multikinase inhibitors used in monotherapy settings for ATC, such as sorafenib[60] and pazopanib,[61] with little to no tumor response observed. Given these results, monotherapy with multikinase inhibitor therapy is not recommended.

GOALS OF CARE CONVERSATION

With several treatment options continuously emerging, the future of ATC care is promising. However, even in the most specialized cancer centers, median OS has only reached 16 months for this disease.[2] The reality remains that ATC has a high mortality rate, often due to its advanced disease presentation with rapid growth and treatment resistance. Having a "goals of care" discussion at an early stage and early involvement of supportive care physicians are therefore important. These conversations include understanding and identifying advanced directives, code status, and surrogate decision makers, while candid discussions where patients understand the prognosis, treatment goals, and side effects of treatment are equally critical. Overall, although prognosis for ATC has improved, most patients with an ATC diagnosis will endure a long (often life-long) treatment course and ultimately still succumb to their disease. Therefore, patients' and their families'/caregivers' expectations must be managed at the outset, with an appropriate awareness of palliative care and hospice care options, should they become necessary.

ACCESS AND COST OF CARE

It is of utmost importance that patients with ATC be managed in highly specialized centers with rapid evaluation and treatment protocols specific to patients with ATC. Physicians in peripheral and/or low-volume ATC centers should establish an efficient rapid-referral process from their respective centers to centers with ATC care expertise to avoid treatment delays. As most novel therapeutics are expensive, patient financial toxicity must also be considered, with clinical trials offering opportunities for some patients to receive drugs. Finally, many targeted therapies have limited to no availability worldwide, or are cost prohibitive, limiting the scope to which novel treatment paradigms can be applied globally.

SUMMARY

ATC is a challenging malignancy to treat on account of advanced presentation, short window of opportunity from diagnosis to treatment commencement, and high rate of treatment resistance. As molecular drivers for tumorigenesis continue to be elucidated for ATC and other aggressive human malignancies, new drugs and drug combinations will hopefully continue to offer life-extending benefit by overcoming treatment resistance. For many patients, ATC treatment has now shifted from a palliative to curative approach, with the goal to offer patients significantly longer survival and quality of life. Ongoing and future studies will continue to refine the role of novel targeted therapies and immunotherapy in ATC management.

CLINICS CARE POINTS

- Patients with ATC often present with rapidly growing neck masses that may involve vital structures such as the trachea and recurrent laryngeal nerve, rendering the patient at risk for airway obstruction and/or aspiration. Evaluation by a head and neck surgeon, with securing of the airway, if necessary, should be performed before any other workup.

- Identification of BRAF mutation status should be prioritized in the initial workup of all patients presenting with a rapidly growing thyroid mass. Immunohistochemistry provides the quickest yield and should be preferentially performed on tissue-based biopsies, with additional specimens sent for NGS. PD-L1 percent analyses should also be conducted to evaluate tumor immunogenicity and potential response to checkpoint inhibitors.

- Stage IVA ATC should be managed with upfront surgery followed by chemoradiation. Stage IVB tumors that are resectable should be treated with upfront surgery or, in select cases, neoadjuvant targeted therapy treatment before surgery, followed by chemoradiation. Stage IVC BRAFV600E-mutated tumors should be treated with BRAF-directed therapy, whereas non-BRAFV600E-mutated tumors should, preferably, be offered a clinical trial when available, immunotherapy-based treatment if PD-L1 score is high, or supportive care/hospice.

DECLARATION OF INTERESTS

A. Maniakas declares no competing interests. M. Zafereo: principal investigator for clinical trials funded by Merck and Eli Lilly. M.E. Cabanillas: research funding from Eisai, Exelixis, Kura Oncology, and Genentech; participated in advisory boards for LOXO, Bayer, and Ignyta.

REFERENCES

1. Lin B, Ma H, Ma M, et al. The incidence and survival analysis for anaplastic thyroid cancer: a SEER database analysis. Am J translational Res 2019;11:5888–96.

2. Maniakas A, Dadu R, Busaidy NL, et al. Evaluation of overall survival in patients with anaplastic thyroid carcinoma, 2000-2019. JAMA Oncol 2020;6:1397–404.

3. Are C, Shaha AR. Anaplastic thyroid carcinoma: biology, pathogenesis, prognostic factors, and treatment approaches. Ann Surg Oncol 2006;13:453–64.

4. Smallridge RC, Marlow LA, Copland JA. Anaplastic thyroid cancer: molecular pathogenesis and emerging therapies. Endocr-related cancer 2009;16:17–44.

5. Smallridge RC, Ain KB, Asa SL, et al. American Thyroid Association guidelines for management of patients with anaplastic thyroid cancer. Thyroid 2012;22: 1104–39.

6. Tuttle RM, Haugen B, Perrier ND. Updated American Joint Committee on Cancer/Tumor-Node-Metastasis Staging System for Differentiated and Anaplastic Thyroid Cancer (Eighth Edition): What Changed and Why? Thyroid 2017;27:751–6.

7. Pozdeyev N, Gay LM, Sokol ES, et al. Genetic Analysis of 779 Advanced Differentiated and Anaplastic Thyroid Cancers. Clin Cancer Res : official J Am Assoc Cancer Res 2018;24:3059–68.

8. Wang JR, Zafereo M, Dadu R, et al. Complete surgical resection following neoadjuvant dabrafenib plus trametinib in BRAFV600E-mutated anaplastic thyroid carcinoma. Thyroid 2019;29(8):1036–43.

9. Xu B, Fuchs T, Dogan S, et al. Dissecting anaplastic thyroid carcinoma: a comprehensive clinical, histologic, immunophenotypic, and molecular study of 360 Cases. Thyroid 2020;30:1505–17.

10. Oishi N, Kondo T, Ebina A, et al. Molecular alterations of coexisting thyroid papillary carcinoma and anaplastic carcinoma: identification of TERT mutation as an independent risk factor for transformation. Mod Pathol 2017;30:1527–37.

11. Bible KC, Kebebew E, Brierley J, et al. 2021 American thyroid association guidelines for management of patients with anaplastic thyroid cancer. Thyroid 2021;31: 337–86.

12. Janz TA, Neskey DM, Nguyen SA, et al. Is the incidence of anaplastic thyroid cancer increasing: A population based epidemiology study. World J Otorhinolaryngol - Head Neck Surg 2019;5:34–40.

13. Iyer PC, Cote GJ, Hai T, et al. Circulating BRAF V600E Cell-Free DNA as a Biomarker in the Management of Anaplastic Thyroid Carcinoma. JCO Precision Oncol 2018;1–11.

14. Cabanillas ME, Williams MD, Gunn GB, et al. Facilitating anaplastic thyroid cancer specialized treatment: A model for improving access to multidisciplinary care for patients with anaplastic thyroid cancer. Head & neck 2017;39:1291–5.

15. Subbiah V, Kreitman RJ, Wainberg ZA, et al. Dabrafenib and trametinib treatment in patients with locally advanced or metastatic braf v600-mutant anaplastic thyroid cancer. J Clin Oncol 2018;36:7–13.

16. Henderson YC, Mohamed ASR, Maniakas A, et al. A high-throughput approach to identify effective systemic agents for the treatment of anaplastic thyroid carcinoma. J Clin Endocrinol Metab 2021;106:2962–78.

17. Maniakas A, Henderson YC, Hei H, et al. Novel anaplastic thyroid cancer PDXs and cell lines: Expanding preclinical models of genetic diversity. J Clin Endocrinol Metab 2021;106(11):e4652–65.

18. Qin Y, Wang JR, Wang Y, et al. Clinical utility of circulating cell-free dna mutations in anaplastic thyroid carcinoma. Thyroid 2021;31:1235–43.

19. Corcoran RB, Chabner BA. Application of Cell-free DNA Analysis to Cancer Treatment. New Engl J Med 2018;379:1754–65.

20. Sandulache VC, Williams MD, Lai SY, et al. Real-time genomic characterization utilizing circulating cell-free dna in patients with anaplastic thyroid carcinoma. Thyroid 2017;27:81–7.

21. Pembrolizumab, Dabrafenib, and Trametinib Before Surgery for the Treatment of BRAF-Mutated Anaplastic Thyroid Cancer. 2020. Available at: https://clinicaltrials.gov/ct2/show/NCT04675710.

22. Wang L, Leite de Oliveira R, Huijberts S, et al. An acquired vulnerability of drug-resistant melanoma with therapeutic potential. Cell 2018;173:1413–25.e14.

23. Facchinetti F, Lacroix L, Mezquita L, et al. Molecular mechanisms of resistance to BRAF and MEK inhibitors in BRAF(V600E) non-small cell lung cancer, 132. Oxford, England: European journal of cancer; 2020. p. 211–23, 1990.

24. Villanueva J, Vultur A, Lee JT, et al. Acquired resistance to BRAF inhibitors mediated by a RAF kinase switch in melanoma can be overcome by cotargeting MEK and IGF-1R/PI3K. Cancer Cell 2010;18:683–95.

25. Poulikakos PI, Persaud Y, Janakiraman M, et al. RAF inhibitor resistance is mediated by dimerization of aberrantly spliced BRAF(V600E). Nature 2011;480:387–90.

26. Van Allen EM, Wagle N, Sucker A, et al. The genetic landscape of clinical resistance to RAF inhibition in metastatic melanoma. Cancer Discov 2014;4:94–109.

27. Danysh BP, Rieger EY, Sinha DK, et al. Long-term vemurafenib treatment drives inhibitor resistance through a spontaneous KRAS G12D mutation in a BRAF V600E papillary thyroid carcinoma model. Oncotarget 2016;7:30907–23.

28. Owen DH, Konda B, Sipos J, et al. KRAS G12V Mutation in Acquired Resistance to Combined BRAF and MEK Inhibition in Papillary Thyroid Cancer. J Natl Compr Cancer Netw 2019;17:409–13.

29. Cabanillas ME, Dadu R, Iyer P, et al. Acquired Secondary RAS Mutation in BRAF(V600E)-Mutated Thyroid Cancer Patients Treated with BRAF Inhibitors. Thyroid 2020;30:1288–96.

30. Kimura ET, Nikiforova MN, Zhu Z, et al. High prevalence of BRAF mutations in thyroid cancer: genetic evidence for constitutive activation of the RET/PTC-RAS-BRAF signaling pathway in papillary thyroid carcinoma. Cancer Res 2003;63:1454–7.

31. Canon J, Rex K, Saiki AY, et al. The clinical KRAS(G12C) inhibitor AMG 510 drives anti-tumour immunity. Nature 2019;575:217–23.

32. Hallin J, Engstrom LD, Hargis L, et al. The KRAS(G12C) Inhibitor MRTX849 Provides Insight toward Therapeutic Susceptibility of KRAS-Mutant Cancers in Mouse Models and Patients. Cancer Discov 2020;10:54–71.

33. Iyer PC, Dadu R, Gule-Monroe M, et al. Salvage pembrolizumab added to kinase inhibitor therapy for the treatment of anaplastic thyroid carcinoma. J Immunother Cancer 2018;6:68.

34. Cabanillas M, Busaidy N, Dadu R, et al. OR27-6 Combination Vemurafenib (BRAF Inhibitor)/Cobimetinib (MEK Inhibitor)/Atezolizumab (Anti-PDL1 Inhibitor) in BRAF-V600E Mutated Anaplastic Thyroid Cancer (ATC): Initial Safety and Feasibility. J Endocr Soc 2019;3(Suppl 1). OR27-6.

35. Chen H, Luthra R, Routbort MJ, et al. Molecular Profile of Advanced Thyroid Carcinomas by Next-Generation Sequencing: Characterizing Tumors Beyond Diagnosis for Targeted Therapy. Mol Cancer Ther 2018;17:1575–84.

36. Dadu R, Rodriguez Canales J, Wistuba I, et al. Targeting immune system in anaplastic thyroid cancer (ATC): a potential treatment approach. Thyroid 2015; Supplement 1:749.

37. Adam P, Kircher S, Sbiera I, et al. FGF-Receptors and PD-L1 in Anaplastic and Poorly Differentiated Thyroid Cancer: Evaluation of the Preclinical Rationale. Front Endocrinol 2021;12:712107.
38. Capdevila J, Wirth LJ, Ernst T, et al. PD-1 Blockade in Anaplastic Thyroid Carcinoma. J Clin Oncol 2020;38:2620–7.
39. Brauner E, Gunda V, Vanden Borre P, et al. Combining BRAF inhibitor and anti PD-L1 antibody dramatically improves tumor regression and anti tumor immunity in an immunocompetent murine model of anaplastic thyroid cancer. Oncotarget 2016;7:17194–211.
40. Zheng L, Li L, He Q, et al. Response to immunotherapy in a patient with anaplastic thyroid cancer: A case report. Medicine 2021;100:e26138.
41. Nabhan F, Kander E, Shen R, et al. Pembrolizumab in a Patient with Treatment-Naïve Unresectable BRAF-Mutation Negative Anaplastic Thyroid Cancer. Case Rep Endocrinol 2021;2021:5521649.
42. Yang SR, Tsai MH, Hung CJ, et al. Anaplastic Thyroid Cancer Successfully Treated With Radiation and Immunotherapy: A Case Report. AACE Clin case Rep 2021;7:299–302.
43. Lorch JH, Barletta JA, Nehs M, et al. A phase II study of nivolumab (N) plus ipilimumab (I) in radioidine refractory differentiated thyroid cancer (RAIR DTC) with exploratory cohorts in anaplastic (ATC) and medullary thyroid cancer (MTC). J Clin Oncol 2020;38:6513.
44. Gunda V, Gigliotti B, Ashry T, et al. Anti-PD-1/PD-L1 therapy augments lenvatinib's efficacy by favorably altering the immune microenvironment of murine anaplastic thyroid cancer. Int J Cancer 2019;144:2266–78.
45. Dierks C, Seufert J, Aumann K, et al. Combination of Lenvatinib and Pembrolizumab Is an Effective Treatment Option for Anaplastic and Poorly Differentiated Thyroid Carcinoma. Thyroid 2021;31:1076–85.
46. Dierks C, Seufert J, Ruf J, et al. 1915P The lenvatinib/pembrolizumab combination induces long lasting and complete responses in patients with metastatic anaplastic or poorly differentiated thyroid carcinoma: Results from a retrospective study and first results from the prospective phase II ATLEP trial. Ann Oncol 2020; 31:S1085.
47. Dierks C, Ruf J, Seufert J, et al. Lenvatinib/Pembrolizumab in Metastasized Anaplastic Thyroid Carcinoma (ATC): Interim results of the ATLEP Trial. Thyroid 2021;31. A-2.
48. Cabanillas ME, Ryder M, Jimenez C. Targeted Therapy for Advanced Thyroid Cancer: Kinase Inhibitors and Beyond. Endocr Rev 2019;40(6):1573–604.
49. Drilon A, Laetsch TW, Kummar S, et al. Efficacy of Larotrectinib in TRK Fusion-Positive Cancers in Adults and Children. New Engl J Med 2018;378:731–9.
50. Kelly LM, Barila G, Liu P, et al. Identification of the transforming STRN-ALK fusion as a potential therapeutic target in the aggressive forms of thyroid cancer. Proc Natl Acad Sci USA 2014;111:4233–8.
51. Santoro M, Moccia M, Federico G, et al. RET Gene Fusions in Malignancies of the Thyroid and Other Tissues. Genes 2020;11.
52. Cabanillas M, Drilon A, Farago A, et al. 1916P Larotrectinib treatment of advanced TRK fusion thyroid cancer. Ann Oncol 2020;31:S1086.
53. Waguespack SG, Drilon A, Lin JJ, et al. Long-term Efficacy and Safety of Larotrectinib in Patients with Advanced TRK Fusion-positive Thyroid Carcinoma. Thyroid 2021;31:A–6.
54. Wirth LJ, Sherman E, Robinson B, et al. Efficacy of Selpercatinib in RET-Altered Thyroid Cancers. New Engl J Med 2020;383:825–35.

55. Subbiah V, Hu MI, Wirth LJ, et al. Pralsetinib for patients with advanced or metastatic RET-altered thyroid cancer (ARROW): a multi-cohort, open-label, registrational, phase 1/2 study. Lancet Diabetes Endocrinol 2021;9:491–501.

56. Isham CR, Bossou AR, Negron V, et al. Pazopanib enhances paclitaxel-induced mitotic catastrophe in anaplastic thyroid cancer. Sci translational Med 2013;5: 166ra3.

57. Sherman EJ, Harris J, Bible KC, et al. 1914MO Randomized phase II study of radiation therapy and paclitaxel with pazopanib or placebo: NRG-RTOG 0912. Ann Oncol 2020;31:S1085.

58. Takahashi S, Kiyota N, Yamazaki T, et al. A Phase II study of the safety and efficacy of lenvatinib in patients with advanced thyroid cancer. Future Oncol (London, England) 2019;15:717–26.

59. Wirth LJ, Brose MS, Sherman EJ, et al. Open-Label, Single-Arm, Multicenter, Phase II Trial of Lenvatinib for the Treatment of Patients With Anaplastic Thyroid Cancer. J Clin Oncol 2021;39:2359–66.

60. Savvides P, Nagaiah G, Lavertu P, et al. Phase II trial of sorafenib in patients with advanced anaplastic carcinoma of the thyroid. Thyroid 2013;23:600–4.

61. Bible KC, Suman VJ, Menefee ME, et al. A multiinstitutional phase 2 trial of pazopanib monotherapy in advanced anaplastic thyroid cancer. J Clin Endocrinol Metab 2012;97:3179–84.

Diagnostic and Treatment Considerations for Thyroid Cancer in Women of Reproductive Age and the Perinatal Period

Evert F.S. van Velsen, MD, MSc[a],*, Angela M. Leung, MD, MSc[b,c],
Tim I.M. Korevaar, MD, PhD[a]

KEYWORDS

- Thyroid cancer • Pregnancy • Fertility • Preconception • Radioactive iodine
- Thyroid hormone

KEY POINTS

- Any woman of reproductive age diagnosed with thyroid cancer should be offered preconception advice on the risks of thyroid cancer progression or recurrence, or adverse obstetric and/or childhood outcomes, and contraception in cases where thyroid cancer treatment contraindicates pregnancy.
- For most cases of differentiated thyroid cancer (DTC) in the perinatal period, treatment can be delayed until after delivery. If surgery is recommended during pregnancy, it should be performed in the second trimester.
- Pregnancy is not associated with clinically meaningful disease progression of previously treated DTC or micropapillary thyroid carcinoma under active surveillance.
- It is recommended to avoid pregnancy for 6 to 12 months after radioactive iodine treatment.
- The need for thyroid hormone therapy to achieve a suppressed serum thyrotropin level during pregnancy is based on the DTC's dynamic risk response, but the harms and benefits of this should be weighed against the risks of adverse pregnancy outcomes.

INTRODUCTION

The worldwide incidence of thyroid cancer has been steadily increasing over the last 2 decades in line with the increased use of imaging modalities.[1,2] Papillary thyroid

[a] Department of Internal Medicine, Academic Center for Thyroid Diseases, Erasmus Medical Center, Dr Molewaterplein 40, 3015 CE, Rotterdam, The Netherlands; [b] Division of Endocrinology, Diabetes, and Metabolism, Department of Medicine, UCLA David Geffen School of Medicine, 100 Medical Plaza, Suite 310, Los Angeles, CA 90095, USA; [c] Division of Endocrinology, Diabetes, and Metabolism, Department of Medicine, VA Greater Los Angeles Healthcare System, 11301 Wilshire Blvd (111D), Los Angeles, CA 90073, USA
* Corresponding author.
E-mail address: e.vanvelsen@erasmusmc.nl

Endocrinol Metab Clin N Am 51 (2022) 403–416
https://doi.org/10.1016/j.ecl.2021.11.021
0889-8529/21/© 2021 The Author(s). Published by Elsevier Inc. This is an open access article under the CC BY license (http://creativecommons.org/licenses/by/4.0/).
endo.theclinics.com

carcinomas (PTC) and follicular thyroid carcinomas (FTC) are referred to as differenti-ated thyroid cancer (DTC) and comprise 80% to 85% of all thyroid carcinomas, whereas the remaining minority is made up of medullary (MTC) and anaplastic thyroid cancer (ATC).

Thyroid cancer occurs more frequently in women than in men and is one of the most common cancers diagnosed in women of reproductive age.[2–4] It is estimated to make up 20% of all diagnosed cancers in the perinatal period, ranking thyroid cancer the second most common cancer after breast cancer.[5,6] About two-thirds of thyroid can-cer diagnoses in the perinatal period are made in the first 12 months postpartum.[5] This is most likely due to reluctance to perform radiographic or invasive procedures during pregnancy and the predominantly absent, mild, or nonacute symptoms of DTCs espe-cially. Importantly, regardless of the type of thyroid cancer that complicates the peri-natal period, specific attention should be paid to psychosocial distress, anticonception strategies, and wish to breastfeed in order to provide optimal care for women with thyroid cancer. The current review focuses on preconception and perinatal-specific clinical considerations predominantly related to the care of patients with thyroid cancer, focusing particularly on DTC.

PREGNANCY AND THYROID CANCER DIAGNOSIS

In the general population, up to 68% of adults have a thyroid nodule detectable by im-aging, and approximately 5% have a palpable thyroid nodule, with the prevalence of both increasing throughout a lifetime.[7,8] During pregnancy, only about 29% of women have a thyroid nodule detectable with imaging, whereas about 5% have a potentially palpable nodule of greater than 1 cm.[9] Although thyroid nodules are more frequent with advancing age, it is not uncommon for thyroid nodules to be first detected in young women during the perinatal period. The goal of thyroid nodule evaluation is the detection of thyroid cancer, which occurs in 7% to 15% of cases. The initial eval-uation of thyroid nodules discovered during pregnancy or postpartum is the same as in the nonpregnant, nonlactating population and includes measuring serum thyroid func-tion and performing an ultrasound.[10] Subsequent fine needle aspiration should be per-formed, if applicable, based on the sonographic pattern and patient preference, but pregnancy is a contraindication for nuclear imaging; during lactation, iodine-123 and technetium pertechnetate can be used if breastmilk for the few days following their administration is discarded.[10]

Several studies have shown decreased quality-of-life (QoL) measures in patients diagnosed with thyroid cancer compared with the general population, with the decrease more pronounced in young women.[11–13] In particular, the lower QoL in young women could be mediated by increased psychosocial distress related to pregnancy planning and/or (future) parenthood.[14–16] A recent study showed that a diagnosis of DTC and its subsequent treatment negatively influenced the desire to have a child in almost 40% of women.[17] The main reasons for these women were that they did not want a child anymore (40%), and fear of medicalization of the upcoming pregnancy (33%), although the outcomes related to family planning were not assessed. As such, the treating physician should have an active role in providing information and support, as is emphasized by the fact that psychological distress is related to suboptimal fertility and pregnancy outcomes.[18,19] Important uncertainties that need to be actively addressed relate to pregnancy-specific thy-roid cancer progression or recurrence, the potential risks of serum thyrotropin (TSH) suppressive therapy, and risks of adverse obstetric and/or childhood outcomes.

IMPACT OF PREGNANCY ON THYROID CANCER

The overall prognosis of most thyroid cancers is excellent, but the remaining reproductive window for many patients, even among younger individuals, is often limited. Therefore, it is important to understand the effects of pregnancy on treated and/or persistent DTC to be able to determine the need for and optimal timing of specific treatments, as well as supporting plans for pregnancy, if desired, in those who received initial treatment or during active surveillance of newly diagnosed DTC.[20]

It should also be considered that normal thyroid physiology during pregnancy complicates the interpretation of serum thyroid test results. During pregnancy, the size of the thyroid gland increases by 10% in iodine-replete areas, but by 20% to 40% in areas of iodine deficiency. Furthermore, serum thyroglobulin (Tg) concentrations, as a marker of thyroid volume and/or remnant DTC, increase during pregnancy, especially in states of insufficient iodine,[21,22] and then normalize postpartum, which may complicate follow-up in women after hemithyroidectomy or with remnant disease following initial therapy for DTC.

Clinical data have refuted the theoretic concept that various pregnancy-specific physiologic changes could promote thyroid cancer (remnant) growth to a clinically meaningful extent (eg, increase in estrogen, placental growth hormone, and human chorionic gonadotropin). Several studies have demonstrated no significant disease recurrence or worsening of structural disease during pregnancy.[23–30] In a study including women with known structural disease, growth was seen in 30% to 50% during pregnancy,[24–26] with 8% requiring additional therapy (neck dissection and tyrosine kinase inhibitor [TKI] treatment) in the first year following pregnancy.[26] However, the interpretation of these studies is limited by the lack of a control group, and therefore, it is unknown what the disease courses would have been in a nonpregnant setting. However, these studies indicate that the American Thyroid Association (ATA) thyroid cancer dynamic risk stratification (DRS) system[8] can also help predict disease progression in pregnant women previously treated for DTC. In women with an excellent response, no additional monitoring is needed during pregnancy, whereas in those with biochemically or structurally incomplete responses, additional monitoring is needed with both serum Tg levels and surveillance neck ultrasounds.[10]

Previous studies have shown that pregnancy does not seem to impact the overall and disease-free survival of newly diagnosed DTC.[10] It must be noted that in most studies, the majority of the patients had stage I disease, which means that there were very few young patients with distant metastasis. For the 2 studies that did show a higher rate of persistent disease and recurrences in women diagnosed with DTC during pregnancy or in the first year thereafter,[28,29] the interpretation of results is limited by the fact that most recurrences (60%) were biochemical,[28] or biochemical and structural disease were shown together.[29] Larger and more detailed studies are needed to better verify the lack of an increased risk of persistent disease (whether biochemical, structural, or both) in patients with DTC that is newly diagnosed during pregnancy. In addition, there would be benefit in studying specific high-risk subgroups, such as women with new lymph node metastases discovered during pregnancy, or persistent disease during pregnancy following history of initial therapy.

Over the past several years, active surveillance for low-risk thyroid papillary carcinomas (mostly <1-cm tumors) has emerged as an acceptable alternative approach to surgery, if no suspicious cervical lymph nodes and no extrathyroidal extension are present.[31] A recent study by Ito and colleagues[32] showed that women with a desire to become pregnant are good candidates for active surveillance. Out of the total of 50 patients, biopsy-proven DTCs grew ≥3 mm in only 4 patients (8%) during the perinatal period. Of these four, 2 patients underwent surgery after delivery and had no recurrence afterward. The others underwent continuous active surveillance because of lack of enlargement after delivery. The current ATA thyroid and pregnancy guidelines advise to monitor these microcarcinomas with a neck ultrasound in each trimester of pregnancy.[10] However, based on the study of Ito and colleagues, as well as an expected physiologic increase in thyroid volume overall during pregnancy, it could be argued that neck ultrasounds may be reasonably performed less frequently in this group (for example, only once in the second trimester).

IMPACT OF THYROID CANCER ON PREGNANCY

It has been shown that general cancer survivors often have a higher risk of adverse obstetric outcomes, such as preterm birth, which is mostly attributed to the long-term effects of cancer treatments like chemotherapy.[3,33–35] The rare occurrence of thyroid cancer in women of reproductive age limits the abilities to perform high-quality prospective studies. Subanalyses of large studies in survivors of any cancer indicate that the risk of adverse obstetric outcomes is not higher in thyroid cancer survivors than controls without a previous diagnosis of any cancer.[3,33–35] In line with such subanalyses, a study of 7734 women showed that those with a history of DTC have similar risks of adverse pregnancy outcomes, such as preeclampsia, preterm birth, or abnormal birth weight, as women without DTC.[36] Furthermore, the available data also do not indicate a higher risk of adverse obstetric outcomes in women diagnosed with DTC during pregnancy.[37] In general, a malignancy is not an absolute risk for preterm birth or indication for cesarean section. Clear communication and reassurance regarding similar risks of adverse pregnancy outcomes are important in this population, as young women in particular exhibit more distress and anxiety related to a thyroid cancer diagnosis,[14,15] which are independent risk factors for adverse pregnancy outcomes.[19,38,39]

DIFFERENTIATED THYROID CANCER TREATMENT-SPECIFIC CONSIDERATIONS IN PREGNANCY

For women with more concerning acute symptoms owing to DTC, or signs of MTC or ATC, pregnancy should not dissuade from recommendations to perform any necessary diagnostics or treatment interventions. The health risks related to these more aggressive types of thyroid cancers in the mother (and thus also risks to the offspring) typically outweigh these necessary procedures. Clinical data on perinatal MTC or ATC are limited to case reports, in comparison to that of DTCs showing that women of reproductive age with DTC have extremely good outcomes (ie, disease-specific survival rates >99%).[40–43] As such, a careful approach to clinical decision making that takes into account the harms and benefits of the timing of diagnostics or treatment interventions, as well as the risks and benefits for future reproductive function and pregnancy, is warranted.

Treatment of DTC is historically based on thyroid surgery followed by radioactive iodine (RAI) ablation. However, in many cases, a less-aggressive therapy seems more appropriate, as DTC-specific mortality has remained very low over the past several decades despite a concurrent increase in its incidence.[1,2,8] For this reason, current ATA guidelines recommend less-extensive surgery and more restricted use of RAI therapy in low-risk tumors,[8] but controversies remain.[44] Nevertheless, postoperative RAI ablation is still one of the cornerstones of the treatment of patients with DTC, particularly in more advanced disease.[8,45] After initial therapy (surgery, plus RAI if needed), patient follow-up strategies can be based on the ATA guidelines, which include regular DRS assessments to determine no evidence of disease, persistent structural and/or biochemical disease, or a recurrence.[8] The need for additional therapy, for example, additional surgery and/or RAI therapy, TKIs, is based on these findings. Reoperative surgery, RAI therapy, and TKI use have different influences on pregnancy planning, reproductive function, and pregnancy course.

Thyroid Surgery

Thyroid surgery for DTC consists of either a hemithyroidectomy or a total thyroidectomy. Thyroid hormone replacement is always necessary following a total thyroidectomy. After hemithyroidectomy for DTC, up to 80% of nonpregnant patients require levothyroxine replacement therapy,[46–48] but this is likely higher during pregnancy because of increased thyroid hormone demands. When taking thyroid hormone replacement therapy, women should be counseled to increase their dose by 25% to 30% upon a positive pregnancy test.[49] After either hemithyroidectomy or total thyroidectomy, serum TSH level should be checked every 3 to 5 weeks during the first and second trimester, and at least once during the third trimester of pregnancy. The indication for TSH suppression is based on the ATA DRS status but should also consider pregnancy-specific risks (see section on Thyrotropin Suppressive Therapy).[10]

After thyroid surgery, permanent hypoparathyroidism may occur in up to 10% of patients.[8,50] Replacement therapy with calcium and/or active vitamin D is then needed, but even when calcium concentrations are normal and stable, episodes of hypocalcemia or hypercalcemia may occur, as pregnancy and lactation affect calcium and vitamin D metabolism. Undertreatment or overtreatment of hypoparathyroidism during pregnancy has been associated with abortion, stillbirth, and perinatal/fetal death.[51] Furthermore, maternal hypocalcemia can cause fetal parathyroid hyperplasia and associated skeletal changes, whereas maternal hypercalcemia can suppress fetal parathyroid hormone production, leading to neonatal hypocalcemia. Therefore, serum calcium levels should be monitored closely during pregnancy (eg, every 3–4 weeks) and during lactation (eg, monthly) with maintaining normocalcemia as the primary goal.[51]

When DTC is discovered during pregnancy, it can be difficult to determine the optimal timing for thyroid surgery. In patients diagnosed with DTC early in pregnancy who have no lymph node or distant metastases, both the current ATA and the British Thyroid Association (BTA) guidelines recommend monitoring with ultrasound.[8,10,52] In cases of rapid tumor growth or the presence/development of lymph node metastases, surgery should be considered in the second trimester. In 2 studies totaling 53 women diagnosed with DTC during pregnancy who underwent thyroid surgery (the majority during the second trimester), there were no pregnancy losses, and neonatal and maternal outcomes were similar to the general population.[53,54] After surgery, thyroid hormone replacement therapy is needed, and serum TSH level should be checked every 3 to 5 weeks during the second trimester, and at least once during the third trimester. In cases of DTC detected in the second half of the pregnancy, surgery after delivery is preferred[8,10] in order to minimize risks of abortion, altered organogenesis, and preterm labor and delivery.[52]

Postoperative Radioactive Iodine Ablation

Multiple studies have examined the effects of RAI ablation on both gonadal function and various pregnancy outcomes. A transient change of the menstrual cycle has been observed in 12% to 31% of women, in addition to a temporary increase of follicle-stimulating hormone levels during the first year after RAI therapy.[55–58] More recent studies have used serum anti-Müllerian hormone (AMH) concentrations as a marker of ovarian reserve.[17,59] AMH is relatively insensitive to intercycle and intracycle variability and oral contraceptives use and gradually declines with age until it becomes undetectable during menopause.[60–62] Systematic reviews have shown a significant decline of serum AMH levels 1 year after RAI therapy, compared with baseline levels.[56,63] One study indicated that women older than age 35 years showed a much stronger decrease in AMH levels than those younger than age 35 years (-71% vs -46%; $P<.001$).[17] These data suggest that, if possible, a less-aggressive RAI treatment strategy should be considered in women over 35 years of age who desire pregnancy.

Several studies have reported that there are no increased infertility rates or adverse obstetric outcomes (eg, spontaneous abortions, stillbirths, preterm births, congenital malformations) in patients after RAI therapy.[57,58,63,64] It must be noted that a recent aggregate data meta-analysis identified a higher risk of abortion (odds ratio, 0.60; 95% confidence interval, 0.53–0.68; $P<.0001$) in women who became pregnant within 1 year of RAI therapy, compared with those who became pregnant greater than 1 year after RAI therapy.[64] Although those results may suggest that pregnancy should be avoided within 1 year of RAI therapy, spontaneous and induced abortions were not distinguished in the aforementioned study. Therefore, it is impossible to identify confounding by indication, in which the decision for an induced abortion is made because of recent RAI use, such as in women with an unexpected pregnancy. More data are required to optimize clinical recommendations on the necessary time between RAI ablation and conception, as is reflected by the current ATA guidelines that recommend avoidance of pregnancy for 6 to 12 months after RAI treatment.[8,10]

As mentioned earlier, RAI therapy is still one of the cornerstones in the treatment of patients with DTC, particularly among patients with more advanced disease.[8,45] However, it is well established that iodine-131 crosses the placenta and accumulates in the fetal thyroid, which may cause fetal/neonatal hypothyroidism, if given after 12 to 13 weeks' gestation.[65] Treatment with iodine-131 during pregnancy is therefore contraindicated and should be deferred to after delivery. After pregnancy, as the lactating breast is very efficient in concentrating iodine, breastfeeding must be stopped 6 weeks before until 3 months after RAI therapy.[66] This protects the mother's breast tissue from irradiation, and also the infant's thyroid gland from ingestion of iodine-131 through breastmilk intake.

Tyrosine Kinase Inhibitors

Currently, 4 TKIs (sorafenib, lenvatinib, pralsetinib, selpercatinib) are approved by the Food and Drug Administration in the United States for use with advanced metastatic DTC. To the authors' knowledge, there are currently no human studies evaluating the effects of these medications on reproductive function and pregnancy course, but associated teratogenicity and embryo toxicity have been shown in animal studies.[10] Because these drugs should be avoided during pregnancy and breastfeeding, contraception strategies and plans for breastfeeding should be actively discussed with every woman of childbearing age in need for treatment with a TKI. For rare cases of advanced DTC diagnosed during pregnancy, it should be recognized that such medications should not be started.

Finally, for any woman of reproductive age who may undergo a treatment that is contraindicated in pregnancy, it is vital to provide detailed advice on contraceptive use. Specifically, the failure risk of commonly used contraceptive techniques, such as barrier methods (condom [13%], diaphragm/cervical cap [up to 27%]), fertility awareness-based methods (2%–23%), and nonadherence to hormonal methods (7%) compared with intrauterine conception or implants (<1%).[67]

Thyrotropin Suppressive Therapy

A large proportion of women who undergo treatment of thyroid cancer will require postoperative levothyroxine replacement and thus require preconception counseling and gestational monitoring, and likely also a levothyroxine dose increase of 25% to 30%.[8] The gestational dose adjustment should be based on the serum TSH concentrations during pregnancy to prevent overtreatment as (athyreotic) women with preconception TSH suppressive therapy are more likely to be overtreated with a standard-dose increase regimen, and a short period of TSH outside the target range is unlikely to affect the risk of thyroid cancer progression.[68]

Based on the ATA DRS status, the recommendation of whether to initiate TSH suppressive therapy, and its extent if so, should be assessed similarly to that of a nonpregnant, nonlactating patient.[10] However, in (prospective) observational studies, a lower serum TSH and higher free thyroxine (FT4) concentration in pregnancy have been associated with preeclampsia, small-for-gestational-age infant, lower child IQ, and less cerebral gray mass.[69–74] These and other data have raised concern for the possibility of levothyroxine overtreatment,[75,76] for example, when it is started for mild thyroid function test abnormalities, but such concerns can be extended to TSH suppressive therapy for thyroid cancer. Therefore, a similar risk assessment as for nonpregnant patients should be made to weigh the harms and benefits of TSH suppressive therapy, while considering the risks of adverse pregnancy outcomes. If surgery is postponed to after delivery, the possible benefits of TSH suppressive therapy during pregnancy, with respect to the prognosis of DTC, are unknown. Current ATA guidelines advise that thyroid hormone replacement therapy be considered to maintain a serum TSH level between 0.4 and 2.0 mU/L,[10] whereas the current BTA guidelines emphasize that there is no evidence for TSH suppression for such cases, and no advise is given.[52]

For women who are considered to not have any active DTC (ie, DRS showing excellent response), iatrogenic hypothyroidism can be approached in the same way as other forms of pregestational hypothyroidism (such as those with Hashimoto disease or congenital hypothyroidism). In this group, the only exception is that levothyroxine treatment should be targeted to a TSH level less than 2.0 mU/L during pregnancy; this is in contrast to the TSH treatment goal of less than 2.5 mU/L in women with Hashimoto disease and no DTC, and the diagnostic threshold for (subclinical) hypothyroidism that is typically less than 4.0 mU/L in women without known thyroid disease.[10] Women with preexisting hypothyroidism before pregnancy who are well controlled on levothyroxine have similar risks of adverse pregnancy outcomes as women without hypothyroidism.[38,77,78]

MEDULLARY THYROID CANCER

MTC is a relatively rare thyroid cancer entity that occurs sporadically or in a hereditary form (all caused by an *RET* germline mutation and may be a component of type 2 multiple endocrine neoplasia [MEN], MEN2A or MEN2B, and the related syndrome, familial MTC). Testing for germline RET mutations is advised in all patients with newly diagnosed MTC. In the case of an RET mutation, it is important to offer genetic counseling to the parents, including possibilities of testing in utero or after delivery. Furthermore, in the case of an *RET* mutation, a pheochromocytoma should be excluded, preferably before pregnancy.[79] Sporadic MTC occurs mainly in the fourth to sixth decade, but those with hereditary MTC may be much younger. Survival in MTC is based on its initial stage, with a 10-year survival rate varying from 100% in stage I to 21% in stage IV.[79] Thyroid surgery, including possible prophylactic lymph node dissection of the central compartment, forms the basis of initial treatment.[79] Afterward, patients will require thyroid hormone replacement with the goal of maintaining serum TSH levels in the euthyroid range, and RAI therapy is typically not administered. In cases of recurrent disease or the presence of neck and/or distant metastases, one might consider surgery, local radiotherapy, or systemic treatment with a TKI.[79]

If MTC is diagnosed during pregnancy, both current ATA and BTA guidelines advise surgery during gestation, because of the more aggressive nature of MTC as compared with DTC.[10,52] To the best of the authors' knowledge, no studies evaluating the benefits of this strategy exist. Women undergoing surgery for MTC should be instructed similarly as those treated for DTC, regarding increasing the dose of their thyroid hormone replacement therapy should they become pregnant (see earlier discussion). There are no studies on disease progression/recurrence during pregnancy in women with MTC. In postoperative women who become pregnant, one might consider performing a thyroid ultrasound and obtaining serum calcitonin and carcinoembryonic antigen (CEA) measurements during the second trimester, in order to rule out recurrence or local disease progression. It should be noted, however, that serum calcitonin concentrations can increase up to 2 to 3 times the upper limit of normal during pregnancy and remain high during the postpartum period, especially in breastfeeding women.[80] For serum CEA, there are no clinically meaningful changes as a result of pregnancy.[81]

Although TKIs should generally be avoided during pregnancy, 1 case report of a woman with metastatic MTC treated with vandetanib until 6 weeks of gestation demonstrated no major pregnancy complications or fetal abnormalities.[82] Although there were no major consequences in this patient, the outcomes of this single case cannot be extracted to other patients, and therefore, pregnancy should be still avoided when on TKI treatment.

ANAPLASTIC THYROID CANCER

ATC is a rare thyroid cancer entity, and in contrast to DTC, is generally extremely aggressive with a disease-specific mortality that approaches 100%. Given its rapid course of disease progression and poor outcome, end-of-life issues and plans for comfort care measure are part of disease management. Recent research from the Netherlands showed a median survival of 2.2 months, and an estimated 1-year survival of 12%.[83] Although the median age in this study was 73 years, the cohort also included patients younger than age 40 years. Immediate therapy is needed, and therefore, in cases of this rare diagnosis made during pregnancy, surgery should not be deferred to after delivery.[10,52] If immediate surgery is not possible, TKI treatment can be considered, but as mentioned earlier, teratogenicity and embryo toxicity have been shown in animals.[10] In general, different treatment options and possibilities impacting both maternal and fetal health should be discussed in a multidisciplinary setting with the patient (and her partner). With respect to the impact of pregnancy on possible recurrence/progression in women successfully treated for ATC, there are no prospective or retrospective studies on this topic to the best of the authors' knowledge.

SUMMARY

Thyroid cancer is one of the most common cancers diagnosed in women of reproductive age and during pregnancy. Studies show that pregnancy is not associated with significant disease progression of previously treated DTC or micro-PTC under active surveillance. Furthermore, there does not seem to be an increased risk of persistent disease in patients with newly diagnosed DTC during pregnancy. Unless DTC has aggressive features, it is usually advised to defer treatment to after delivery, as this delay will not pose a threat to both the patient and the fetus. However, if surgery is necessary during pregnancy, it should be performed in the second trimester. With respect to RAI treatment, it should be noted that a less-aggressive RAI treatment strategy in women over 35 years of age who have desire for pregnancy should be considered. It is recommended to avoid pregnancy for 6 to 12 months after RAI ablation for DTC, but further research is needed to be better define this period. The need for TSH suppressive therapy during pregnancy is based on the ATA DRS status, but the harms and benefits of TSH suppressive therapy should be weighed against the risks of adverse pregnancy outcomes. Finally, preconception and perinatal management and surveillance should be based on careful discussion of thyroid cancer prognosis and recommended treatment, fertility issues, and the risk for adverse pregnancy or child outcomes within a multidisciplinary team with the woman and her partner.

CLINICS CARE POINTS

- Advice should be given on the risks of progression, adverse pregnancy outcomes, and contraception.
- Women should contact their doctor upon a positive pregnancy test.
- Radioactive iodine treatment should not be given during pregnancy.
- Breastfeeding should be stopped 6 weeks before until 3 months after radioactive iodine treatment.
- In women over 35 years of age with the desire for pregnancy and without high-risk tumor features, a less-aggressive radioactive iodine strategy should be considered.
- Pregnancy should be avoided for 6 to 12 months after radioactive iodine treatment.
- Levothyroxine dose should be increased by 25% to 30% upon a positive pregnancy test.
- The need for thyrotropin suppressive therapy during pregnancy is based on the American Thyroid Association dynamic risk stratification response, but the harms and benefits of this should be weighed against the risks of adverse pregnancy outcomes.
- For DTC, in the case of an excellent response, no additional monitoring is needed during pregnancy.
- For DTC, in those with biochemical or structural incomplete response, monitoring with both serum thyroglobulin levels and surveillance neck ultrasounds is needed.
- In micro-papillary thyroid carcinomas under active surveillance, a neck ultrasounds should be performed in the second trimester.
- For most women, treatment DTC can be delayed until after delivery. If surgery is recommended, it should be performed in the second trimester.

DISCLOSURE

The authors declare no conflicts of interest, and no competing financial interests exist.

REFERENCES

1. La Vecchia C, Malvezzi M, Bosetti C, et al. Thyroid cancer mortality and incidence: a global overview. Int J Cancer 2015;136(9):2187–95.
2. Davies L, Welch HG. Increasing incidence of thyroid cancer in the United States, 1973-2002. JAMA 2006;295(18):2164–7.

3. Anderson C, Engel SM, Mersereau JE, et al. Birth outcomes among adolescent and young adult cancer survivors. JAMA Oncol 2017;3(8):1078–84.

4. Araque DVP, Bleyer A, Brito JP. Thyroid cancer in adolescents and young adults. Future Oncol 2017;13(14):1253–61.

5. Smith LH, Danielsen B, Allen ME, et al. Cancer associated with obstetric delivery: results of linkage with the California Cancer Registry. Am J Obstet Gynecol 2003; 189(4):1128–35.

6. Cottreau CM, Dashevsky I, Andrade SE, et al. Pregnancy-associated cancer: a U.S. population-based study. J Womens Health (Larchmt) 2019;28(2):250–7.

7. Burman KD, Wartofsky L. Thyroid nodules. N Engl J Med 2016;374(13):1294–5.

8. Haugen BR, Alexander EK, Bible KC, et al. 2015 American Thyroid Association management guidelines for adult patients with thyroid nodules and differentiated thyroid cancer: the American Thyroid Association Guidelines Task Force on thyroid nodules and differentiated thyroid cancer. Thyroid 2016;26(1):1–133.

9. Ollero MD, Toni M, Pineda JJ, et al. Thyroid function reference values in healthy iodine-sufficient pregnant women and influence of thyroid nodules on thyrotropin and free thyroxine values. Thyroid 2019;29(3):421–9.

10. Alexander EK, Pearce EN, Brent GA, et al. 2017 Guidelines of the American Thyroid Association for the diagnosis and management of thyroid disease during pregnancy and the postpartum. Thyroid 2017;27(3):315–89.

11. Aschebrook-Kilfoy B, James B, Nagar S, et al. Risk factors for decreased quality of life in thyroid cancer survivors: initial findings from the North American Thyroid Cancer Survivorship study. Thyroid 2015;25(12):1313–21.

12. Van Velsen EFS, Massolt E, Heersema H, et al. Longitudinal analysis of quality of life in patients treated for differentiated thyroid cancer. Eur J Endocrinol 2019; 181(6):671–9.

13. Papaleontiou M, Reyes-Gastelum D, Gay BL, et al. Worry in thyroid cancer survivors with a favorable prognosis. Thyroid 2019;29(8):1080–8.

14. Bresner L, Banach R, Rodin G, et al. Cancer-related worry in Canadian thyroid cancer survivors. J Clin Endocrinol Metab 2015;100(3):977–85.

15. Roerink SH, de Ridder M, Prins J, et al. High level of distress in long-term survivors of thyroid carcinoma: results of rapid screening using the distress thermometer. Acta Oncol 2013;52(1):128–37.

16. Logan S, Perz J, Ussher JM, et al. Systematic review of fertility-related psychological distress in cancer patients: informing on an improved model of care. Psychooncology 2019;28(1):22–30.

17. van Velsen EFS, Visser WE, van den Berg SAA, et al. Longitudinal analysis of the effect of radioiodine therapy on ovarian reserve in females with differentiated thyroid cancer. Thyroid 2020;30(4):580–7.

18. Rooney KL, Domar AD. The relationship between stress and infertility. Dialogues Clin Neurosci 2018;20(1):41–7.

19. Ding XX, Wu YL, Xu SJ, et al. Maternal anxiety during pregnancy and adverse birth outcomes: a systematic review and meta-analysis of prospective cohort studies. J Affect Disord 2014;159:103–10.

20. Haymart MR, Pearce EN. How much should thyroid cancer impact plans for pregnancy? Thyroid 2017;27(3):312–4.

21. Bath SC, Pop VJ, Furmidge-Owen VL, et al. Thyroglobulin as a functional biomarker of iodine status in a cohort study of pregnant women in the United Kingdom. Thyroid 2017;27(3):426–33.

22. Zhang X, Li C, Mao J, et al. Gestation-specific changes in maternal thyroglobulin during pregnancy and lactation in an iodine-sufficient region in China: a longitudinal study. Clin Endocrinol (Oxf) 2017;86(2):229–35.

23. Rosario PW, Barroso AL, Purisch S. The effect of subsequent pregnancy on patients with thyroid carcinoma apparently free of the disease. Thyroid 2007;17(11): 1175–6.

24. Leboeuf R, Emerick LE, Martorella AJ, et al. Impact of pregnancy on serum thyroglobulin and detection of recurrent disease shortly after delivery in thyroid cancer survivors. Thyroid 2007;17(6):543–7.

25. Hirsch D, Levy S, Tsvetov G, et al. Impact of pregnancy on outcome and prognosis of survivors of papillary thyroid cancer. Thyroid 2010;20(10):1179–85.

26. Rakhlin L, Fish S, Tuttle RM. Response to therapy status is an excellent predictor of pregnancy-associated structural disease progression in patients previously treated for differentiated thyroid cancer. Thyroid 2017;27(3):396–401.

27. Driouich Y, Haraj NE, El Aziz S, et al. Impact of pregnancy on papillary thyroid carcinoma prognosis. Pan Afr Med J 2021;38:261.

28. Vannucchi G, Perrino M, Rossi S, et al. Clinical and molecular features of differentiated thyroid cancer diagnosed during pregnancy. Eur J Endocrinol 2010; 162(1):145–51.

29. Messuti I, Corvisieri S, Bardesono F, et al. Impact of pregnancy on prognosis of differentiated thyroid cancer: clinical and molecular features. Eur J Endocrinol 2014;170(5):659–66.

30. Chen AC, Livhits MJ, Du L, et al. Recent pregnancy is not associated with high-risk pathological features of well-differentiated thyroid cancer. Thyroid 2018; 28(1):68–71.

31. Sugitani I, Ito Y, Takeuchi D, et al. Indications and strategy for active surveillance of adult low-risk papillary thyroid microcarcinoma: consensus statements from the Japan Association of Endocrine Surgery Task Force on management for papillary thyroid microcarcinoma. Thyroid 2021;31(2):183–92.

32. Ito Y, Miyauchi A, Kudo T, et al. Effects of pregnancy on papillary microcarcinomas of the thyroid re-evaluated in the entire patient series at Kuma Hospital. Thyroid 2016;26(1):156–60.

33. Hartnett KP, Ward KC, Kramer MR, et al. The risk of preterm birth and growth restriction in pregnancy after cancer. Int J Cancer 2017;141(11):2187–96.

34. Madanat-Harjuoja LM, Malila N, Lahteenmaki PM, et al. Preterm delivery among female survivors of childhood, adolescent and young adulthood cancer. Int J Cancer 2010;127(7):1669–79.

35. Stensheim H, Klungsoyr K, Skjaerven R, et al. Birth outcomes among offspring of adult cancer survivors: a population-based study. Int J Cancer 2013;133(11): 2696–705.

36. Cho GJ, Kim SY, Lee HC, et al. The risk of adverse obstetric outcomes and the abnormal growth of offspring in women with a history of thyroid cancer. Thyroid 2019;29(6):879–85.

37. Yasmeen S, Cress R, Romano PS, et al. Thyroid cancer in pregnancy. Int J Gynaecol Obstet 2005;91(1):15–20.

38. Taylor PN, Minassian C, Rehman A, et al. TSH levels and risk of miscarriage in women on long-term levothyroxine: a community-based study. J Clin Endocrinol Metab 2014;99(10):3895–902.

39. Haddow JE, Palomaki GE, Allan WC, et al. Maternal thyroid deficiency during pregnancy and subsequent neuropsychological development of the child. N Engl J Med 1999;341(8):549–55.

40. van Velsen EFS, Stegenga MT, van Kemenade FJ, et al. Comparing the prognostic value of the eighth edition of the American Joint Committee on Cancer/Tumor Node Metastasis Staging System between papillary and follicular thyroid cancer. Thyroid 2018;28(8):976–81.

41. Ganly I, Nixon IJ, Wang LY, et al. Survival from differentiated thyroid cancer: what has age got to do with it? Thyroid 2015;25(10):1106–14.

42. Moosa M, Mazzaferri EL. Outcome of differentiated thyroid cancer diagnosed in pregnant women. J Clin Endocrinol Metab 1997;82(9):2862–6.

43. van Velsen EFS, Peeters RP, Stegenga MT, et al. The influence of age on disease outcome in 2015 ATA high risk differentiated thyroid cancer patients. Eur J Endocrinol 2021;185(3):421–9.

44. Luster M, Aktolun C, Amendoeira I, et al. European perspective on 2015 American Thyroid Association management guidelines for adult patients with thyroid nodules and differentiated thyroid cancer: proceedings of an interactive international symposium. Thyroid 2019;29(1):7–26.

45. van Velsen EFS, Stegenga M, van Kemenade FJ, et al. Evaluating the 2015 American Thyroid Association risk stratification system in high risk papillary and follicular thyroid cancer patients. Thyroid 2019;29(8):1073–9.

46. Verloop H, Louwerens M, Schoones JW, et al. Risk of hypothyroidism following hemithyroidectomy: systematic review and meta-analysis of prognostic studies. J Clin Endocrinol Metab 2012;97(7):2243–55.

47. Ahn D, Lee GJ, Sohn JH. Levothyroxine supplementation following hemithyroidectomy: incidence, risk factors, and characteristics. Ann Surg Oncol 2019; 26(13):4405–13.

48. Schumm MA, Lechner MG, Shu ML, et al. Frequency of thyroid hormone replacement after lobectomy for differentiated thyroid cancer. Endocr Pract 2021;27(7): 691–7.

49. Alexander EK, Marqusee E, Lawrence J, et al. Timing and magnitude of increases in levothyroxine requirements during pregnancy in women with hypothyroidism. N Engl J Med 2004;351(3):241–9.

50. Orloff LA, Wiseman SM, Bernet VJ, et al. American Thyroid Association statement on postoperative hypoparathyroidism: diagnosis, prevention, and management in adults. Thyroid 2018;28(7):830–41.

51. Lebrun B, De Block C, Jacquemyn Y. Hypocalcemia after thyroidectomy and parathyroidectomy in a pregnant woman. Endocrinology 2020;161(7):bqaa067.

52. Perros P, Boelaert K, Colley S, et al. Guidelines for the management of thyroid cancer. Clin Endocrinol (Oxf) 2014;81(Suppl 1):1–122.

53. Boucek J, de Haan J, Halaska MJ, et al. Maternal and obstetrical outcome in 35 cases of well-differentiated thyroid carcinoma during pregnancy. Laryngoscope 2018;128(6):1493–500.

54. Uruno T, Shibuya H, Kitagawa W, et al. Optimal timing of surgery for differentiated thyroid cancer in pregnant women. World J Surg 2014;38(3):704–8.

55. Cho GJ, Kim SY, Lee HC, et al. Risk of adverse obstetric outcomes and the abnormal growth of offspring in women with a history of thyroid cancer. Thyroid 2019;29(6):879–85.

56. Anagnostis P, Florou P, Bosdou JK, et al. Decline in anti-Mullerian hormone concentrations following radioactive iodine treatment in women with differentiated thyroid cancer: a systematic review and meta-analysis. Maturitas 2021;148:40–5.

57. Clement SC, Peeters RP, Ronckers CM, et al. Intermediate and long-term adverse effects of radioiodine therapy for differentiated thyroid carcinoma–a systematic review. Cancer Treat Rev 2015;41(10):925–34.

58. Sawka AM, Lakra DC, Lea J, et al. A systematic review examining the effects of therapeutic radioactive iodine on ovarian function and future pregnancy in female thyroid cancer survivors. Clin Endocrinol (Oxf) 2008;69(3):479–90.

59. Nies M, Cantineau AEP, Arts E, et al. Long-term effects of radioiodine treatment on female fertility in survivors of childhood differentiated thyroid carcinoma. Thyroid 2020;30(8):1169–76.

60. de Vet A, Laven JS, de Jong FH, et al. Antimullerian hormone serum levels: a putative marker for ovarian aging. Fertil Steril 2002;77(2):357–62.

61. Dewailly D, Andersen CY, Balen A, et al. The physiology and clinical utility of anti-Mullerian hormone in women. Hum Reprod Update 2014;20(3):370–85.

62. Depmann M, Eijkemans MJC, Broer SL, et al. Does AMH relate to timing of menopause? Results of an individual patient data meta-analysis. The Journal of Clinical Endocrinology & Metabolism 2018;103(10):3593–600.

63. Piek MW, Postma EL, van Leeuwaarde R, et al. The effect of radioactive iodine therapy on ovarian function and fertility in female thyroid cancer patients: a systematic review and meta-analysis. Thyroid 2021;31(4):658–68.

64. Zhang L, Huang Y, Zheng Y, et al. The effect of I-131 therapy on pregnancy outcomes after thyroidectomy in patients with differentiated thyroid carcinoma: a meta-analysis. Endocrine 2021;73(2):301–7.

65. Gorman CA. Radioiodine and pregnancy. Thyroid 1999;9(7):721–6.

66. American Thyroid Association Taskforce On Radioiodine Safety, Sisson JC, Freitas J, McDougall IR, et al. Radiation safety in the treatment of patients with thyroid diseases by radioiodine 131I : practice recommendations of the American Thyroid Association. Thyroid 2011;21(4):335–46.

67. Peragallo Urrutia R, Polis CB, Jensen ET, et al. Effectiveness of fertility awareness-based methods for pregnancy prevention: a systematic review. Obstet Gynecol 2018;132(3):591–604.

68. Yassa L, Marqusee E, Fawcett R, et al. Thyroid hormone early adjustment in pregnancy (the THERAPY) trial. J Clin Endocrinol Metab 2010;95(7):3234–41.

69. Medici M, Korevaar TI, Schalekamp-Timmermans S, et al. Maternal early-pregnancy thyroid function is associated with subsequent hypertensive disorders of pregnancy: the generation R study. J Clin Endocrinol Metab 2014;99(12): E2591–8.

70. Derakhshan A, Peeters RP, Taylor PN, et al. Association of maternal thyroid function with birthweight: a systematic review and individual-participant data meta-analysis. Lancet Diabetes Endocrinol 2020;8(6):501–10.

71. Jansen TA, Korevaar TIM, Mulder TA, et al. Maternal thyroid function during pregnancy and child brain morphology: a time window-specific analysis of a prospective cohort. Lancet Diabetes Endocrinol 2019;7(8):629–37.

72. Haddow JE, Craig WY, Neveux LM, et al. Implications of high free thyroxine (FT4) concentrations in euthyroid pregnancies: the FaSTER trial. J Clin Endocrinol Metab 2014;99(6):2038–44.

73. Zhang C, Yang X, Zhang Y, et al. Association between maternal thyroid hormones and birth weight at early and late pregnancy. J Clin Endocrinol Metab 2019; 104(12):5853–63.

74. Lemieux P, Yamamoto JM, Nerenberg KA, et al. Thyroid laboratory testing and management in women on thyroid replacement before pregnancy and associated pregnancy outcomes. Thyroid 2021;31(5):841–9.

75. Hales C, Taylor PN, Channon S, et al. Controlled antenatal thyroid screening II: effect of treating maternal suboptimal thyroid function on child behavior. J Clin Endocrinol Metab 2020;105(3):dgz098.

76. Maraka S, Mwangi R, McCoy RG, et al. Thyroid hormone treatment among pregnant women with subclinical hypothyroidism: US national assessment. BMJ 2017; 356:i6865.
77. Bryant SN, Nelson DB, McIntire DD, et al. An analysis of population-based prenatal screening for overt hypothyroidism. Am J Obstet Gynecol 2015;213(4): 565.e1–6.
78. Turunen S, Vaarasmaki M, Mannisto T, et al. Pregnancy and perinatal outcome among hypothyroid mothers: a population-based cohort study. Thyroid 2019; 29(1):135–41.
79. Wells SA Jr, Asa SL, Dralle H, et al. Revised American Thyroid Association guidelines for the management of medullary thyroid carcinoma. Thyroid 2015;25(6): 567–610.
80. Ardawi MS, Nasrat HA, BA'Aqueel HS. Calcium-regulating hormones and parathyroid hormone-related peptide in normal human pregnancy and postpartum: a longitudinal study. Eur J Endocrinol 1997;137(4):402–9.
81. Sarandakou A, Protonotariou E, Rizos D. Tumor markers in biological fluids associated with pregnancy. Crit Rev Clin Lab Sci 2007;44(2):151–78.
82. Thomas N, Glod J, Derse-Anthony C, et al. Pregnancy on vandetanib in metastatic medullary thyroid carcinoma associated with multiple endocrine neoplasia type 2B. Clin Endocrinol (Oxf) 2018;88(5):754–6.
83. de Ridder M, Nieveen van Dijkum E, Engelsman A, et al. Anaplastic thyroid carcinoma: a nationwide cohort study on incidence, treatment and survival in the Netherlands over 3 decades. Eur J Endocrinol 2020;183(2):203–9.

Preconception Counseling and Care for Pregnant Women with Thyroid Disease

Rima K. Dhillon-Smith, MBChB, PhD, MRCOG[a],
Kristien Boelaert, MD, PhD, FRCP[b],*

KEYWORDS

- Thyroid disease • Preconception • Pregnancy • Thyroid autoimmunity

KEY POINTS

- Women with overt thyroid disease should receive preconception counseling regarding the risks to pregnancy and fetal outcomes and be monitored regularly during pregnancy using appropriate reference ranges for thyroid function testing.
- Universal screening for thyroid dysfunction preconception or in early pregnancy is not currently recommended.
- Antithyroid drugs are the main treatment modality for hyperthyroidism in pregnancy and the dose and choice of medication requires careful consideration.
- Treatment strategies for subclinical hypothyroidism and isolated hypothyroxinemia and thyroid autoimmunity are still debated.
- Current evidence indicates that levothyroxine administration to euthyroid TPO antibody–positive women does not improve fertility and pregnancy outcomes.

BACKGROUND

Thyroid disorders are among the most prevalent medical conditions in women of reproductive age. Normal functioning of the thyroid gland is essential for optimal conception and pregnancy.

PHYSIOLOGIC CHANGES OF THYROID FUNCTION IN PREGNANCY

Pregnancy induces dynamic changes in thyroid function throughout the course of pregnancy, designed to provide adequate concentrations of thyroid hormone to the

[a] Institute of Metabolism and Systems Research, Tommy's National Centre for Miscarriage Research, University of Birmingham, Birmingham, B15 2TT, UK; [b] Institute of Applied Health Research, Room 232 Murray Learning Centre, University of Birmingham, Birmingham, B15 2FG, UK
* Corresponding author.
E-mail address: k.boelaert@bham.ac.uk

Endocrinol Metab Clin N Am 51 (2022) 417–436
https://doi.org/10.1016/j.ecl.2021.12.005

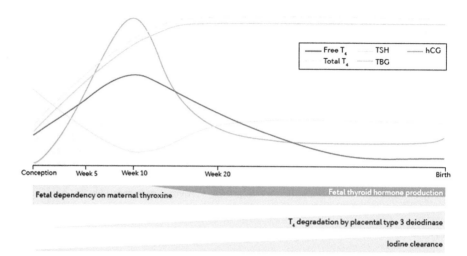

Fig. 1. Changes in thyroid physiology during pregnancy. hCG, human chorionic gonadotrophin; T4, thyroxine; TBG, thyroid-binding globulin; TSH, thyroid-stimulating hormone. (*From* Korevaar TIM, Medici M, Visser TJ, Peeters RP. Thyroid disease in pregnancy: new insights in diagnosis and clinical management. Nat Rev Endocrinol. 2017 Oct;13(10):610-622.)

mother and fetus (**Fig. 1**).[1–5] Overall, the demands on maternal thyroid hormone production increase by approximately 50% during pregnancy[6]; this requires an adequate supply of iodine for the biosynthesis of thyroid hormones and the absence of significant thyroid disease.

Elevated estrogen in pregnancy leads to increases in thyroid binding globulin concentrations, starting early in pregnancy, and plateauing by approximately 18 to 20 weeks of gestation. To maintain adequate free thyroid hormone concentrations, thyroxine (T4) and triiodothyronine (T3) production by the thyroid gland increases during the first half of pregnancy. By midgestation, a new steady state is reached and the synthesis of thyroid hormones returns to around prepregnancy rates. The first trimester sees increases in human chorionic gonadotrophin (hCG), which because of its weak thyroid-stimulating activity, transiently increases free T4 (fT4) and free T3 (fT3) and decreases thyrotropin (thyroid-stimulating hormone [TSH]). From midgestation, as hCG declines, serum fT4 and fT3 concentrations decline gradually, whereas serum TSH concentrations rise slightly.[7]

Iodine requirements increase considerably during pregnancy. In the mother, there is increased consumption of iodine for thyroid hormone synthesis and increased renal iodine clearance.[8] The placenta may also be an organ of storage for iodine.[9] The fetal thyroid begins to take up iodine from 10 to 12 weeks of gestation and fetal thyroid function commences at 18 to 22 weeks' gestation. Breastmilk production begins to rise from the second half of gestation, adding to further maternal iodine demand.[10]

Maternal thyroid hormones are essential for the maintenance of pregnancy and may influence placental development. Transplacental passage of maternal T4 is essential for normal fetal development, especially neurodevelopment during the first half of gestation.[11,12] The fetus is completely dependent on maternal T4 before commencement of its own thyroid hormone production, but remains reliant on maternal supply of iodine[1] and continues to receive maternal T4 until delivery.[13]

It is recommended that population-, trimester-, and manufacturer-specific reference ranges are used for the correct interpretation of thyroid function during pregnancy. The use of reference ranges determined in similar populations, free from thyroid disease and iodine sufficient, using the same assay, is advised when specific ranges are not available. In the absence of such information it is reasonable to set an upper limit of TSH of 4.0 mIU/L in pregnancy.[14]

THYROID DYSFUNCTION: DEFINITIONS, EPIDEMIOLOGY, AND EFFECTS ON PREGNANCY

Overt Hyperthyroidism

Overt hyperthyroidism is diagnosed on the finding of a reduced serum TSH concentration with high fT4 and/or fT3 levels, using trimester- and laboratory-specific reference ranges. Overt hyperthyroidism is present in around 0.1% to 0.4% of pregnant women and the most common cause is autoimmune Graves disease.[15,16] Uncontrolled Graves thyrotoxicosis has been associated with miscarriage, preeclampsia, preterm birth, placental abruption, and fetal hyperthyroidism.[17–19]

Overt Hypothyroidism

The diagnosis of overt hypothyroidism is based on confirmation of a low fT4 concentration in combination with an elevated serum TSH concentration. The prevalence of overt hypothyroidism in pregnancy is around 0.2% to 0.6%.[4,5,20] Overt hypothyroidism is most commonly caused by autoimmune Hashimoto thyroiditis and has been associated with adverse pregnancy outcomes, such as miscarriage, hypertensive disorders of pregnancy, placental abruption, preterm delivery, and higher rates of neonates being admitted to intensive care units and lower intelligence scores in the offspring.[5,14,21]

Subclinical Thyroid Disease

Subclinical hyperthyroidism (SCHyper) and subclinical hypothyroidism (SCHypo) are biochemical diagnoses based on abnormal serum TSH concentrations in combination with normal fT4 levels. These conditions may represent the earliest stages of thyroid dysfunction and SCHypo in particular may progress to overt disease, although reversion to euthyroidism is common.[22,23] The prevalence of SCHypo (TSH higher than the reference range and fT4 within the reference range) varies widely because of inconsistent definitions and is reported to range from 3% up to 18% in pregnant women.[14,24] There is mounting evidence that SCHypo is linked to negative pregnancy outcomes, such as miscarriage, preterm birth, preeclampsia, gestational hypertension, and perinatal mortality.[25,26] The effects seem to be augmented by the presence of thyroid antibodies.[26] There is insufficient evidence to suggest a causal association between SCHypo and infertility. There is, however, consensus that subfertile women are more likely to have mildly raised TSH concentrations.

There are no known harmful effects of SCHyper in pregnancy.[27] However, fT4 concentrations that remain higher than the upper limit of the normal range, and even those at the higher end of normal, might have unfavorable effects. Studies have shown that higher fT4 concentrations are associated with lower birth weight; reduced child neurocognition; and increased risks of autism, attention-deficit/hyperactivity disorder, and epilepsy.[28–31]

Isolated Hypothyroxinemia

Isolated hypothyroxinemia is defined as serum concentrations of fT4 lower than the reference range in combination with normal TSH concentrations. It is considered a form of mild thyroid dysfunction and is predominantly associated with adverse neurobehavioral outcomes in the child.[32–34] It has a prevalence of approximately 1% to 2%

of pregnant women in iodine-sufficient populations with a higher prevalence in countries with more severe iodine deficiency.[35]

Gestational Thyrotoxicosis

Gestational hyperthyroidism, biochemically defined by elevated concentrations of fT4 and suppressed TSH, is diagnosed in approximately 1% to 3% of pregnancies. Most cases of the disease occur secondary to high hCG concentrations and in 50% of cases it coexists with hyperemesis gravidarum.[15,16,36] Patients with gestational hyperthyroidism have a higher risk of low birth weight and a higher risk of preeclampsia than patients with euthyroid pregnancies.[5]

Thyroid Autoimmunity

Thyroid autoimmunity describes the presence of circulating antithyroid autoantibodies that are targeted against the thyroid and can occur with or without affecting thyroid function. The three most clinically important antibodies are thyroid peroxidase antibodies (TPOAb), thyroglobulin antibodies, and TSH receptor antibodies (TRAb).

TPOAb are the most common antithyroid autoantibody, present in 90% of cases of Hashimoto thyroiditis, 75% of Graves disease, and 10% to 20% of nodular goiter or thyroid carcinoma. However, around 10% to 15% of biochemically euthyroid individuals also have elevated TPOAb titers.[37,38] The prevalence observed among unselected pregnant women ranges from 2% to 17%, with higher prevalence seen in iodine-deficient populations.[39] Some studies have reported higher rates of TPOAb positivity in women considered to be "high risk" (eg, with subfertility or history of recurrent pregnancy loss).[40] However, a large prevalence study of more than 19,000 women with history of miscarriage or subfertility showed no difference in prevalence whether women had one or two miscarriages, three or more miscarriages, or if they had subfertility (9.8%, 9.7%, and 9.5% prevalence of TPOAb, respectively).[41]

Studies have shown that the presence of thyroid autoantibodies leads to significantly increased odds of miscarriage and preterm birth for women from low- and high-risk obstetric populations compared with women without thyroid autoantibodies.[26,40] Associations between TPOAb positivity and subfertility, and increased risks of postpartum thyroiditis, have also been established.[42] Euthyroid women who are positive for TPOAb are more likely to develop impaired thyroid function during pregnancy and are particularly at risk of developing SCHypo.[43,44]

PRECONCEPTION CARE

In view of the known adverse effects of overt thyroid disease on pregnancy outcomes, it is crucial for women with preexisting thyroid disease to be counseled on the importance of having a normal thyroid function before conception. Women with poorly controlled thyroid disease should be managed by the relevant endocrinologists and such women should also receive prepregnancy counseling from obstetric specialists.

Preconception Counseling for Women with Known Overt Hyperthyroidism

All women of reproductive age who develop thyrotoxicosis should have a discussion regarding potential future pregnancy. The risks and benefits of all treatment options including antithyroid drugs, radioactive iodine (^{131}I) administration, or surgery should be discussed. Thyroid function should be controlled and stable on two measurements 2 months apart before conception. If the woman is on levothyroxine (LT4) replacement following definitive thyroid ablation or thyroidectomy, then optimal TSH and fT4 concentrations (TSH <2.5 mU/L with normal fT4) should be achieved preconception.[14]

Following radioiodine treatment TRAb concentrations may rise, increasing the risk of fetal Graves disease caused by transplacental passage of maternal TRAb, even when maternal thyroid function tests are normal.[45,46] It is advised that following ^{131}I, pregnancy should be delayed by 6 months.[47] Surgery may be the better option in women with high TRAb concentrations because antibody levels usually normalize within months after a thyroidectomy,[48] and cure is immediate. However, the risks of surgery and lifelong need for LT4 replacement have to be considered.

For women who continue on antithyroid drugs, propylthiouracil (PTU) is the preferred drug preconception and during the first trimester, because this has a lower teratogenic risk than methimazole (MMI). The lowest possible dose of antithyroid drugs to maintain euthyroidism should be used.[49–51] Consideration should be given to discontinuation preconception once euthyroidism is achieved for at least 6 months.[14,52] Early discontinuation to reduce teratogenic risks needs to be weighed against risks of a hyperthyroid flare in the periconception period, which has the attendant risks of increased adversity in pregnancy.

Preconception Counseling for Women with Known Overt Hypothyroidism

In women with hypothyroidism, preconception encouragement of treatment compliance and adequate replacement may reduce the risk of early pregnancy hypothyroidism. A preconception target TSH less than or equal to 2.5 mU/L is recommended.[52,53] In pregnancy, the required LT4 dose increment may vary depending on the cause of hypothyroidism and the prepregnancy TSH concentrations. A self-initiated empirical dose increase by approximately 25% to 30% as soon as there is a positive pregnancy test can significantly reduce the risk of developing hypothyroidism in pregnancy, without any adverse consequences on the pregnancy provided regular thyroid function monitoring in pregnancy is performed. This empirical dose increase is usually recommended as doubling of the dose on 2 days of the week[14] or alternatively implementing a dose increment of 25 µg per day for women taking 100 µg or less T4 daily and a dose increment of 50 µg per day for women taking greater than 100 µg T4 daily.

Preconception Counseling for Women with Subclinical Hypothyroidism with or without Thyroid Peroxidase Antibodies

There is a universal consensus that women with SCHypo who have TSH levels higher than 10 mIU/L should be treated preconception with LT4, aiming for a target TSH of less than 2.5 mIU/L before pregnancy. There is also a general agreement that women with moderately raised levels of TSH that is higher than the laboratory assay range (usually 4–5 mIU/L) and 10 mIU/L should receive LT4 treatment. As for overt hypothyroidism, it is recommended that women with SCHypo have an empirical dose increase following a positive pregnancy test in view of the risk of progression to overt hypothyroidism as a consequence of increased demands on T4 requirements.

The area of uncertainty is regarding the management of women who are actively seeking pregnancy from certain high-risk populations. For women undergoing assisted-reproductive technologies the 2017 American Thyroid Association guideline recommends the following: "subclinically hypothyroid women undergoing in vitro fertilization or intracytoplasmic sperm injection should be treated with LT4. The goal of treatment is to achieve a TSH concentration less than 2.5 mU/L."[14] This has led to widespread practice in many countries of initiating LT4 treatment in any subfertile woman undergoing in vitro fertilization or intracytoplasmic sperm injection treatment with a TSH value greater than 2.5 mIU/L; however, the evidence of benefit with this management strategy is limited.

The Endocrine Society Clinical Practice Guideline also makes the recommendation of aiming for a preconception TSH of less than 2.5 mIU/L for all subfertile women, and extends this to women with history of miscarriage or preterm birth.[53] This strategy is controversial, because data showing evidence of benefit are conflicting and often do not consider thyroid antibody status. Furthermore, there is insufficient evidence suggesting reduced fertility outcomes or higher miscarriage rates exist in women with mild thyroid dysfunction.

In summary, there is wide variation in clinical practice in the management of mild thyroid dysfunction, in particular in women with history of subfertility or pregnancy loss. The ongoing controversy is regarding the initiation of LT4 treatment in women with high normal/mildly raised thyroid dysfunction, that is, TSH levels 2.50 to 5.00 mIU/L, especially for women considered high risk with a history of subfertility or miscarriage or who are positive for thyroid antibodies.

Finally, there is no evidence of benefit with LT4 treatment, commenced preconception, in euthyroid women who are positive for TPOAb. The evidence is discussed in detail later.

Universal Preconception Screening for Thyroid Disease

There is great debate regarding the need and the cost-effectiveness of routinely screening for thyroid disease and for thyroid autoimmunity in women who are planning for pregnancy.

Proponents of universal screening have argued that a case for screening for overt hypothyroidism can be made because it is a condition that has serious adverse consequences in pregnancy and on the newborn.[54] Furthermore, it is detectable by a safe and simple thyroid function test, and is treated with LT4 to reduce the chances of adverse outcomes. A large prevalence study of thyroid disease in asymptomatic preconception women from "high-risk" populations (women with history of miscarriage or subfertility) found that 0.4% of women had undiagnosed overt hypothyroidism[41]; this demonstrates that a proportion of women will be missed without universal screening. However, the overall cost-effectiveness remains debatable.

If a universal thyroid function screening approach is adopted, overt thyroid disease will constitute only a small proportion of the abnormal thyroid function detected. Most will fall into the gestational hyperthyroidism, SCHypo, and isolated hypothyroxinemia groups, where the benefit of treatment remains controversial.

Targeted Preconception Screening for Thyroid Disease in High-Risk Populations

There is a lack of consensus on what factors should trigger thyroid function screening and risk-based thyroid function screening remains controversial.[55] The American Thyroid Association 2017 guidelines recommend that all patients seeking pregnancy who have any of the following risk factors should undergo clinical evaluation and have serum TSH testing (**Box 1**).[14]

The guideline also states that there is insufficient evidence to recommend for or against universal screening for abnormal TSH concentrations preconception, with the exception of women planning assisted reproduction or those known to have TPOAb positivity.[14] The European Society for Human Reproduction and Embryology (ESHRE) guideline for recurrent pregnancy loss recommends routine thyroid function testing in women who have suffered two or more previous miscarriages.[56]

One of the criteria that a screening test should meet, in accordance with World Health Organization guidance, is that there should be an accepted and proven treatment of the disease.[54,55] Regarding TPOAb, there is currently no evidence in support of any treatment, which can improve pregnancy outcomes for women with TPOAb. At

---

Box 1
American Thyroid Association 2017 guidance on high-risk populations who require preconception TSH testing

Risk factors that warrant preconception TSH screening
- A history of hypothyroidism/hyperthyroidism or current symptoms/signs of thyroid dysfunction
- Known thyroid antibody positivity or presence of a goiter
- History of head or neck radiation or prior thyroid surgery
- Age greater than 30 years
- Type 1 diabetes or other autoimmune disorders
- History of pregnancy loss, preterm delivery, or infertility
- Multiple prior pregnancies (two or more)
- Family history of autoimmune thyroid disease or thyroid dysfunction
- Morbid obesity (body mass index $\geq$40 kg/m^2)
- Use of amiodarone or lithium, or recent administration of iodinated radiologic contrast
- Residing in an area of known moderate to severe iodine insufficiency

---

present the ESHRE guideline recommends routine testing of TPOAb in women with recurrent pregnancy loss,[56] but this was based on the potential benefit with LT4 treatment suggested by two small studies. The ESHRE guideline predates the results of two of the biggest trials on the subject.[57,58]

An important counterargument in favor of TPOAb testing is that the presence of TPOAb represents the primary cause leading to hypothyroidism in pregnant women. Thus, knowing TPOAb status allows identification and stratification of the women at higher risk of progression to thyroid disease in pregnancy, consequently requiring thyroid function monitoring. This is particularly important for women undergoing ovarian stimulation within the process of assisted-reproductive technologies. TSH levels have been shown to be maintained at high levels for prolonged periods in women with TPOAb undergoing ovarian stimulation. However, there is a need for detailed clinical and cost-effectiveness analyses to determine whether routine testing for TPOAb is beneficial, or whether routine thyroid function testing in pregnancy should be performed instead.

MANAGEMENT OF THYROID DISEASE IN PREGNANCY
Overt Hyperthyroidism

Treatment with antithyroid drugs represents the mainstay of treatment of active hyperthyroidism in pregnancy. Minor adverse effects of antithyroid drugs, including skin rash, occur in 3% to 5% of patients. Serious adverse effects are rare and include agranulocytosis occurring in 0.15% with either drug and liver failure in 0.1%, the latter pertaining almost exclusively to PTU.[59]

If a woman has been euthyroid for 6 months or more on a low dose of an antithyroid drug (<10 mg MMI daily or <200 mg PTU daily), consideration should be given to discontinuing antithyroid drugs, before the period of highest teratogenic risk (6–10 weeks of gestation).[14,60,61] This period of time also coincides with rising hCG concentrations, which may exacerbate any residual hyperthyroidism, thus it is recommended that there is close monitoring of thyroid function from early gestation until the midtrimester of pregnancy.

The lowest effective dose of antithyroid drugs should be used targeting serum fT4 at the upper end, or slightly higher than the normal reference range, or total T4 at 1 to 1.5 times the upper limit of the nonpregnant reference range to minimize the risk of fetal hypothyroidism from transplacental passage of the drug.[51,62] Titration should not be primarily based on TSH concentrations, and there is no role for fT3 and total T3 measurements.

Large population studies have indicated that the use of PTU during early pregnancy is associated with a slightly lower risk of adverse reactions and outcomes, and less severe fetal anomalies, compared with MMI.[36,49,51] Therefore, it is advised that women who are receiving MMI and are in need of continuing therapy during pregnancy are switched to PTU as early as possible and remain treated with PTU up until the 16th week of pregnancy.[14]

Even with successful antithyroid drug therapy, there is a relapse rate of Graves disease of around 30% to 50% in the nonpregnant population.[63] It has been observed that women whose Graves disease is biochemically controlled prepregnancy with stable low doses of MMI (5–10 mg) or PTU (100–200 mg) have a lower chance of relapse than women with uncontrolled disease. If a relapse has occurred following cessation of antithyroid medication this usually occurs after a few months in those women who are susceptible.[61] To minimize the potential harmful effects of antithyroid drugs on the fetus, clinicians can discuss the possibility of stopping treatment in women who wish to become pregnant or at the point of a first positive pregnancy test in unplanned pregnancies. However, if antithyroid drugs are discontinued, it is recommended that clinicians monitor thyroid function closely at regular intervals (eg, every 1–2 weeks).[14]

Monitoring for the fetus

Clinicians should perform a baseline assessment of concentrations of TRAb in patients with Graves hyperthyroidism. If TRAb concentrations are elevated, the fetus should be monitored every 4 to 6 weeks by assessing the fetal heart rate, fetal growth, and/or fetal thyroid appearance via ultrasonography from midpregnancy until birth. Together with maternal thyroid function, these measures are a reflection of the fetal thyroid hormone status.[64,65]

Gestational Thyrotoxicosis

It is important to differentiate gestational thyrotoxicosis from Graves disease. New-onset Graves disease requires prompt treatment in pregnancy and is far less common than gestational thyrotoxicosis. The clinical features, including palpitations, tremor, anxiety, and tachycardia, are seen in both conditions and therefore diagnosis cannot be determined by symptoms alone. However, the lack of symptoms of thyrotoxicosis and weight loss before a pregnancy, the absence of a goiter, ophthalmopathy or a personal/family history of thyroid disease, and the presence of significant nausea and vomiting are more suggestive of gestational hyperthyroidism. Serum blood tests are done for TRAb and serum T3 concentrations, because these are raised in Graves disease but generally not in gestational hyperthyroidism.[15,36] Serum hCG concentrations are not useful in distinguishing the two conditions.[66] Where there is doubt, a repeat thyroid function test 2 weeks from the initial test, demonstrating a declining fT4 concentration without antithyroid treatment, is suggestive of gestational hyperthyroidism. TSH concentrations take longer to recover, and often remain suppressed, making this a less useful test.

Management of gestational hyperthyroidism is predominantly supportive with symptomatic relief through antiemetics, rehydration, and correction of electrolyte imbalances if the woman has hyperemesis gravidarum. There may be a need for temporary treatment with β-blockers to control symptoms of thyrotoxicosis and tachycardia.[16,36] There is no evidence that treatment with antithyroid drugs improves obstetric and fetal outcomes in women with transient gestational hyperthyroidism.[67]

Overt Hypothyroidism

There have not been any randomized controlled trials investigating the effect of LT4 treatment of overt hypothyroidism during pregnancy. However, in view of the well-established adverse effects of overt hypothyroidism on pregnancy outcomes and fetal development, the general consensus is that overt hypothyroidism during pregnancy should be treated as early as possible.[14] The placental transfer of maternal T4 to the fetus is essential for optimal fetal brain development, and because LT4 supplementation is the treatment of choice for overt hypothyroidism, the therapy should be initiated as soon as possible. Patients using LT4 and liothyronine combination therapy or desiccated thyroid extracts often have a T4/T3 ratio that is lower than that of patients with normal thyroid function. Therefore, in these patients, the placental transfer of maternal T4 to the fetal brain might be insufficient. These findings indicate that patients using combination therapy or desiccated thyroid extracts who desire to become pregnant should be switched to LT4.

Following the initial empirical dose increase in women taking LT4 preconception, up to 40% may require further dose adjustments in either direction.[14,68] Hence regular thyroid function monitoring is required, especially in the first half of the pregnancy. This is the period over which thyroid-binding globulin concentrations are rising, in conjunction with the other previously outlined physiologic changes in pregnancy. The ultimate LT4 dose increments depend on the underlying cause of hypothyroidism. Studies have shown that there are higher dose requirements in subjects with radioiodine- or surgery-induced hypothyroidism[69] compared with patients with autoimmune thyroiditis.[70] The aim of dose titration is to maintain euthyroidism by replicating the normal dynamic changes of pregnancy that affect thyroid hormone requirements.

Subclinical Hypothyroidism, Isolated Hypothyroxinemia, and Thyroid Peroxidase Antibodies Positivity

Thyroid hypofunction

Because of the association between adverse pregnancy outcomes and SCHypo (defined as serum TSH higher than the pregnancy-specific reference range), it is recommended that SCHypo is treated preconception, and during pregnancy, with LT4 therapy (**Table 1**). In contrast, evaluation of the effects of isolated hypothyroxinemia on maternal and fetal outcomes has yielded conflicting data. Some studies have shown an association between hypothyroxinemia and poor cognitive development of the offspring.[28,32-34] Effects on prematurity and low birth weight are uncertain[26,28,32] and results from observational studies of isolated hypothyroxinemia on pregnancy outcomes are conflicting.[7,71]

It remains unclear if treatment of SCHypo and isolated hypothyroxinemia with thyroid hormone-replacement therapy is beneficial. The two separate large randomized controlled trials evaluating treatment of SCHypo and isolated hypothyroxinemia with T4, regardless of anti-TPO status, commencing at a median gestation beyond 12 weeks of gestation, demonstrated no benefit to offspring intelligence scores and obstetric and neonatal outcomes. However, these studies were limited by the late timing of the intervention, that is, after completion of the first trimester of pregnancy.[72,73] Moreover there is mounting evidence that overzealous replacement with LT4 may be associated with adverse pregnancy outcomes.[74,75]

A post hoc analysis of the randomized controlled trial by Negro and colleagues[76] demonstrated a potential benefit in reducing adverse pregnancy outcomes with LT4 intervention starting in the first trimester in TPOAb-positive women with very mild

Table 1
A summary of all the published and ongoing randomized studies on management of subclinical hypothyroidism, isolated hypothyroxinemia, and TPOAb-positive euthyroidism in preconception and pregnancy

Author/Year/ Country	Population/Number of Participants in Trial	Thyroid Dysfunction Group of Interest	TSH Ref Range (mIU/L)	Intervention	Comparison	Main Findings
Negro et al,[77] 2005 Italy	Women undergoing assisted reproduction N = 72	Euthyroid TPOAb positive	0.27–4.2	LT4 1 mg/kg/d	Placebo	No difference in pregnancy rate between the groups. TPOAb-positive women had higher miscarriage rate than TPOAb-negative. LT4 treatment in TPOAb-positive women did not affect delivery rate.
Negro et al,[43] 2006 Italy	Pregnant women in first trimester N = 115	Euthyroid TPOAb positive	0.27–4.2	LT4: dose dependent on TSH	No treatment	At baseline, TPOAb-positive women had higher TSH compared with TPOAb-negative. LT4 treatment may be able to lower the chance of miscarriage and premature delivery.

Study/Country	Population	Thyroid status	Reference range	Intervention	Control	Findings
Negro et al,[76] 2010 Italy	Pregnant women (natural conception) in first trimester N = 4562 randomized to universal or case finding screening	High-normal TSH/mild SCHypo Mixed TPOAb positive and negative	0.27–4.2	LT4 (if TSH >2.5 mIU/L and TPOAb positive)	No treatment if TSH <2.5 mIU/L	Universal screening compared with case finding did not result in a decrease in adverse outcomes. Treatment of hypothyroidism or hyperthyroidism identified by screening a low-risk group was associated with a lower rate of adverse outcomes.
Lazarus et al,[73] 2012 United Kingdom	Pregnant women ≤15+6 wk with subclinical hypothyroidism (median gestation 12 + 3 wk) N = 794	SCHypo and isolated hypothyroxinemia Mixed TPOAb positive and negative	>97.5th centile (>3.3 mIU/L)	Being screened and detected as SCHypo LT4 commenced 150 μg/d Dose titrated to maintain TSH level 0.1–1.0 mIU/L	Control group, not screened	Antenatal screening and maternal treatment of hypothyroidism did not result in improved cognitive function in children at 3 y of age.
Negro et al,[80] 2016 Italy	Pregnant women in first trimester N = 413	Euthyroid and TPOAb positive	0.2–2.5 mIU/L	LT4; women with TSH 0.5–1.5 mIU/L were begun on 0.5 μg/kg/d, women with a TSH 1.5–2.5 mIU/L were begun on 1 μg/kg/d	No treatment in first trimester	LT4 intervention had no impact on the rate of miscarriage and preterm delivery in euthyroid thyroid antibody–positive women.
Casey et al,[72] 2017 United States	Pregnant women with a singleton pregnancy <20 wk gestation (median gestation 17 wk) N = 677	SCHypo (n = 677) isolated hypothyroxinemia (n = 526) Mixed TPOAb positive and negative	>4.0 mIU/L	LT4 100 μg/d	Placebo	No significant effect of T4 replacement therapy, compared with placebo, on child cognitive function and other indexes of neurodevelopment up to 5 y of age.

(continued on next page)

Table 1
(continued)

Author/Year/ Country	Population/Number of Participants in Trial	Thyroid Dysfunction Group of Interest	TSH Ref Range (mIU/L)	Intervention	Comparison	Main Findings
Wang et al,[58] 2017 China	Women being treated for infertility N = 600	Euthyroid and TPOAb positive	0.50–4.78	LT4, dose dependent on TSH	Placebo	Treatment with LT4, compared with no LT4 treatment, did not reduce miscarriage rates or increase live-birth rates.
Nazarpour et al,[81] 2017 Iran	Pregnant women in first trimester N = 131	SCHypo and TPOAb positive	2.5–10	LT4, dose dependent on TSH	No treatment	Treatment with LT4 decreases the risk of preterm delivery in women who are positive for TPOAb.
Nazarpour et al,[82] 2018 Iran	Pregnant women in first trimester N = 366	SCHypo and TPOAb negative	2.5–10	LT4, morning dose of 1 μg/kg/d	No treatment	Using the TSH cutoff of 2.5 mIU/L, no significant difference in preterm delivery was observed. However, analysis based on a cutpoint of 4.0 mIU/L demonstrated a significantly lower rate of preterm delivery in LT4-treated women compared with those who received no treatment.

| Dhillon-Smith et al,[57] 2019 United Kingdom | Women with history of miscarriage or subfertility N = 952 | Euthyroid and TPOAb positive | 0.44–3.63 | LT4 50 µg/d | Placebo | LT4 treatment, compared with placebo, showed no improvement in live birth at or beyond 34 wk or any secondary pregnancy, maternal or neonatal outcomes. |
| Vissenberg et al (publication awaited) Netherlands | Women with history of recurrent pregnancy loss N = 240 | Euthyroid and TPOAb positive | 0.5–5.0 | LT4, dose dependent on weight | Placebo | Not available. |

hypothyroidism (defined as a TSH >2.5 mIU/L). However this was a small sample size (n = 83 treated vs n = 34 untreated) and adverse pregnancy outcome was not the primary outcome of this trial.

Thyroid peroxidase antibodies–positive euthyroidism

Evidence from older published studies suggested benefit with LT4 treatment in euthyroid TPOAb-positive women.[43,77] However, newer evidence from much larger studies has contested this.

The POSTAL trial randomized 600 euthyroid TPOAb-positive women undergoing assisted reproduction.[58] In contrast to the previous studies, this study reported no difference in clinical pregnancy or miscarriage rates between women who received LT4 therapy and those that did not.

In the most recent and largest trial on the subject, the TABLET trial, there was no improvement in live birth outcome at or beyond 34 weeks in those taking LT4 and no difference in any secondary pregnancy or neonatal outcomes, including pregnancy rates and miscarriage. Subgroup analyses were performed looking at individual populations; no difference was seen for those with a history of miscarriage or those with subfertility.[57]

Previous studies have shown the presence of thyroid antibodies can increase the risk of progression from euthyroid to subclinical or overt hypothyroidism in pregnancy.[78] Overall, data from the TABLET trial found 7% of euthyroid women with TPOAb developed SCHypo, either before or during pregnancy. In view of this, women found to be TPOAb positive should have regular monitoring (at least once per trimester) of their thyroid function during pregnancy, starting from around 7 to 9 weeks' gestation.

The results of the T4Life trial, which focuses on LT4 treatment for euthyroid TPOAb-positive women with history of recurrent pregnancy loss, are eagerly awaited.[79]

Given the lack of benefit shown with LT4 in euthyroid TPOAb-positive women, across all populations, this treatment strategy should not be implemented routinely into clinical practice.

DISCUSSION

There is international consensus on the management of overt thyroid disease preconception and during pregnancy. However, as highlighted in this review there are many areas of controversy within thyroid disease and pregnancy. **Box 2** highlights the key areas with ongoing uncertainty and that require further research.

Box 2
Areas for further research

Screening
- Cost effectiveness of preconception or early pregnancy universal screening of thyroid dysfunction
- In select high-risk groups, such as subfertile women with recurrent pregnancy loss, routine preconception TPOAb testing to identify and monitor those at risk of disease progression versus routine TSH measurements in each trimester of pregnancy

Management
- Effect of LT4 commenced preconception or early pregnancy on obstetric outcomes in women with mild SCHypo/isolated hypothyroxinemia
- Effect of LT4 on obstetric outcomes in women with SCHypo and raised TPOAb; with particular focus on women undergoing assisted conception

Research Collaborative for Thyroid Disease and Pregnancy

An international consortium, led by thyroid specialists in the Netherlands, has been set up to produce large scale individual-participant data meta-analyses by collating data from all relevant clinical studies into thyroid disease and pregnancy. The work generated by this group will add significantly to the knowledge of thyroid disease and pregnancy and help to identify areas where new primary research is needed. Examples of work published by this group include an individual-participant data meta-analysis demonstrating the association of thyroid function test abnormalities and thyroid autoimmunity with preterm birth.[26] Another study published in 2020, found that high-normal levels of fT4 in pregnancy are associated with low birthweight, adding to the argument that there may be harm from LT4 overtreatment.[83]

SUMMARY

This review provides an overview of the latest evidence-based recommendations for management of women with thyroid disease preconception and during pregnancy. In addition, we have highlighted areas of controversy and areas for future research.

CLINICS CARE POINTS

- Population-, trimester-, and laboratory-specific reference ranges for serum TSH and fT4 should be used when determining thyroid function in pregnancy.
- Women with overt thyroid disease should receive preconception counseling from the appropriate specialists, regarding the risks of their condition in pregnancy. Such women should have a stable thyroid function for at least 2 months before trying for a pregnancy.
- There is currently insufficient evidence to recommend universal screening for all women trying for pregnancy.
- Routine preconception thyroid function tests should be offered to women with identified risk factors for thyroid disease, in particular women with history of recurrent pregnancy loss and women undergoing fertility treatment.
- Women with overt thyroid disease require regular thyroid function monitoring in pregnancy and should be managed jointly by endocrinologists and obstetricians.
- New-onset hyperthyroidism during pregnancy requires differentiation between Graves disease and transient gestational thyrotoxicosis.
- Graves disease in pregnancy should be treated with antithyroid drugs and the lowest possible dose should be administered; PTU is the preferred medication preconception and in the first trimester of pregnancy.
- Women positive for TRAb antibodies need increased fetal surveillance.
- Untreated moderate SCHypo (TSH 4.0–10.0 mIU/L) is associated with early pregnancy loss and other adverse pregnancy outcomes.
- Evidence for reducing adverse outcomes in women with SCHypo with LT4 therapy is limited; however, best practice is still to treat preconception and during pregnancy.
- There is insufficient evidence of adverse pregnancy outcomes for women with high-normal TSH levels (2.5–4.0 mIU/L) and therefore insufficient evidence of LT4 therapy in this group.
- There is conflicting evidence that isolated hypothyroxinemia is harmful in pregnancy.
- There is no benefit from LT4 treatment in improving pregnancy outcomes for euthyroid TPOAb-negative women.
- Knowing TPOAb status allows for stratification of women who will require thyroid function monitoring during pregnancy. The options of performing TPOAb testing for "high-risk"

women (eg, undergoing assisted reproductive technologies) versus routine early pregnancy thyroid function testing are both acceptable strategies, until clinical and cost-effectiveness analyses are available.

- If a woman is known to be TPOAb-positive, measurement of serum TSH concentration should be taken at 7 to 9 weeks and then in each subsequent trimester, because of the risk of progression to SCHypo and overt hypothyroidism.

- Further studies are needed to determine the role of LT4 therapy in women with mildly elevated TSH levels with or without raised TPOAb.

DISCLOSURE

The authors have nothing to disclose.

REFERENCES

1. Glinoer D. The regulation of thyroid function during normal pregnancy: importance of the iodine nutrition status. Best Pract Res Clin Endocrinol Metab 2004; 18(2):133–52.
2. Hershman JM. Physiological and pathological aspects of the effect of human chorionic gonadotropin on the thyroid. Best Pract Res Clin Endocrinol Metab 2004;18(2):249–65.
3. McNeil AR, Stanford PE. Reporting thyroid function tests in pregnancy. Clin Biochem Rev 2015;36(4):109–26.
4. Medici M, Korevaar TI, Visser WE, et al. Thyroid function in pregnancy: what is normal? Clin Chem 2015;61(5):704–13.
5. Korevaar TIM, Medici M, Visser TJ, et al. Thyroid disease in pregnancy: new insights in diagnosis and clinical management. Nat Rev Endocrinol 2017;13(10):610–22.
6. Alexander EK, Marqusee E, Lawrence J, et al. Timing and magnitude of increases in levothyroxine requirements during pregnancy in women with hypothyroidism. N Engl J Med 2004;351:241–9.
7. Chan S, Boelaert K. Optimal management of hypothyroidism, hypothyroxinaemia and euthyroid TPO antibody positivity preconception and in pregnancy. Clin Endocrinol (Oxf) 2015;82(3):313–26.
8. Glinoer D. The importance of iodine nutrition during pregnancy. Public Health Nutr 2007;10(12a):1542–6.
9. Burns R, O'Herlihy C, Smyth PP. The placenta as a compensatory iodine storage organ. Thyroid 2011;21(5):541–6.
10. Zimmermann MB. The effects of iodine deficiency in pregnancy and infancy. Paediatr Perinat Epidemiol 2012;26(Suppl 1):108–17.
11. Williams GR. Neurodevelopmental and neurophysiological actions of thyroid hormone. J Neuroendocrinol 2008;20(6):784–94.
12. de Escobar GM, Obregón MJ, del Rey FE. Maternal thyroid hormones early in pregnancy and fetal brain development. Best Pract Res Clin Endocrinol Metab 2004;18(2):225–48.
13. Vulsma T, Gons MH, de Vijlder JJ. Maternal-fetal transfer of thyroxine in congenital hypothyroidism due to a total organification defect or thyroid agenesis. N Engl J Med 1989;321(1):13–6.
14. Alexander EK, Pearce EN, Brent GA, et al. 2017 Guidelines of the American Thyroid Association for the diagnosis and management of thyroid disease during pregnancy and the postpartum. Thyroid 2017;27(3):315–89.

15. Andersen SL, Knøsgaard L. Management of thyrotoxicosis during pregnancy. Best Pract Res Clin Endocrinol Metab 2020;34(4):101414.

16. Nguyen CT, Mestman JH. Graves' hyperthyroidism in pregnancy. Curr Opin Endocrinol Diabetes Obes 2019;26(5):232–40.

17. Pillar N, Levy A, Holcberg G, et al. Pregnancy and perinatal outcome in women with hyperthyroidism. Int J Gynaecol Obstet 2010;108(1):61–4.

18. Millar LK, Wing DA, Leung AS, et al. Low birth weight and preeclampsia in pregnancies complicated by hyperthyroidism. Obstet Gynecol 1994;84(6):946–9.

19. Aggarawal N, Suri V, Singla R, et al. Pregnancy outcome in hyperthyroidism: a case control study. Gynecol Obstet Invest 2014;77(2):94–9.

20. Krassas GE, Poppe K, Glinoer D. Thyroid function and human reproductive health. Endocr Rev 2010;31(5):702–55.

21. Abalovich M, Amino N, Barbour LA, et al. Management of thyroid dysfunction during pregnancy and postpartum: an Endocrine Society Clinical Practice Guideline. J Clin Endocrinol Metab 2007;92(8 Suppl):S1–47.

22. Surks MI, Ortiz E, Daniels GH, et al. Subclinical thyroid disease: scientific review and guidelines for diagnosis and management. JAMA 2004;291(2):228–38.

23. Meyerovitch J, Rotman-Pikielny P, Sherf M, et al. Serum thyrotropin measurements in the community: five-year follow-up in a large network of primary care physicians. Arch Intern Med 2007;167(14):1533–8.

24. Dong AC, Stagnaro-Green A. Differences in diagnostic criteria mask the true prevalence of thyroid disease in pregnancy: a systematic review and meta-analysis. Thyroid 2019;29(2):278–89.

25. Maraka S, Ospina NM, O'Keeffe DT, et al. Subclinical hypothyroidism in pregnancy: a systematic review and meta-analysis. Thyroid 2016;26(4):580–90.

26. Korevaar TIM, Derakhshan A, Taylor PN, et al. Association of thyroid function test abnormalities and thyroid autoimmunity with preterm birth: a systematic review and meta-analysis. JAMA 2019;322(7):632–41.

27. Casey BM, Dashe JS, Wells CE, et al. Subclinical hyperthyroidism and pregnancy outcomes. Obstet Gynecol 2006;107(2 Pt 1):337–41.

28. Medici M, Timmermans S, Visser W, et al. Maternal thyroid hormone parameters during early pregnancy and birth weight: the Generation R Study. J Clin Endocrinol Metab 2013;98(1):59–66.

29. Hales C, Taylor PN, Channon S, et al. Controlled antenatal thyroid screening ii: effect of treating maternal suboptimal thyroid function on child behavior. J Clin Endocrinol Metab 2020;105(3):dgz098.

30. Korevaar TI, Muetzel R, Medici M, et al. Association of maternal thyroid function during early pregnancy with offspring IQ and brain morphology in childhood: a population-based prospective cohort study. Lancet Diabetes Endocrinol 2016;4(1):35–43.

31. Ge GM, Leung MTY, Man KKC, et al. Maternal thyroid dysfunction during pregnancy and the risk of adverse outcomes in the offspring: a systematic review and meta-analysis. J Clin Endocrinol Metab 2020;105(12):dgaa555.

32. Korevaar TI, Schalekamp-Timmermans S, de Rijke YB, et al. Hypothyroxinemia and TPO-antibody positivity are risk factors for premature delivery: the generation R study. J Clin Endocrinol Metab 2013;98(11):4382–90.

33. Henrichs J, Ghassabian A, Peeters RP, et al. Maternal hypothyroxinemia and effects on cognitive functioning in childhood: how and why? Clin Endocrinol (Oxf) 2013;79(2):152–62.

34. Julvez J, Alvarez-Pedrerol M, Rebagliato M, et al. Thyroxine levels during pregnancy in healthy women and early child neurodevelopment. Epidemiology 2013;24(1):150–7.

35. Berbel P, Mestre JL, Santamaría A, et al. Delayed neurobehavioral development in children born to pregnant women with mild hypothyroxinemia during the first month of gestation: the importance of early iodine supplementation. Thyroid 2009;19(5):511–9.

36. Cooper DS, Laurberg P. Hyperthyroidism in pregnancy. Lancet Diabetes Endocrinol 2013;1(3):238–49.

37. Saravanan P, Dayan CM. Thyroid autoantibodies. Endocrinol Metab Clin North Am 2001;30(2):315–37, viii.

38. Chardès T, Chapal N, Bresson D, et al. The human anti-thyroid peroxidase autoantibody repertoire in Graves' and Hashimoto's autoimmune thyroid diseases. Immunogenetics 2002;54(3):141–57.

39. Dhillon-Smith RK, Coomarasamy A. TPO antibody positivity and adverse pregnancy outcomes. Best Pract Res Clin Endocrinol Metab 2020;34(4):101433.

40. Thangaratinam S, Tan A, Knox E, et al. Association between thyroid autoantibodies and miscarriage and preterm birth: meta-analysis of evidence. Bmj 2011;342:d2616.

41. Dhillon-Smith RK, Tobias A, Smith PP, et al. The prevalence of thyroid dysfunction and autoimmunity in women with history of miscarriage or subfertility. J Clin Endocrinol Metab 2020;105(8):dgaa302.

42. van den Boogaard E, Vissenberg R, Land JA, et al. Significance of (sub)clinical thyroid dysfunction and thyroid autoimmunity before conception and in early pregnancy: a systematic review. Hum Reprod Update 2011;17(5):605–19.

43. Negro R, Formoso G, Mangieri T, et al. Levothyroxine treatment in euthyroid pregnant women with autoimmune thyroid disease: effects on obstetrical complications. J Clin Endocrinol Metab 2006;91(7):2587–91.

44. Negro R, Formoso G, Coppola L, et al. Euthyroid women with autoimmune disease undergoing assisted reproduction technologies: the role of autoimmunity and thyroid function. J Endocrinol Invest 2007;30(1):3–8.

45. Schneider DF, Sonderman PE, Jones MF, et al. Failure of radioactive iodine in the treatment of hyperthyroidism. Ann Surg Oncol 2014;21(13):4174–80.

46. Laurberg P, Wallin G, Tallstedt L, et al. TSH-receptor autoimmunity in Graves' disease after therapy with anti-thyroid drugs, surgery, or radioiodine: a 5-year prospective randomized study. Eur J Endocrinol 2008;158(1):69–75.

47. Royal College of Physicians. Radioiodine in the management of benign thyroid disease. 2007.

48. Laurberg P, Bournaud C, Karmisholt J, et al. Management of Graves' hyperthyroidism in pregnancy: focus on both maternal and foetal thyroid function, and caution against surgical thyroidectomy in pregnancy. Eur J Endocrinol 2009; 160(1):1–8.

49. Andersen SL, Olsen J, Wu CS, et al. Birth defects after early pregnancy use of antithyroid drugs: a Danish nationwide study. J Clin Endocrinol Metab 2013; 98(11):4373–81.

50. Yoshihara A, Noh J, Yamaguchi T, et al. Treatment of graves' disease with antithyroid drugs in the first trimester of pregnancy and the prevalence of congenital malformation. J Clin Endocrinol Metab 2012;97(7):2396–403.

51. Seo GH, Kim TH, Chung JH. Antithyroid drugs and congenital malformations: a nationwide Korean Cohort Study. Ann Intern Med 2018;168(6):405–13.

52. Stagnaro-Green A, Abalovich M, Alexander E, et al. Guidelines of the American Thyroid Association for the diagnosis and management of thyroid disease during pregnancy and postpartum. Thyroid 2011;21(10):1081–125.

53. De Groot L, Abalovich M, Alexander EK, et al. Management of thyroid dysfunction during pregnancy and postpartum: an Endocrine Society clinical practice guideline. J Clin Endocrinol Metab 2012;97(8):2543–65.

54. Stagnaro-Green A, Dong A, Stephenson MD. Universal screening for thyroid disease during pregnancy should be performed. Best Pract Res Clin Endocrinol Metab 2020;34(4):101320.

55. van der Spek AH, Bisschop PH. Universal screening for thyroid disease SHOULD NOT be recommended before and during pregnancy. Best Pract Res Clin Endocrinol Metab 2020;34(4):101429.

56. Bender Atik R, Christiansen OB, Elson J, et al. ESHRE guideline: recurrent pregnancy loss. Hum Reprod Open 2018;2018(2):hoy004.

57. Dhillon-Smith RK, Middleton LJ, Sunner KK, et al. Levothyroxine in women with thyroid peroxidase antibodies before conception. N Engl J Med 2019;380(14): 1316–25.

58. Wang H, Gao H, Chi H, et al. Effect of levothyroxine on miscarriage among women with normal thyroid function and thyroid autoimmunity undergoing in vitro fertilization and embryo transfer: a randomized clinical trial. JAMA 2017; 318(22):2190–8.

59. Taylor PN, Vaidya B. Side effects of anti-thyroid drugs and their impact on the choice of treatment for thyrotoxicosis in pregnancy. Eur Thyroid J 2012;1(3): 176–85.

60. Laurberg P, Andersen SL. Therapy of endocrine disease: antithyroid drug use in early pregnancy and birth defects: time windows of relative safety and high risk? Eur J Endocrinol 2014;171(1):R13–20.

61. Nedrebo BG, Holm PI, Uhlving S, et al. Predictors of outcome and comparison of different drug regimens for the prevention of relapse in patients with Graves' disease. Eur J Endocrinol 2002;147(5):583–9.

62. Patil-Sisodia K, Mestman JH. Graves hyperthyroidism and pregnancy: a clinical update. Endocr Pract 2010;16(1):118–29.

63. Ross DS, Burch HB, Cooper DS, et al. 2016 American Thyroid Association guidelines for diagnosis and management of hyperthyroidism and other causes of thyrotoxicosis. Thyroid 2016;26(10):1343–421.

64. Momotani N, Noh J, Oyanagi H, et al. Antithyroid drug therapy for Graves' disease during pregnancy. Optimal regimen for fetal thyroid status. N Engl J Med 1986;315(1):24–8.

65. Korevaar TI, Chaker L, Jaddoe VW, et al. Maternal and birth characteristics are determinants of offspring thyroid function. J Clin Endocrinol Metab 2016; 101(1):206–13.

66. Yoshihara A, Noh JY, Mukasa K, et al. Serum human chorionic gonadotropin levels and thyroid hormone levels in gestational transient thyrotoxicosis: is the serum hCG level useful for differentiating between active Graves' disease and GTT? Endocrinol Jpn 2015;62(6):557–60.

67. Bouillon R, Naesens M, Van Assche FA, et al. Thyroid function in patients with hyperemesis gravidarum. Am J Obstet Gynecol 1982;143(8):922–6.

68. Yassa L, Marqusee E, Fawcett R, et al. Thyroid hormone early adjustment in pregnancy (the THERAPY) trial. J Clin Endocrinol Metab 2010;95(7):3234–41.

69. Verga U, Bergamaschi S, Cortelazzi D, et al. Adjustment of L-T4 substitutive therapy in pregnant women with subclinical, overt or post-ablative hypothyroidism. Clin Endocrinol (Oxf) 2009;70(5):798–802.
70. Loh JA, Wartofsky L, Jonklaas J, et al. The magnitude of increased levothyroxine requirements in hypothyroid pregnant women depends upon the etiology of the hypothyroidism. Thyroid 2009;19(3):269–75.
71. Ramezani Tehrani F, Nazarpour S, Behboudi-Gandevani S. Isolated maternal hypothyroxinemia and adverse pregnancy outcomes: a systematic review. J Gynecol Obstet Hum Reprod 2021;50(7):102057.
72. Casey BM, Thom EA, Peaceman AM, et al. Treatment of subclinical hypothyroidism or hypothyroxinemia in pregnancy. N Engl J Med 2017;376(9):815–25.
73. Lazarus JH, Bestwick JP, Channon S, et al. Antenatal thyroid screening and childhood cognitive function. N Engl J Med 2012;366(6):493–501.
74. Maraka S, Mwangi R, McCoy RG, et al. Thyroid hormone treatment among pregnant women with subclinical hypothyroidism: US national assessment. Bmj 2017; 356:i6865.
75. Lemieux P, Yamamoto JM, Nerenberg KA, et al. Thyroid laboratory testing and management in women on thyroid replacement before pregnancy and associated pregnancy outcomes. Thyroid 2021;31(5):841–9.
76. Negro R, Schwartz A, Gismondi R, et al. Universal screening versus case finding for detection and treatment of thyroid hormonal dysfunction during pregnancy. J Clin Endocrinol Metab 2010;95(4):1699–707.
77. Negro R, Mangieri T, Coppola L, et al. Levothyroxine treatment in thyroid peroxidase antibody-positive women undergoing assisted reproduction technologies: a prospective study. Hum Reprod 2005;20(6):1529–33.
78. Vanderpump MP, Tunbridge WM, French JM, et al. The incidence of thyroid disorders in the community: a twenty-year follow-up of the Whickham Survey. Clin Endocrinol (Oxf) 1995;43(1):55–68.
79. N T Register. T4Life trial. Available at: trialregister.nl/trialreg/admin/rctview.asp? TC=3364. Accessed 2012.
80. Negro R, Schwartz A, Stagnaro-Green A. Impact of levothyroxine in miscarriage and preterm delivery rates in first trimester thyroid antibody-positive women with TSH less than 2.5 mIU/L. J Clin Endocrinol Metab 2016;101(10):3685–90.
81. Nazarpour S, Ramezani Tehrani F, Simbar M, et al. Effects of levothyroxine treatment on pregnancy outcomes in pregnant women with autoimmune thyroid disease. Eur J Endocrinol 2017;176(2):253–65.
82. Nazarpour S, Ramezani Tehrani F, Simbar M, et al. Effects of levothyroxine on pregnant women with subclinical hypothyroidism, negative for thyroid peroxidase antibodies. J Clin Endocrinol Metab 2018;103(3):926–35.
83. Derakhshan A, Peeters RP, Taylor PN, et al. Association of maternal thyroid function with birthweight: a systematic review and individual-participant data meta-analysis. Lancet Diabetes Endocrinol 2020;8(6):501–10.

Printed and bound by CPI Group (UK) Ltd, Croydon, CR0 4YY

08/05/2025

01864713-0002